METABOLIC PROCESSES
IN THE FOETUS AND NEWBORN INFANT

Nutricia Symposium

METABOLIC PROCESSES IN THE FOETUS AND NEWBORN INFANT

Rotterdam 22—24 October 1970

EDITORS:

J. H. P. JONXIS M.D., H. K. A. VISSER M.D. AND

J. A. TROELSTRA M.D.

1971

H. E. STENFERT KROESE N.V. — LEIDEN

SOLE DISTRIBUTOR FOR THE UNITED STATES OF AMERICA AND CANADA
THE WILLIAMS AND WILKINS COMPANY / BALTIMORE

ISBN-13:978-94-010-2953-7 e-ISBN-13:978-94-010-2951-3
DOI: 10.1007/978-94-010-2951-3

Library of Congress Catalog Card number 70-153468

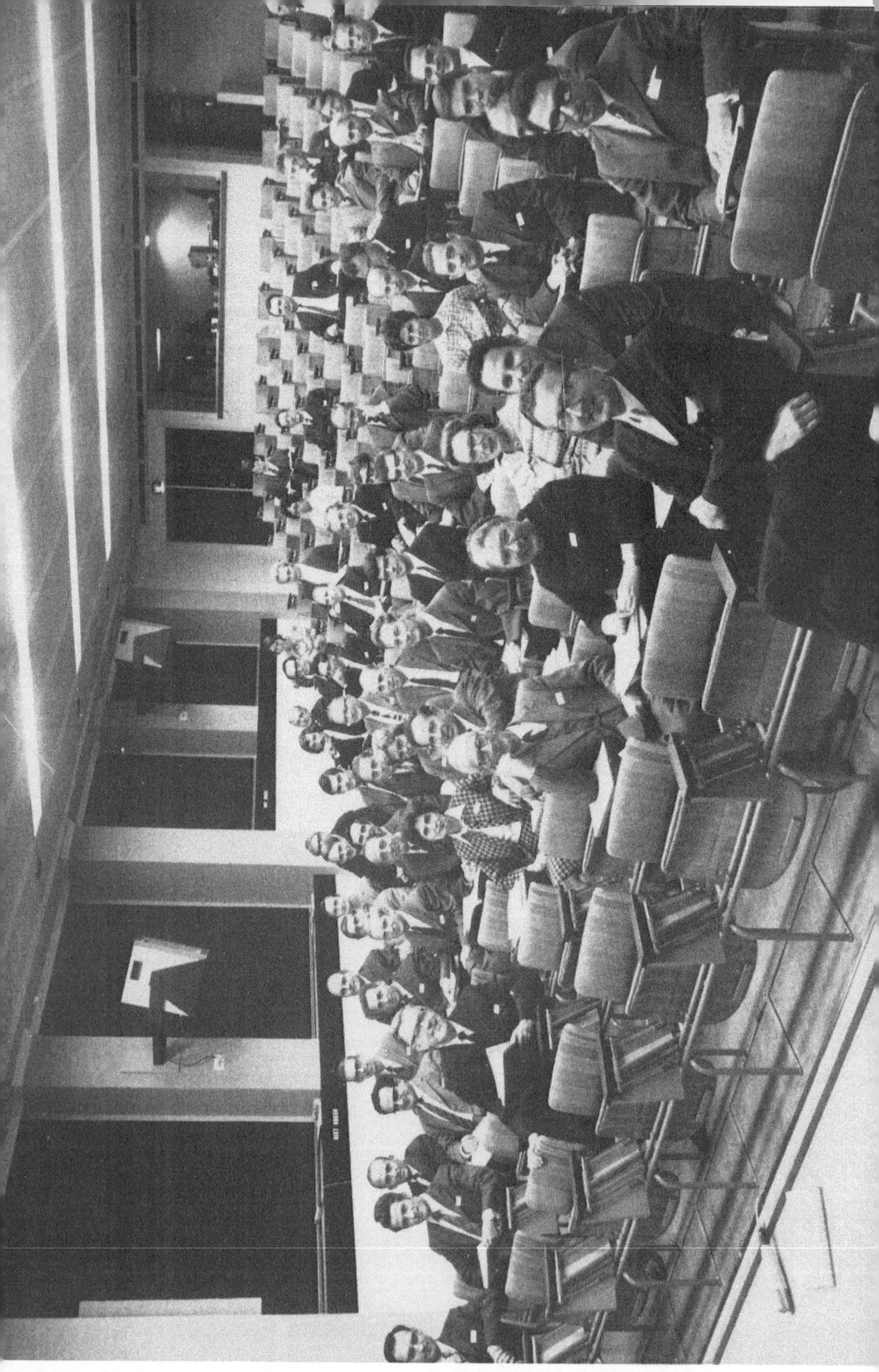

PARTICIPANTS

LEGEND*

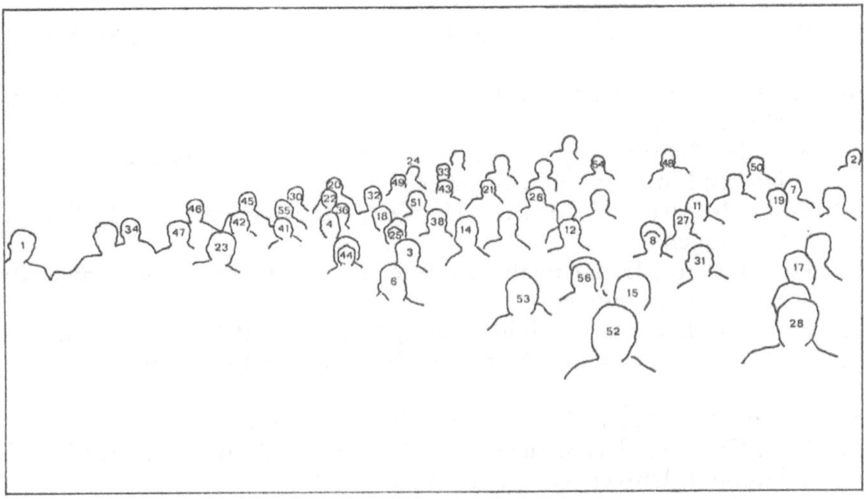

1 R. Assan, Medical Faculty of Paris, Department of Metabolic Diseases, Paris
2 G. A. Atallah, Pediatrician, Amman
3 H. Bickel, University Children's Hospital, Heidelberg
4 J. I. de Bruyne, Department of Physiology and Pathology of the Newborn, University of Amsterdam
5 F. Bravo Icaza, Pediatrician, Panama
6 R. A. McCance, Dunn Nutritional Laboratory, Infant Nutrition Research Division, University of Cambridge and Medical Research Council
7 D. Carton, Department of Pediatrics, University Hospital, Ghent
8 J. Dodion-Fransen, Department of Obstetrics and Gynecology, Free University of Brussels, University Hospital St.-Pierre
9 F. Diaz Dominguez, Pediatrician, Santo Domingo
10 A. C. Drogendijk, Department of Obstetrics and Gynecology, Free University of Amsterdam
11 R. Eeckels, Department of Pediatrics, University Hospital St.-Rafaël, Louvain
12 E. Eggermont, Department of Pediatrics, University Hospital St.-Rafaël, Louvain

* Some participants do not appear on the photograph.

13 J. Engelhardt, Department of Pediatrics, Zuiderziekenhuis, Rotterdam
14 J. Fernandes, Department of Pediatrics, Sophia Children's Hospital and Neonatal Unit, Medical School of Rotterdam, Rotterdam
15 S. J. Fomon, University Hospitals, Department of Pediatrics, Iowa City, Iowa
16 H. H. van Gelderen, Department of Pediatrics, University Hospital, Leiden
17 P. Gerard, Department of Pediatrics, University Hospital St.-Rafaël, Louvain
18 R. H. Gevers, Department of Obstetrics and Gynecology, University Hospital, Leiden
19 S. G. H. Hensen, Department of Obstetrics and Gynecology, University Hospital St.-Radboud, Nijmegen
20 F. A. Hommes, University Hospital, Department of Pediatrics, Groningen
21 H. J. Huisjes, Department of Obstetrics and Gynecology, University Hospital, Groningen
22 D. Hull, Institute of Child Health, University of London, London
23 J. H. P. Jonxis, University Hospital, Department of Pediatrics, Groningen
24 C. Kassimos, Pediatric Clinic of Athens University, Athens
25 B. E. Kingma, Department of Pediatrics, Wilhelmina Children's Hospital, University of Utrecht, Utrecht
26 G. J. Kloosterman, Department of Obstetrics and Gynecology, Wilhelmina Gasthuis, University of Amsterdam, Amsterdam
27 B. S. Lindblad, Medical Faculty of Stockholm, Department of Pediatrics, St.-Görans Children's Hospital, Stockholm
28 H. Loeb, Department of Pediatrics, University Hospital, Brussels
29 N. S. Matsaniotis, Pediatric Clinic of Athens University, Athens
30 G. Meeuwisse, University Hospital, Department of Pediatrics, Lund
31 R. de Meyer, University Hospital St.-Rafaël, Department of Pediatrics, Louvain
32 R. D. G. Milner, University of Manchester, Department of Child Health, St -Mary's Hospital, Manchester
33 D. Nicolopoulos, Pediatric clinic of Athens University, Athens
34 C. Papadatos, Pediatric clinic of Athens University, Athens
35 N. Räihä, University Central Hospital, Department of Pediatrics, Helsinki
36 R. Rappaport, Hôpital des Enfants Malades, Medical faculty of Paris, Paris
37 B. C. Reyes, Department of Pediatrics, Far Eastern University, Manila
38 J. H. Ruys, Department of Pediatrics, University Hospital, Leiden
39 A. L. C. Schmidt, Department of Obstetrics and Gynaecology University Hospital 'Dijkzigt', Rotterdam
40 E. D. A. M. Schretlen, Department of Pediatrics, University Hospital St.-Radboud, Nijmegen

41 W. Schröter, University Hospital, Department of Pediatrics, Hamburg
42 F. Sereni, University of Milan, Department of Pediatrics, Clinica Pediatrica 'G. e D. de Marchi', Milan
43 H. G. Sie, Department of Pediatrics, University Hospital of the Free University of Amsterdam, Amsterdam
44 S. E. Snyderman, New York University Medical Center, Department of Pediatrics, New York
45 W. Teller, University Children's Hospital, Ulm
46 J. A. Troelstra, Department of Pediatrics, University Hospital, Groningen
47 T. Valaes, The Anne-Marie Institute of Child Health, Athens
48 W. Veeger, Department of Internal Medicine, University Hospital, Groningen
49 G. Vergonet, University Hospital, Department of Pediatrics, Groningen
50 W. Verhoeven, Nutricia Comp., Zoetermeer
51 C. A. Villee Jr., Harvard Medical School, Department of Biological Chemistry, Boston
52 H. K. A. Visser, Sophia Children's Hospital and Neonatal Unit, Department of Pediatrics Medical School of Rotterdam, Rotterdam
53 E. M. Widdowson, University of Cambridge and Medical Research Council Infant Nutrition Research Division, Dunn Nutrional Laboratory, Cambridge
54 G. Wiseman, University of Sheffield, Physiology Department, Sheffield
55 H. Wolf, University Hospital, Department of Pediatrics, Göttingen
56 M. Young, Departmentt of Gynecology, St.-Thomas' Hospital Medical School, London

CONTENTS

SESSION I

THE DEVELOPMENT OF ENZYME SYSTEMS IN THE MAMMAL

SESSION II

AMINOACID METABOLISM

SESSION III

CARBOHYDRATE-FAT METABOLISM

OPENING

PROF. DR. H. K. A. VISSER

Ladies and Gentlemen,

It is a great honour and pleasure to welcome all of you at this third Nutricia Symposium. The first Nutricia Symposium was held in Groningen at the end of February 1964. The title of the symposium was 'the adaptation of the newborn infant to extra-uterine life' and the four sessions were on 'food reserves and food requirements of the newborn; water and electrolyte metabolism of the newborn infant; respiratory problems in the newborn infant, and temperature control of the newborn'.

The second Nutricia Symposium was also held in Groningen, May 1967. The subject was 'aspects of prematurity and dysmaturity'. Sessions were on 'role of the placenta; assessment of foetal development; experimental aspects of dysmaturity; hereditary and environmental aspects of low birthweight; adaptation of the low birthweight-infant to extra-uterine life, obstetrical and preventive aspects of dysmaturity, and developmental aspects'.

One might say that the first symposium dealt with some of the most important clinical problems of the newborn period; at the second symposium the main emphasis was on those factors which influence foetal growth.

Today we are here to discuss another aspect of perinatal pathofysiology: the metabolism of the foetus and newborn, with emphasis on developmental aspects of aminoacid and carbohydrate-fat metabolism. I am very happy to welcome many old friends; several of you have participated in the other two symposia. It is also a privilege to welcome so many young participants. This symposium, which again has been so generously supported by Nutricia Ltd., brings together a small group of people from different disciplines. All of us, pediatricians, obstetricians, biologists and biochemists are deeply interested in the problems of fysiology and pathology of the foetus and newborn.

I sincerely hope that this meeting will be as successful as the other two symposia, which means good spirit, good friendship and good discussions.

SESSION I

THE DEVELOPMENT OF ENZYME SYSTEMS IN THE MAMMAL

DEVELOPMENT OF ENZYME SYSTEMS IN GLYCOLYSIS

F. A. HOMMES*

INTRODUCTION

The control of any metabolic pathway depends on the concentration of the participating enzymes and the allosteric properties of these enzymes. Energy production as it takes place in glycolysis and oxidative phosphorylation of the fetal rat liver differs in some aspects from that of the adult rat liver. The concentration of glycolytic enzymes is different (1, 2, 3) as well as the ratio of L- and M-type isozymes of pyruvate kinase (4, 5) and aldolase (6). Also the number of mitochondria per cell is smaller in the hepatocyte of the fetal liver than in that of the adult liver (7) and rather large differences can be observed in the enzymic equipment of the mitochondria. Fetal rat liver mitochondria have no glycerophosphate oxidase (8, 9), a low activity of succinic dehydrogenase (9) and a low activity of aconitase relative to citrate synthase (10).

These differences will be reflected in the flux of energy production and in the contrast of this process. It is the purpose of this contribution to analyse some of the differences in the mechanism of control of energy production.

MATERIALS AND METHODS

The rats used in this study were of the TNO (Dutch organization of Applied Science) strain and had unlimited access to food and water. The food consisted of the normal laboratory diet.

Samples of aerobic and anaerobic rat liver were taken by the freeze

* Department of Pediatrics, University of Groningen, School of Medicine, Groningen, The Netherlands.

clamping technique described by Wollenberger et al. (11). The sample was pulverized in a mortar at liquid nitrogen temperature, weighed and thawed under 18% $HClO_4$. The extract was neutralized with 1 M KOH to pH 7.0. After standing for 60 min at 0 °C, the mixture was centrifuged and the supernatant used for analysis.

Pregnant rats were anaesthesized with aether and the liver and the livers of the embryo's were exposed. Aerobic samples were taken *in situ*. Anaerobic samples of the adult liver were taken 2 min. after clamping of the liver veins and arteries. Anaerobic samples of the fetal rat liver were taken 2 min. after clamping of the umbilical cord.

Analysis of glycolytic intermediates and adenine nucleotides was carried out fluorometrically as described by Estabrook and Maitra (12), with minor modifications. Adenosine triphosphate was assayed according to Lamprecht and Trautschold (13). Homogenates of liver were prepared in a 5 fold volume of icecold 0.25 M sucrose with a Potter-Elvejhem homogenizer. Mitochondria were prepared as described by Schneider (14). Adenylate kinase was assayed according to Adam (15) in the presence of oligomycin (10γ per ml) to inhibit mitochondrial ATP-ase. The cytoplasmic adenylate kinase was assayed in the supernatant obtained after centrifugation of the homogenate for 1 hr at 20.000 × g at 0 °C.

RESULTS AND DISCUSSION

The results of an analysis of glycolytic intermediates and adenine nucleotides of aerobic and anaerobic fetal rat liver are shown in table 1.

In contrast to the adult rat liver (16) the fetal rat liver maintains even under aerobic conditions near equilibrium for the adenylate kinase system. Brosnan et al. (17) have shown that this is the case for the adult rat liver under anaerobic conditions, that is under conditions where oxidative phosphorylation has been cut off (see also table 2).

Therefore, if the mitochondrial ATP synthesis cannot contribute to the total ATP synthesis, the activity of the adenylate kinase is high enough to maintain near equilibrium. The adenylate kinase activity of the adult rat liver is one of the highest activities of energy metabolism (18). The question arises now whether the activity of this enzyme in the fetal liver is high enough to maintain near equilibrium in this tissue as well. The development of adenylate kinase of rat liver has

Table 1. *Analysis of glycolytic intermediates and adenine nucleotides during aerobic and anaerobic glycolysis of fetal rat liver (3 days before birth). Values are given in μ moles per gram wet weight.*

	Aerobic	Anaerobic
Glucose-6-phosphate	0,36	0,39
Glucose-1-phosphase	0,02	0,02
Fructose-6-phosphate	0.06	0.07
Fructose-1 6-diphosphate	0.06	0.13
Dihydroxyacetone-phosphate	0.13	0.20
Glyceraldehyde-3-phosphate	0.15	0.13
3-Phosphoglycerate	0.30	0.19
2-Phosphoglycerate	0.18	0.11
Phosphoenolpyruvate	0.33	0.13
Pyruvate	0.63	0.25
ATP	1.90	1.71
ADP	1.22	1.20
AMP	0.50	0.64
Σ adeninenucleotides	3.62	3.55
$\frac{[ATP][AMP]}{[ADP]^2}$	0.64	0.76

Table 2. *Analysis of glycolytic intermediates and adenine nucleotides during anaerobic glycolysis of adult rat liver. Values are given in μ moles per gram wet weight.*

Glucose-6-phosphate	0.74
Glucose-1-phosphate	0.09
Fructose-6-phosphate	0.15
Fructose-1, 6-diphosphate	0.05
Dihydroxyacetonephosphate	0.10
Glyceraldehyde-3-phosphate	0.04
3-Phosphoglycerate	0.39
2-Phosphoglycerate	0.14
Phosphoenolpyruvate	0.18
Pyruvate	0.14
ATP	1.10
ADP	1.50
AMP	0.93
Σ adenine nucleotides	3.53
$\frac{[ATP][AMP]}{[ADP]^2}$	0.45

therefore been studied, in the cytoplasmic and mitochondrial compartments. The results are shown in fig. 1. The activity of this enzyme increases considerably in both cell compartments upon maturation.

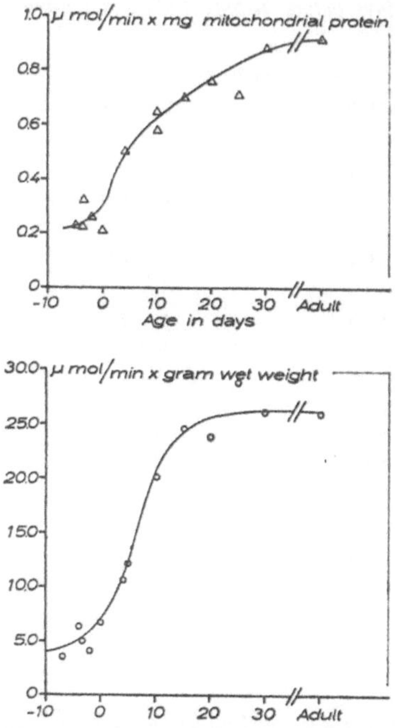

Fig. 1. Adenylate kinase activity of the mitochondrial compartment of rat liver (top) and supernatant fraction of rat liver homogenate (bottom) as a function of age.

Table 1 demonstrates however that, despite the lower activity, the fetal liver can establish near equilibrium under anaerobic conditions for the adenylate kinase reaction.

As is illustrated in table 1, the adenylate kinase system of the fetal liver operates in near equilibrium under aerobic conditions as well. It is known that this is not the case in the adult rat liver (16). The adenylate kinase cannot keep pace with the process of oxidative phosphorylation where ATP is synthesized. The conclusion must be that in the fetal rat liver the process of oxidative phosphorylation does not contribute in the same degree to the total ATP production as it does in the adult liver.

This can easily be understood because at 3 days before birth the fetal hepatocyte has only one third of the number of mitochondria in the hepatocyte of the adult rat liver (7, 19). The oxidative capacity of the fetal rat liver is lower than that of the adult rat liver, as has also been demonstrated by MÄENPÄÄ and RÄIHÄ (20).

A second reason is the lower activity per mitochondrion of succinic dehydrogenase (9) and the lower activity of aconitase relative to citrate synthase (10) of the fetal rat liver mitochondria, resulting in a lower turnover of the tricarboxylic acid cycle. This lower turnover of the tricarboxylic acid cycle and the lower number of mitochondria per hepatocyte of the fetal liver result in a smaller contribution of mitochondrial ATP synthesis to the total ATP synthesis as compared to the adult liver. It seems therefore that the fetal rat liver is less dependent on oxidative reactions for ATP synthesis.

An increased glycolytic flux is always associated with a decreased concentration of glucose-6-phosphate. This has been demonstrated for many tissues (16, 21, 22). Table 1 demonstrates that the concentration of glucose-6-phosphate is virtually the same under aerobic and anaerobic conditions, which seems to indicate that no change in glycolytic flux has occurred after the aerobic-anaerobic transition. An increased rate of glucose-6-phosphate production cannot originate from glycogen because at this stage of development there is very little, if any, glycogen (23). An increase in the rate of glucose-6-phosphate production from glucose by the hexokinase reaction cannot be expected either because the serum and liver glucose concentrations are well above the saturation level of hexokinase (23) and the glucokinase has not yet developped (24).

The other possible cause for a change in the glucose-6-phosphate concentration – resulting in a decrease in concentration – would be an increased utilization. Fig. 2 shows the relative changes of glycolytic

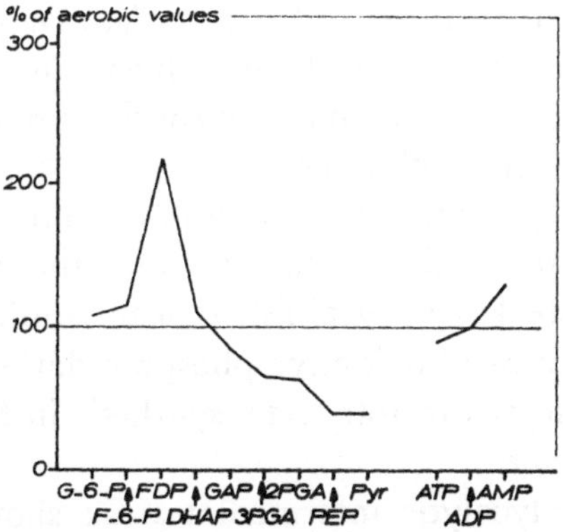

Fig. 2. Changes of glycolytic intermediates and adenine nucleotides in anaerobic fetal rat liver, relative to the values of aerobic fetal rat liver.

intermediates and adenine nucleotides, 2 min. after clamping of the umbilical cord. The changes are small which indicate that the tissue is relatively insensitive to anaerobiosis. This is in agreement with the above derived conclusions from the adenylate kinase system.

A slight activation of phosphofructokinase can however be observed, as is illustrated by the rise in FDP. In many tissues where a true control of glycolysis by phosphofructokinase has been demonstrated (see f.i. ref. 22) the changes in fructose-1, 6-diphosphate are one order of magnitude higher. There is furthermore an inhibition further down the glycolytic pathway, presumably at the glyceraldehyde-3-phosphate dehydrogenase step, resulting in lower concentrations of the 3-carbon intermediates. The increase in FDP may be – at least partly – due to this inhibition.

It can therefore be concluded that phosphofructokinase does not control glycolysis in the fetal rat liver. It may exert fine control, as illustrated by the slight rise in FDP upon anaerobiosis. The pace of glycolysis in fetal rat liver is however set by a step preceeding the phosphofructokinase reaction. This is presumably the glucose phosphorylating system, a conclusion which would be in agreement with computer simulations of this system (25, 26).

SUMMARY

The development of adenylate kinase in the mitochondrial and 'cell-sap' compartments of rat liver has been studied. Despite a considerable lower activity of this enzyme in the fetal liver, the enzyme establishes near equilibrium for the adenine nucleotides under anaerobic conditions, as it does in the adult liver.

Analysis of glycolytic intermediates and adenine nucleotides in the aerobic and anaerobic fetal liver demonstrated that also under aerobic conditions adenylate kinase establishes near equilibrium. It is concluded that the process of oxidative phosphorylation does not contribute in the same degree to total ATP synthesis in fetal rat liver as it does in the adult liver.

The analysis of glycolytic intermediates has shown that phosphofructokinase does only exert fine control on glycolysis, the main rate determining step being at glucose phosphorylation.

ACKNOWLEDGEMENT

The expert technical assistance of Miss A. Beere is grateful acknowledged. The investigations were supported (in part) by the Netherlands Foundation for Chemical Research (SON) with financial aid from the Netherlands Organization for the Advancement of Pure Research (ZWO).

REFERENCES

1. Burch H. B., O. H. Lowry, A. M. Kuhlmans, J. Skerjance, E. J. Diamont, S. R. Lowry and P. van Dippe, (1963) *J. Biol. Chem.* 238:2267.
2. Stawe U., (1964) *Biol. Neonat.* 6:128.
3. Hommes F. A. and C. W. Wilmink, (1968) *Biol. Neonat.* 12:181.
4. Tanaka F., Y. Harano, F. Sue and H. Morimuro, (1967) *J. Biochem.*, Tokyo, 62:71.
5. Tepper T. and F. A. Hommes, (1970) In: *Enzymes and isozymes, structure, properties and function*, Shugar D. ed., Acad. Press, London, (1970) p. 209.
6. Hommes F. A. and M. I. Draisma, (1970) *Biochim. Biophys. Acta*, 222:251.
7. Hommes F. A. and A. R. Richters, (1969) *Biol. Neonat.* 14:359.
8. Hemon P., (1967) *Biochim. Biophys. Acta*, 132:175.
9. De Vos M. A., C. W. Wilmink and F. A. Hommes, (1968) *Biol. Neonat.* 133:83.
10. Hommes F. A., G. Luit-De Haan and A. R. Richters, (1971) *Biol. Neonat.* 17:15.
11. Wollenberger A., E. C. Krause and B. E. Walker, (1958) *Naturwiss.* 45:294.
12. Estabrook R. A. and P. K. Maitra, (1962) *Anal. Biochem.* 3:369.
13. Lamprecht W. and I. Trautschold, (1965) In: *Methods in enzymatic analysis*, Bergmeyer H. U. ed., Acad. Press, New York, p. 543.
14. Schneider W. C., (1948) *J. Biol. Chem.* 176:259.
15. Adam H., (1963) In: *Methods in enzymatic analysis*, Bergmeyer H. U. ed., Acad. Press, London, p. 573.
16. Bücher Th., K. Krejci, W. Rüssmann, H. Schnitger and W. Wesemann, (1964) In: *Rapid mixing and sampling techniques in biochemistry*, Chance B., R. H. Eisenhardt, Q. H. Gibson and K. K. Lonberg-Holm eds., Acad. Press, New York, p. 255.
17. Brosnan J. T., H. A. Krebs and D. H. Williamson, (1970) *Biochem. J.* 117:91.
18. Adelman R. C., C. H. Lo and S. Weinhouse, (1968) *Adv. Enzyme Reg.* 6:425.
19. Vergonet G., F. A. Hommes and I. Molenaar, (1970) *Biol. Neonat.* 16:273.
20. Mäenpää P. M. and N. C. R. Räihä, (1968) *Scand. J. Clin. Lab. Invest.* 21. Suppl. 101.7.
21. Goldberg N. D., J. V. Passoneau and O. H. Lowry, (1965) In: *Control of energy metabolism*, Chance B., R. Estabrook and J. R. Williamson, Acad. Press, New York, p. 321.
22. Williamson J. R., (1965) In: *Control of energy metabolism*, Chance B., R. W. Estabrook and J. R. Williamson, Acad. Press, New York, p. 333.
23. Burch H. B., (1965) *Adv. Enzyme Reg.* 3:185.

24. Walker D. G., H. H. Khan and S. W. Eaton, (1966) *Biol. Neonat.* 9:224.
25. Vergonet G. and F. A. Hommes, (1970) In: *Metabolic pathways in mammalian embryo's during organogenesis and its modification by drugs*, Merker H. J. and D. Neubert eds., Berlin, in press.
26. Vergonet G., (1970) this volume, p. 14.

DISCUSSION

Dr. Sereni: I would like to know on which kind of liver cells you made your very interesting experiments. It is well known that in foetal rat liver the per cent of parenchymous cells increases very much during the last three days of gestation, mainly because the total amount of hemopoietic cells drops sharply.

Dr. Hommes: We have not isolated the hepatocytes. We just worked with whole liver. In other words this applies to a mixture of the cells. Also the adult liver is not a homogeneous tissue. We have recently succeeded in isolating suspensions of rat hepatocytes.* This method can also be applied to foetal liver. Sofar we have only done some preliminary experiments. This will enable us to look more precisely at the hepatocytes.

Dr. Sereni: There is no doubt that we will reach a better understanding on development of enzyme activities in foetal and newborn liver, if we will succeed working on hepatocytes suspensions. JACQUOT, in Rennes, has already obtained very interesting results on glycogen metabolism of foetal hepatocytes. We are now working using the same technique, looking for factors controlling tyrosine aminotransferase and glucose-6-phosphatase activity.

Dr. Hommes: It is true that we are working with a mixture of cells. Again this applies to all studies using whole tissues. The only way out is to prepare hepatocytes by tissue culture techniques or by isolating the cells you want to study.

Prof. Villee: I would like to express my admiration of these studies you have carried out. You have done a great deal to show precisely where there are changes during early development. My own studies

* F. A. HOMMES, M. J. DRAISMA and J. MOLENAAR, (1970) *Biochim. Biophys. Acta* 222, 361.

with whole slices are consistent with your results. You may remember that I showed that the course of enzymatic development in human foetal liver is a little different from that in rat liver. I hope it is part of your plan to do studies such as these with human foetal liver at an early opportunity.

Dr. Räihä: There is an old observation that foetal and newborn animals withstand complete oxygen deficiency much better than adults. In your experiments you probably found the same thing. You showed clearly that the ATP concentration during anaerobic conditions was higher or stayed higher in the foetus than in the adult. I should like to show a slide from our study on the ATP levels in the rat heart during anoxia. The results are consisting with your findings. The ATP concentration is shown in μ moles per gram fresh weight. The animals have been kept during different times in 100% nitrogen. In the adult the ATP level dropped very quickly during anoxia. In the foetus the ATP concentration stays much longer on a higher level.

Dr. Hommes: There is a difference between heart and liver. The enzymatic equipment of the heart mitochondria is different from that of liver. I don't think there is in foetal heart such a relative deficiency of succinic-dehydrogenase as compared to the adult.

Secondly the foetal rat heart does have a beta-hydroxybutyrate dehydrogenase. I don't know what the meaning of this is but the foetal liver mitochondria do not.

I don't know anything about the adenylate-kinase in heart. I think it should be pretty high in heart compared to the liver.

One should also measure the cytochrome content. The situation in heart is about the same as it is in liver: a much higher contribution to total ATP synthesis from glycolysis than from oxydative phosphorylation.

Dr. Räihä: Your explanation for the survival of the foetus during prolonged anoxia would be a higher rate of glycolysis in the foetus.

Dr. Hommes: I would not say a higher rate, because in absolute terms the rate is lower.

Dr. Räihä: Its lactate production is lower.

Dr. Hommes: It is not so much a higher rate. You have to take into account the ATP utilization as well. All these factors determine the steady state level of ATP. It does make much difference where you generate the ATP: from glycolysis which is independent of oxygen or from oxydative phosphorylation. If you cut off the oxydative phosphorylation by anoxia in the adult liver the ATP level drops rapidly. If the contribution in the foetal liver to total ATP synthesis by oxydative phosphorylation is low and you cut off this little part, you don't see large changes.

Dr. Schröter: I should like to ask a question concerning the rate-limiting enzyme of glycolysis in the foetal liver. You have shown that the activity of hexokinase is about two third of the activity of adults. You mentioned that the hexokinase activity includes the activity of glucokinase in the adult liver. In the newborn liver glucokinase activity is zero. I think we can assume that the hexokinase activity is true hexokinase activity.

Do you think that the hexokinase is a rate-limiting enzyme in the foetal liver or the phosphofructokinase or any other enzyme?

A second question. Is the same enzyme rate limiting under aerobic and anaerobic conditions?

Dr. Hommes: It is the hexokinase which is rate limiting in the foetal liver. This does not exclude phosphofructokinase as a fine control and in fact you could see (fig. 2) that beyond the point of glyceraldehyde-phosphate it drops to below the 100 percent level, in other words there must be another control point. The situation is of course different in the adult tissue. There you can under anaerobic conditions by-pass the glucose-phosphorylating step by generating glucose-6-phosphate from glycogen, which actually takes place. Then the phosphofructokinase becomes rate limiting. That is something like a safety-device.

COMPUTER REPRESENTATION OF GLYCOLYSIS IN ADULT AND FETAL RAT LIVER

G. VERGONET*

INTRODUCTION

It is well known that fetal tissue is more able to survive an anoxious period than more mature tissue. From a biochemical point of view, this means that fetal tissue is better equipped to maintain a certain ATP level under anaerobic conditions than the adult tissue. Because glycolysis is under anaerobic conditions the main producer of ATP, computer studies are made in order to evaluate differences in control of this process in fetal and adult rat liver.

THE MODEL

In order to carry out these computations it is necessary to construct a kinetic model of glycolysis. The model used is essentially a model proposed by GARFINKEL (1) for the ascites tumor cell, but differs from this in some important aspects.

A blockdiagram is shown in fig. 1. Enzymes are represented as 'black-boxes' with in- and output of fluxes of the concerned substrates, products and coenzymes. The use of this symbolism gives us a framework for a convenient description of multi-enzyme systems.

Important differences with the ascites cell model are:

1. It is not assumed that ATP is compartmented between cytosol and mitochondria, because the available experimental evidence is not found to be sufficient (2, 3, 4).
2. A fructosediphosphate (FDP) activation of the enzyme pyruvate kinase (5) is introduced for the adult system.

* Department of Paediatrics, University of Groningen School of Medicine, Groningen, The Netherlands.

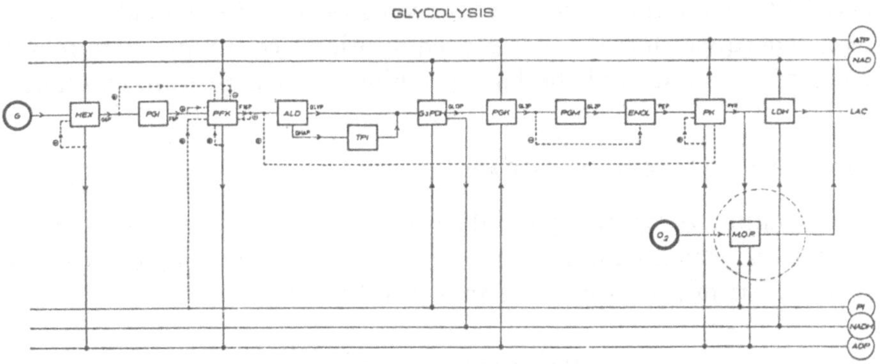

Fig. 1. Model of glycolysis. The enzymes are represented by squares. The interrupted lines indicate if an intermediate inhibits (—sign) or activates (+ sign). For abbreviations see table II.

3. It is not accepted that a complex is formed between the enzymes aldolase and triosephosphate isomerase in order to explain the anomal ratio of the concentrations of glyceraldehydephosphate and dihydroxyacetonephosphate. Ultracentrifuge experiments with the two enzymes in the presence and in the absence of the substrate did not show the existence of such a complex.
4. A hexomonophosphate shunt (HMP) is introduced being always 1% of the glucose-6-phosphate flux (6).
5. The allosteric properties of phosphofructokinase as far as inhibition by ATP and activation by ADP, G-6-P, F-6-P and FDP are concerned, have been accounted for (7).

METHODS

The concentrations of the enzymes were determined in adult and fetal liver using the specific activities from the literature. The enzymes were assayed under the same conditions as specified in the literature (8). Glycolytic enzymes of liver were also assayed at pH 7.4 and 22 °C in a buffer containing 50 mM TRA, 10 mM KCl and 2 mM $MgCl_2$.

The activities measured in this way were compared with the activities which can be calculated from the inserted kinetics, used in the glycolytic model. If deviations occurred corrections were applied in order to obtain agreement between the measured activities and the activities used in the model. Also the kinetics of the individual enzymes were checqued for the correct equilibrium constants, MICHAELIS MENTEN constants and the known inhibition or activation constants.

THE STEADY STATE PROGRAM

Two computerprograms were developed to simulate glycolysis. First a program which computes the steady state of the complete system. A flowchart of this program is shown in fig. 2.

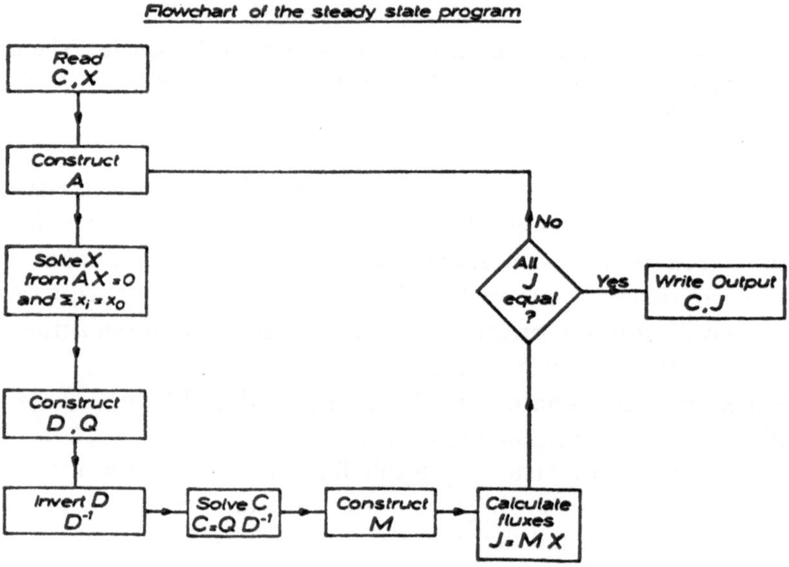

Fig. 2. C, Xo are arrays representing the concentrations of substrates, products and coenzymes resp. the total enzyme concentrations. A, D and Q are matrices describing relationships between concentration values of intermediates and time.

This program is based on an iteration procedure. The input consists of concentration values of substrates, products and coenzymes represented by a vector C and the total enzyme concentrations represented by a vector Xo. From these data and the known velocity constants a matrix A is constructed for each individual enzyme system, giving the time dependency of the enzyme and the enzyme-substrate complexes. The steady state values of these enzyme forms represented by a vector X belonging to the given set of initial concentrations of substrates and products can be calculated if this time dependency is set zero.

The same calculations can be carried out according to the rules of King & Altman (9). The matrices D and Q are constructed for the complete system, giving the time-dependency of the concentrations of substrates and products (C). D and Q are functions of the enzyme species. The calculated values of the enzyme species are used to derive a new set of concentration values C for steady state conditions. Finally the fluxes are calculated with the aid of the constructed flux matrices M. If the fluxes are not equal throughout the glycolytic system, taking into account a factor of 2 for the 3-carbon intermediates, the procedure is repeated, untill the fluxes in and out of each individual enzyme system are equal. Then steady state has been reached.

Another program is developed which simulates the transition from aerobic to anaerobic glycolysis. This program especially developed for systems containing stiff equations is based on a steady state assumption of the enzyme forms, which are in general responsable for the stiffness of the system (10).

A correction procedure is incorporated. A complete description of this method of calculation has recently been published (11). The advantage of the first program is that no integration procedures are used, so the program is very fast, which makes it possible to do many runs in order to analize the steady state behaviour of the system thoroughly.

RESULTS AND DISCUSSION

The calculated concentrations of the substrates, products and coenzymes are shown in table 1. Also the fluxes are given for the aerobic steady state in adult and fetal rat liver.

The adult flux is about three times higher than the fetal flux. Also the hexokinase concentrations differ about a factor 3. It seems that the hexokinase concentration determines the flux under these conditions that is when glucose is the substrate.

The purpose of these investigations was to analize the rate of ATP production and consumption under aerobic and anaerobic conditions. Because the anaerobic glycolytic flux determines the rate of ATP production, it is important to know, how the flux depends on the ATP and ADP level.

Table 1. *Calculated steady state concentrations of glycolytic intermediates of the fetal and adult rat liver*

Substrates	Fetal liver	Adult liver
Glucose	10 mM	10 mM
Glucose-6-phosphate	0.62 mM	1.45 mM
Fructose-6-phosphate	0.16 mM	0.36 mM
Fructose-1, 6-diphosphate	0.08 mM	0.38 mM
Glyceraldehyde-3-phosphate	0.005 mM	0.008 mM
Dihydroxy acetonephosphate	0.12 mM	0.40 mM
1, 3 diphosphoglycerate	0.002 mM	0.0016 mM
3-phosphoglycerate	0.037 mM	0.074 mM
2-phosphoglycerate	0.007 mM	0.008 mM
Phosphoenolpyruvate	0.04 mM	0.046 mM
Pyruvate	0.17 mM	0.15 mM
Lactate	2.37 mM	3.86 mM
ATP	3.31 mM	2.82 mM
ADP	0.29 mM	0.68 mM
Pi	1.10 mM	1.10 mM
NAD	3.00 mM	3.00 mM
NADH	0.004 mM	0.0075 mM
glycolytic flux:	0.63 μMol/min/gr	1.74 μMol/min/gr

In fig. 3 are shown the fluxes which are involved in aerobic ATP production and consumption. Glycolysis proceeds up to pyruvate yielding a net synthesis of 2 ATP and 1 NADH. The pyruvate produced enters the mitochondria and is metabolized to CO_2 and H_2O. An ener-

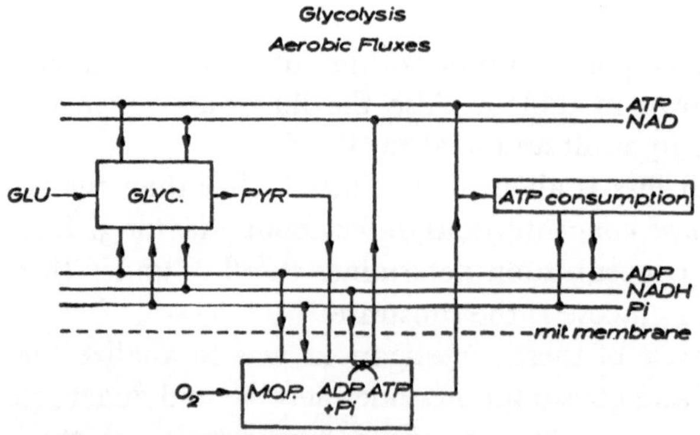

Fig. 3. Aerobic fluxes. It is assumed that pyruvate is consumed by the mitochondria and completely metabolized into CO_2 and water according the equation.
$pyr + 15\,ADP + 15\,Pi + 3\,O_2 \rightarrow 15\,ATP + 3\,CO_2 + 3\,H_2O$

gy, equivalent to 15 ATP is thus available for the cell. The mitochondrial membrane is not impermeable for NADH. However by interference of reducible substrates it is possible that the NADH formed cytoplasmatically is reoxidized by the respiratory chain, localized in the mitochondria.

For this transfer various mechanisms have been postulated (12, 13, 14). Per NADH oxidized 3 ATP are formed. Steady state implies that no changes in concentration occur. Therefore the NAD/NADH ratio has to remain constant and the effect of an assumed transfer mechanism is that the same quantity of NADH as is formed in the cytosol is reoxidized to NAD. From these steady state assumptions the ATP production can be calculated.

In order to obtain the relation between fluxes and the ATP and ADP levels, glycolytic fluxes are calculated at various ATP and ADP levels. This is shown in fig. 4.

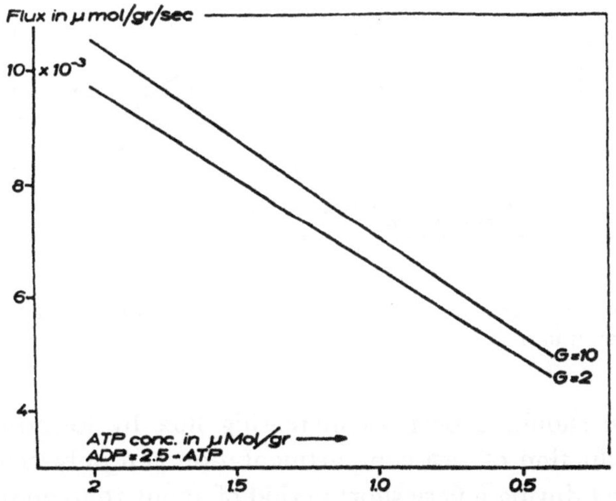

Fig. 4. Glycolytic fluxes calculated with the steady state program by various ATP and ADP concentrations. The total amount of ATP, ADP and Pi has been kept constant.

It can be seen that the fluxes decrease with lowering ATP level if glucose is used as substrate for glycolysis. This means that in this model the hexokinase reaction controls the flux and phosphofructokinase acts as fine control only.

Control by hexokinase is clearly illustrated in fig. 5, where the flux through the hexokinase system is calculated as a function of the ATP concentration. Comparison of the behaviour of the glycolytic flux with the flux produced by the hexokinase system shows that the fluxes behave in the same way. Variation of glucose-6-phosphate has little effect. This behaviour of the flux cannot explain the Pasteur effect,

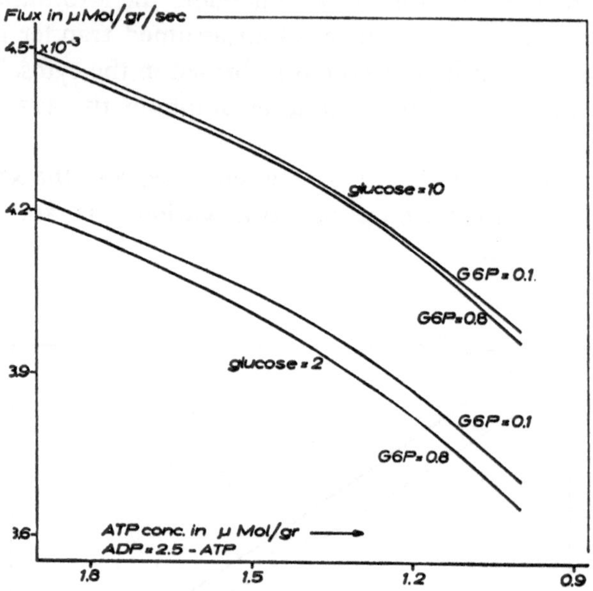

Fig. 5. Fluxes of glucose-6-phosphate produced by the hexokinase mechanism under steady state conditions.

because one should expect an increasing flux by lowering the ATP level. Introduction of ATP compartmentation can only account for a Pasteur effect during a very short period of about 10 to 20 seconds (1). However from the properties of phosphofructokinase it is obvious that a Pasteur effect can be explained with this model.

In fig. 6 is shown that the percentage phosphofructokinase (PFK) in the active form is increasing strongly with lowering of the ATP level. If the ATP concentration switches from 2 to 1 the percentage of PFK which is in the active state is increased 50 times and the flux through PFK increases by about a factor of 5, as is illustrated in fig. 7. The

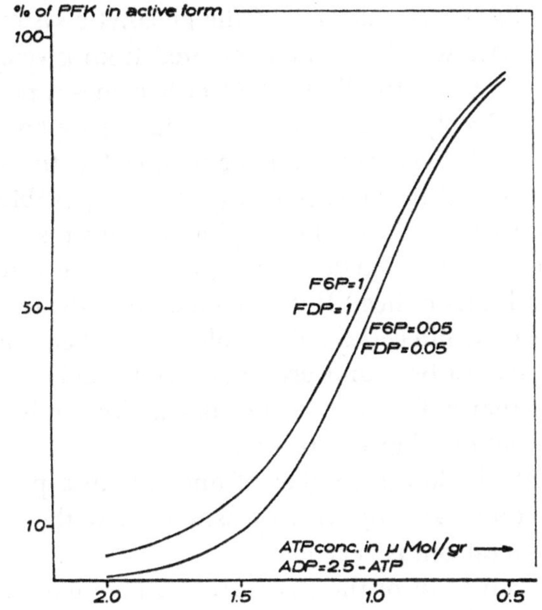

Fig. 6. Percentage of phosphofructokinase in the active form as function of the ATP level.

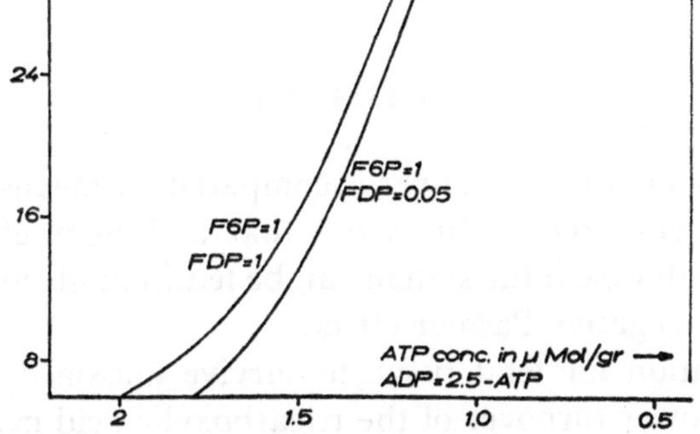

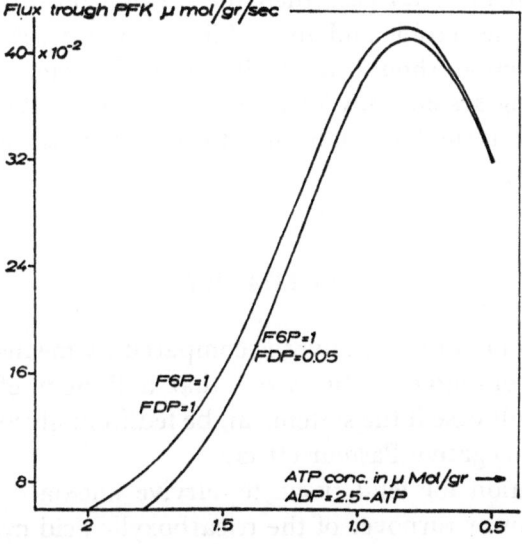

Fig. 7. The calculated flux of FDP produced by the enzyme phosphofructokinase as function of the ATP level.

conclusion can be drawn that only if the glycolytic system is fed with glucose-6-phosphate which can be generated from glycogen, PFK can act as control point and the Pasteur effect becomes a possible feature of this model of glycolysis. This supply of glucose-6-phosphate can be realized in the adult liver. However the fetal cell at three days before birth contains very little glycogen (15). So we possibly can expect here a negative Pasteur effect. The fact that fetal liver is more equipped to survive an anoxious period does not agree very well with the existence of a negative Pasteur effect. If it is assumed that the model is correct for the fetal tissue within certain allowable errors, then the explanation of this feature has to be found elsewhere. A possible explanation on enzyme level is that in fetal liver some enzymes of the Krebs cycle are practically not yet developed (16, 17).

Together with the lower number of mitochondria per cell as compared to the adult case (8) we can assume that the mitochondrial capacity of the fetal cell is very low.

This means that most of the pyruvate is converted via acetyl-CoA into fatty acids, or is converted into lactate.

It is known that the synthesis of fatty acids in the fetal cell is considerably (18). If one should assume that pyruvate does not enter the Krebs cycle in the fetal case then there exists no difference in ATP production in the aerobic and anaerobic steady state. A small decrease in ATP production should result if pyruvate enters the oxidative phosphorylating system only to a minor degree. If this difference in ATP production is small enough, then the organism is well equipped to survivc anoxia.

SUMMARY

Glycolysis in fetal and adult liver is compared by means of simulation on a digital computer. It turns out that a Pasteur effect can exist only in the adult case if the system can be fed from glycogen. The fetal tissue shows a negative Pasteur effect.

An explanation for fetal tissue to survive anoxia can possibly be found in the lower turnover of the tricarboxylic acid cycle.

AKNOWLEDGEMENT

This work was carried out under the auspices of the Netherlands Foundation for Chemical Research (SON) and with financial aid from the Netherlands Organization for the Advancement of Pure Research (ZWO).

REFERENCES

1. GARFINKEL D. and B. HESS, (1964) *J. Biol. Chem.* 239: 971.
2. SIEKEVITZ P., (1961) *Proc. Vth Intern. Congr. of Biochemistry*, Moscow.
3. HOMMES F. A., (1962) *Fed. Proc.* 21: 142.
4. HESS B. and B. CHANCE, (1961) *J. Biol. Chem.* 236: 239.
5. TAYLOR C. B., E. BAILY, (1967) *Biochem. J.* 102: 32C.
6. KÖHLER E., (1970) In: NEUBERT D. and H. MERKER, *Metabolic pathways in mammalian Embryo's during organogenesis and its modification by Drugs*, Berlin, (in press).
7. GARFINKEL D., (1966) *J. Biol. Chem.* 241: 286.
8. VERGONET G., F. A. HOMMES and I. MOLENAAR, (1970) *Biol. Neonat.* 16: 297.
9. KING E. L. and C. ALTMAN, (1956) *J. Phys. Chem.*, Ithaca, 60: 1375.
10. GARFINKEL D., S. CHING, M. ADELMAN, P. CLARK, (1966) *Ann. N.Y. Acad. Sci.* 128: 1054.
11. VERGONET G. and H. J. C. BERENDSEN, (1970) *J. Theoret. Biol.* 28: 155.
12. KLINGENBERG M. and TH. BÜCHER, (1960) *Ann. Rev. Biochem.* 29: 669.
13. DEVLIN T. H. and B. BEDELL, *J. Biol. Chem.* 235: 2134.
14. BORST P., (1962) *Funktionelle und Morphologische Organization der Zelle*, Springer Verlag, Heidelberg, p. 137.
15. BURCH H. B., (1965) *Adv. Enzyme Reg.* 3: 185.
16. DE VOS M. A., C. W. WILMINK and F. A. HOMMES, (1968) *Biol. Neonat.* 13: 83.
17. HOMMES F. A., G. LUIT-DE HAAN and A. R. RICHTERS, (1970), (in press).
18. BALLARD F. J. and R. W. HANSON, (1967) *Biochem. J.* 102: 952.

Table 2. *List of abbreviations:*

HK	: hexokinase
PGI	: phosphogluco isomerase
PFK	: phosphofructokinase
ALD	: aldolase
TPI	: triosephosphate isomerase
GAPDH	: glyceraldehyde-3-phosphate dehydrogenase
PGK	: phosphoglycerokinase
PGM	: phosphoglyceromutase
EN	: enolase
PK	: pyruvatekinase
LDH	: lactate dehydrogenase
MK	: myokinase
HMP	: hexosemonophosphate shunt

DISCUSSION

Dr. Schröter: You have shown relatively high concentrations of glucose-6-phosphate and low concentrations of fructose-6-phosphate in foetal liver.

Dr. Vergonet: The glucose-6-phosphate concentration is lower in foetal liver because the enzyme hexokinase is three times lower here in concentration.

Dr. Hommes: I may add that in the foetal liver as well as in the adult liver the ratio of G-6-P over F-6-P are according to the isomerase equilibrium. This is comparable to other enzyme systems for example 3-phosphoglycerate over 2-phosphoglycerate and 2-phosphoglycerate over phosphoenol pyruvate. Those are the three enzymes who are very high in activity, in fact so high that they can easily bring the whole system in near equilibrium. And if you calculate this it is according to the thermodynamic equilibrium.

Dr. Young: I wonder if I could ask the biochemist a very simple question. It always seems to me a little strange that the fetus has exactly the same oxygen consumption per kilo as the adult.

Dr. Hommes: I don't think it is a simple question. I think it is an embarrasing question. All the fetal tissues per gram wet weight so far examined have a lower cytochrome oxydase activity than the adult tissues. This is the terminal oxygen acceptor. This will give you the maximum capacity for oxygen uptake per gram wet weight.

Prof. Villee: This must mean then that cytochrome oxydase is not the rate limiting step, perhaps the rate limiting step is the rate at which the electrons are passed through the electron transport system to the final cytochrome oxydase. If there is a rate limiting step further down the electrons cannot get up any faster. In constructing your models,

Dr. VERGONET, you really made two models, one for foetal livers and one for adult livers, is that right?

Dr. Vergonet: It is about the same model, but with different enzyme concentrations.

Prof. Villee: To get the number to use in each model you used I suppose the numbers of Dr. HOMMES for the foetal liver and for the adult liver. The model is the same but the individual components of the model are different.

Does this also take account possible differences in the isozymes present in the two systems?

Dr. Vergonet: For instance pyruvatekinase is in the adult liver activated by fructosediphosphate and not in the foetal case.

Prof. Villee: Now I ask you a very unfair question. It looks as though with a computer-model you can carry out your calculation and if you don't like the number that comes out the first time you run it through a second time. Do you really do this? What happens?

Dr. Vergonet: I have tried to make this model as correct as possible. Then I do a run and I realise very well that the concentrations I find are not completely in agreement with the concentration you can measure. We did not try to obtain a complete fit between measured and calculated concentrations.

Dr. Hommes: There is in fact a very fundamental deficiency in the model. The ratio of di-hydroxy-acetone-phosphate and glyceraldehydephosphate in vivo is, as far as I remember, 1:1. According to the triosephosphate-isomerase equilibrium it should be 22:1.

In our model it is nearer to this number than to 1:1. Others have solved this problem by introducing a complex between aldolase and triosephosphate-isomerase. If one wants to solve this problem one has to use two different thermodynamic equilibrium constants for the triosephosphate-isomerase reaction. I think that this is simply not permissible, and furthermore there is no experimental evidence for such a complex. We just don't know what is going on there. In regard to this aspect the model is deficient.

THE DEVELOPMENT OF SOME ENZYMES OF AMINOACID METABOLISM IN THE HUMAN LIVER

N. C. R. RÄIHÄ*

Besides problems concerned with specific inborn errors of metabolism the enzymes of aminoacid metabolism have a twofold interest to the pediatrician. The fundamental question of mammalian enzyme development and regulation of enzyme 'induction' has been studied intensively during recent years with respect to some of the enzymes involved in amino-acid metabolism such as tyrosine-transaminase (1, 2, 3). Furthermore from a nutritional and clinical point of view the maturity of enzymes involved in aminoacid synthesis and metabolism is of importance during the perinatal and neonatal period, since it has become apparent that the fetus and the newborn infant are metabolically different than the mature older organism of the same species and consequently the young organism cannot synthesize and metabolize some aminoacids as effectively as later. This leads to problems of differential diagnosis during early postnatal life especially with respect to premature infants which may show high levels of e.g. tyrosine in their blood due to transient low activity in the liver of enzymes oxidizing tyrosine (4). Furthermore the immaturity of some aminoacid synthesizing enzymes must be kept in mind with respect to artificial nutrition of premature infants. It has been known for some time that histidine is essential during human infancy (5). Recently it has been shown that also cyst(e)ine may be essential in the human fetus and premature infant (6).

During the last two years our laboratory has been involved in studies concerning the development of enzymes of tyrosine and cysteine metabolism in *human* liver. The studies involving the development of tyrosine-transaminase have been carried out in collaboration

* Departments of Medical Chemistry and Obstetrics and Gynecology, University of Helsinki, Finland.

with Drs. M. LINDROOS of Helsinki University and A. SCHWARTZ of Case Western Reserve University in Cleveland, Ohio, and the studies on the transsulfuration pathway in collaboration with Drs. G. GAULL and J. STURMAN of the Institute for Basic Research in Mental Retardation, Staten Island, New York.

In the following I will outline some of these experiments and their results.

INDUCTION OF TYROSINE-TRANSAMINASE IN FETAL RAT AND FETAL HUMAN LIVER IN ORGAN CULTURE

Tyrosine transaminase (L-tyrosine: 2 oxoglutarate aminotransferase), the first enzyme in the tyrosine oxidizing system (fig. 1) has a very

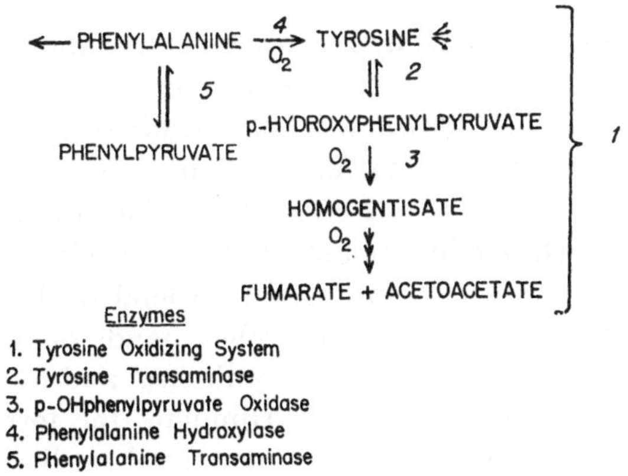

Fig. 1. Pathways of phenylalanine and tyrosine metabolism.

low activity in fetal rat liver but beginning with the 2nd hour after birth there is a rapid increase in activity reaching a maximum at ca. 12 hours (1). Our studies have confirmed this and we find the following developmental curve in the rat using the tyrosine transaminase assay described by DIAMONDSTONE (7) (fig. 2). The activity of tyrosine transaminase in human fetal liver at 14 to 26 weeks of gestation was somewhat variable and was approximately twice that found in fetal rats. In adult human liver the tyrosine transaminase activity was much higher and a postnatal increase as in the rat seems to occur since the

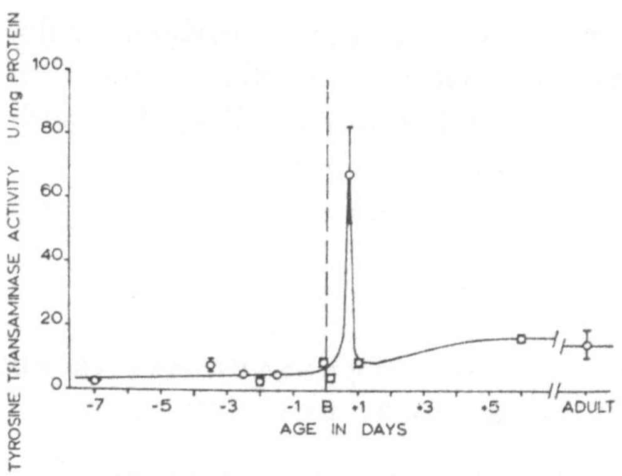

Fig. 2. Development of tyrosine transaminase activity in the rat. Each point represents the mean ± S.E. of at least three animals.

activity in the livers of some newborn infants who died at 12–24 hours of age showed considerably more activity than the fetal livers.

GREENGARD (8) has shown that the administration of glucagon, adrenaline and cyclic AMP to fetal rats during the last 2 days of gestation stimulated the appearance of tyrosine transaminase *in vivo* although hydrocortisone injected into rat fetuses *in utero* did not effect this enzyme activity (1). *In vitro* studies on fetal rat liver maintained in organ culture (2) have, on the other hand, demonstrated that tyrosine transaminase is elevated by cyclic AMP and by the hormones glucagon and catecholamine which stimulate the formation of this nucleotide, as well as by hydrocortisone in fetal rat liver near term.

No studies on regulatory mechanisms involved in the development of tyrosine-transaminase in human liver have been presented. Since artificial stimulation of enzyme development during fetal life may in the future facilitate certain metabolic adjustments of the premature and fullterm newborn infant to extrauterine life, we decided to undertake a comparative study of the development of tyrosine transaminase in fetal rat and fetal human liver maintained in organ culture with reference to the stage of development at which hormonal enzyme 'induction' can be evoked.

Fresh explants of fetal rat and fetal human liver of different gestational ages were cultured in Eagles minimal essential medium with Hank's balanced salt solution containing twice the normal concentration of glucose and bicarbonate and with 100 units of penicillin and 100 μg of streptomycin per ml. The dishes containing the explants (fig. 3) were placed in high humidity chambers and maintained at +37° with a circulating gas phase of 95% air +5% CO_2. All explants were kept in culture at least for 40 hours before the experiments. The viability of the liver explants was evaluated as follows: histological appearance after staining with hematoxylin – eosin and incorporations of radioactive precursors for protein (^{3}H-leucine), RNA (^{14}C-orotic acid) and DNA (^{3}H-thymidine). All incorporations were performed with one hour pulses in each culture dish. Figs. 5 and 6 show fetal rat and human liver explants in culture after 72 hours as compared to a fresh preparation of term fetal rat liver (fig. 4). As can be noted from the figures the appearance of the hepatocytes does not change markedly during the culture period although a dissappearance of erythrocytes and hematopoetic cells can be seen. As seen from table 1 the in-

Table 1. *Incorporation of ^{14}C-orotic acid, ^{3}H-leucine and ^{3}H-thymidine into fetal rat and fetal human liver in organ culture. Mean ± S.E., with number of observations in pa renthesis.*

	^{14}C-orotic acid	^{3}H-leucine	^{3}H-thymidine
		cpm/mg protein	
Fetal Rat (48 hours in culture)	3480 ± 650(12)	2260 ± 600(10)	582 ± 199(5)
Fetal Human (39–48 hours in culture)	1020 ± 147(12)	1393 ± 185(15)	36 ± 20(7)

corporation of radioactive precursors for protein, RNA and DNA indicate that the tissue explants remained functional during the period of the experiment. Very little ^{3}H-thymidine was incorporated into the fetal tissue during a 1-hour pulse, however when the labelling time was extended a considerable incorporation was found. In general the incorporation was somewhat greater into the rat tissue than into the human.

The activity of fetal rat liver tyrosine transaminase increased slightly during the culture period of the explants, this pattern was also evident in the fetal human liver explants. When term rat liver explants were cultured with hydrocortisone (10 $^{-6}$ M) for 24 h the tyrosine transaminase activity was markedly elevated as seen in fig. 7. This response was not evident under identical conditions in liver explants from fetal rats less than 14–15 days (fig. 7).

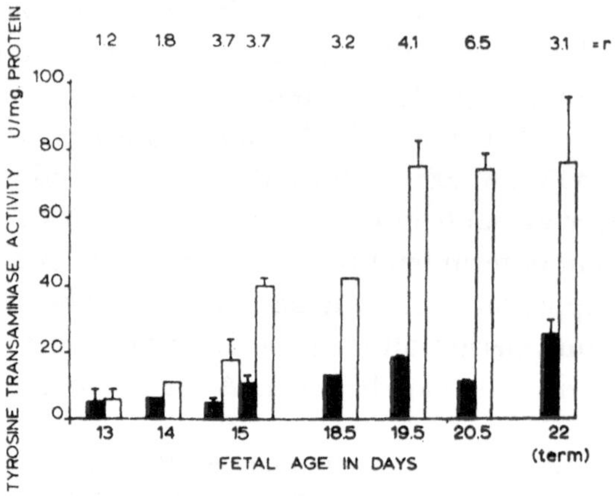

Fig. 7. Development of hydrocortisone induction of rat-liver tyrosine transaminase in culture. Open bars-hydrocortisone; closed bars-controls. Standard deviations are given for more than 2 determinations. Ages are ± 8 hours; r = hydrocortisone/control. All experiments began after 40 hours in culture and lasted 20–24 hours. Both sets of data at day 15 have identical r values.

Addition of actinomycin D (25 μg/ml) to the culture medium inhibited completely the hydrocortisone induced increase in tyrosine /transaminase activity (fig. 8). Cycloheximide (10 μg/ml) was also a potent inhibitor.

In addition to hydrocortisone glucagon and insulin had an increasing effect on tyrosine transaminase activity. When term fetal rat liver explants were incubated with these hormones a doubling of the enzyme activity could be noted in 20 hours.

No increase in tyrosine transaminase activity could be produced by any of the three hormones tested in liver explants from 14 to 24 weeks old human fetuses under identical conditions. However, at 26 weeks, human fetal liver explants responded to the glucocorticoid triamnicolone (10 $^{-4}$ M) by a 4-fold increase in tyrosine transaminase activity after an incubation of 24 hours with the hormone. This fetal liver was obtained from a fetus who died traumatically at spontaneous breech

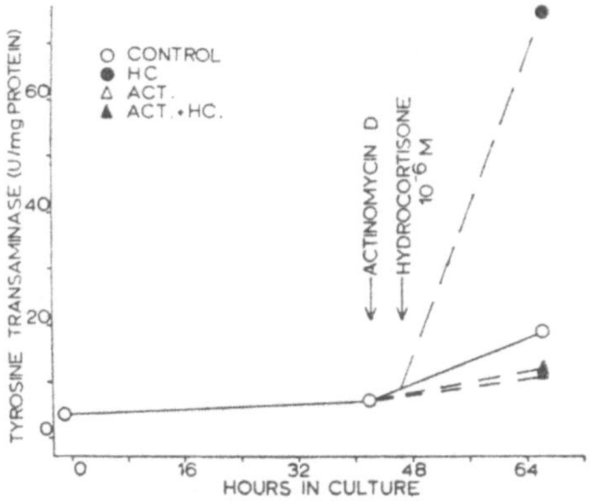

Fig. 8. Effect of Actinomycin D on hydrocortisone-induced tyrosine transaminase activity in term fetal rat liver explants. Each point represents the average of two parallel determinations. The experiments were begun after 40 hours in culture O-control, ●-hydrocortisone, Δ-Actinomycin D, ▲-Actinomycin D followed by hydrocortisone

delivery at 26 weeks of gestation. The control values for tyrosine transaminase were 14.7 and 17.4 U/mg protein and after incubation with the glucocorticoid the values were 50.0 and 63.0 U/gm protein. The histological appearance of the hepatocytes after the incubation period was good.

The development of tyrosine transaminase in human liver seems to have a similar course as that found in rat liver, and becomes inducible by corticosteroid hormone when ca. 60% of gestation is completed. These studies support the hypothesis that mammalian liver is incompetent to respond to hormone induced enzyme synthesis before a certain developmental stage is reached.

DEVELOPMENT OF THE TRANSSULFURATION PATHWAY IN HUMAN FETAL LIVER

In the adult mammal, including the human, ingested methionine is converted to cystine or cysteine in the transsulfuration pathway (fig. 9). The activities of methionine activating enzyme, cystathionine synthase and cystathionase were assayed during the development of the rat and the human using methods described previously (9). 24 livers from

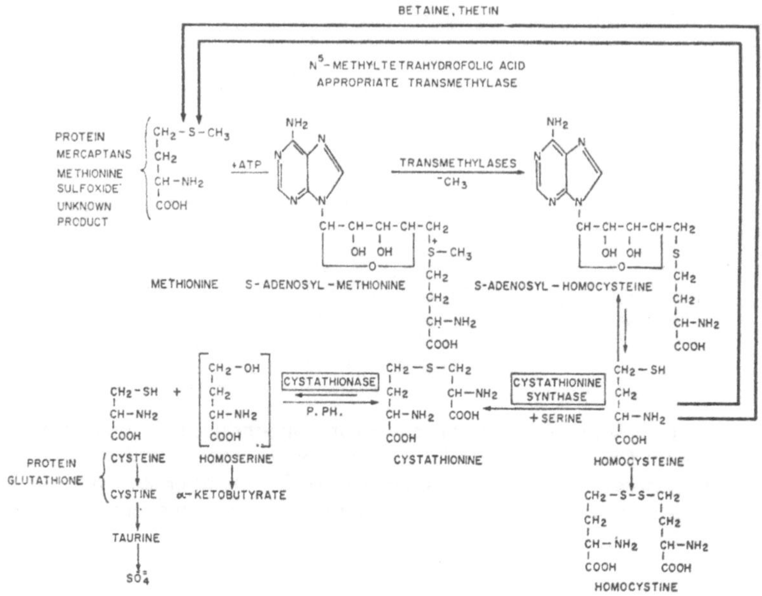

Fig. 9. Transsulfuration pathway.

human fetuses (2.5 to 20.5 cm, crown-rump length) obtained at therapeutic abortion, 5 premature infants (birth weights between 830–1500 g) and two fullterm newborns were studied. The control material consisted of 9 human adults and children (minimum age 2½ years). The results of these studies are seen in tables 2 and 3. The most striking finding is that cystathionase activity is absent in the liver of all the 24 fetuses and all the premature infants who died at less than 24 hours of age. In the fullterm infant less than 24 hours of age the cystathionase activity is barely measurable. In the one premature infant at 96 hours of age and in the other full-term infant at 72 hours of age considerable cystathionase activity is already present. The results seem to indicate that both gestational age and time after birth effects the cystathionase activity in the human liver. Further studies on the regulation of cystathionase activity in human fetal liver are being carried out in our laboratory. The finding that cystathionine, the substrate of cystathionase, is present in relatively high concentration in the liver of the human fetuses and premature infants in contrast

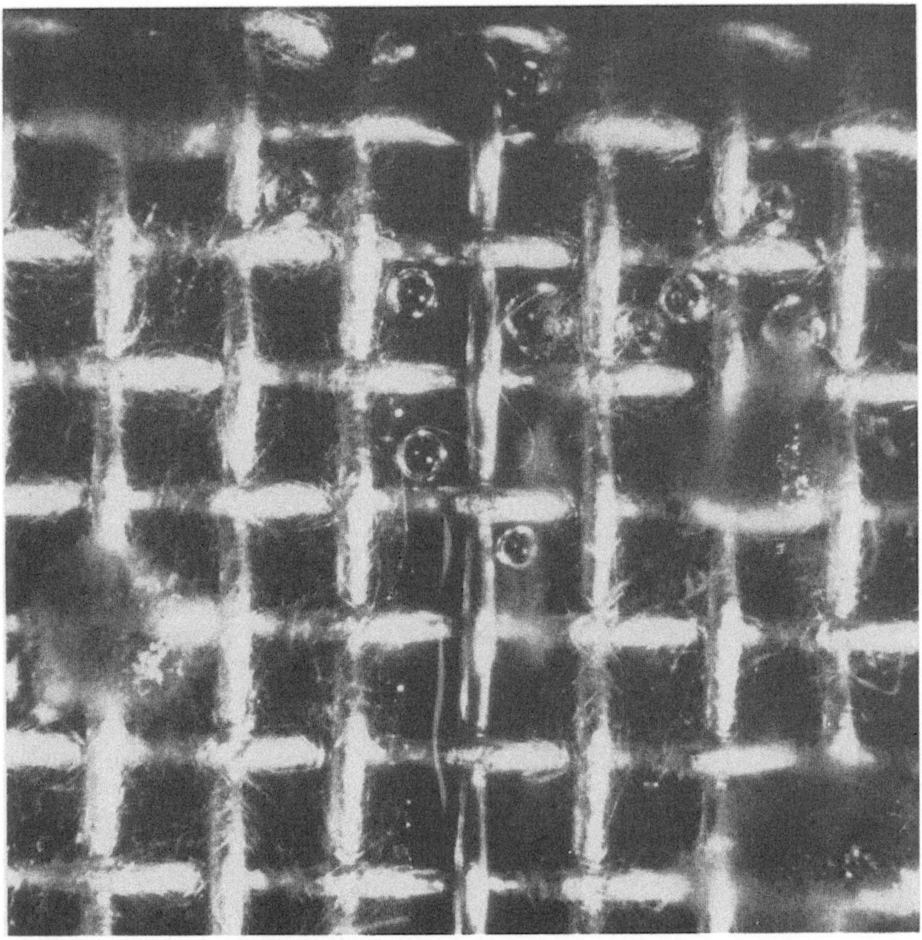

Fig. 3.

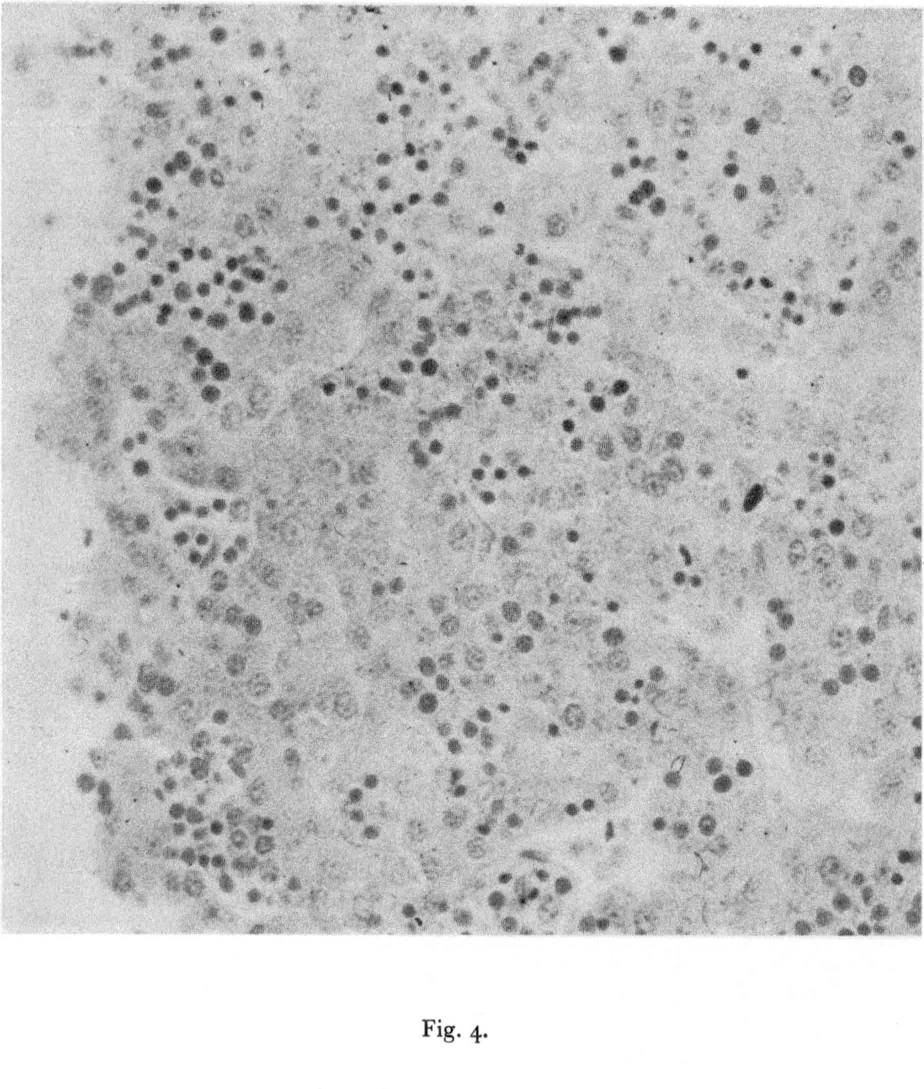

Fig. 4.

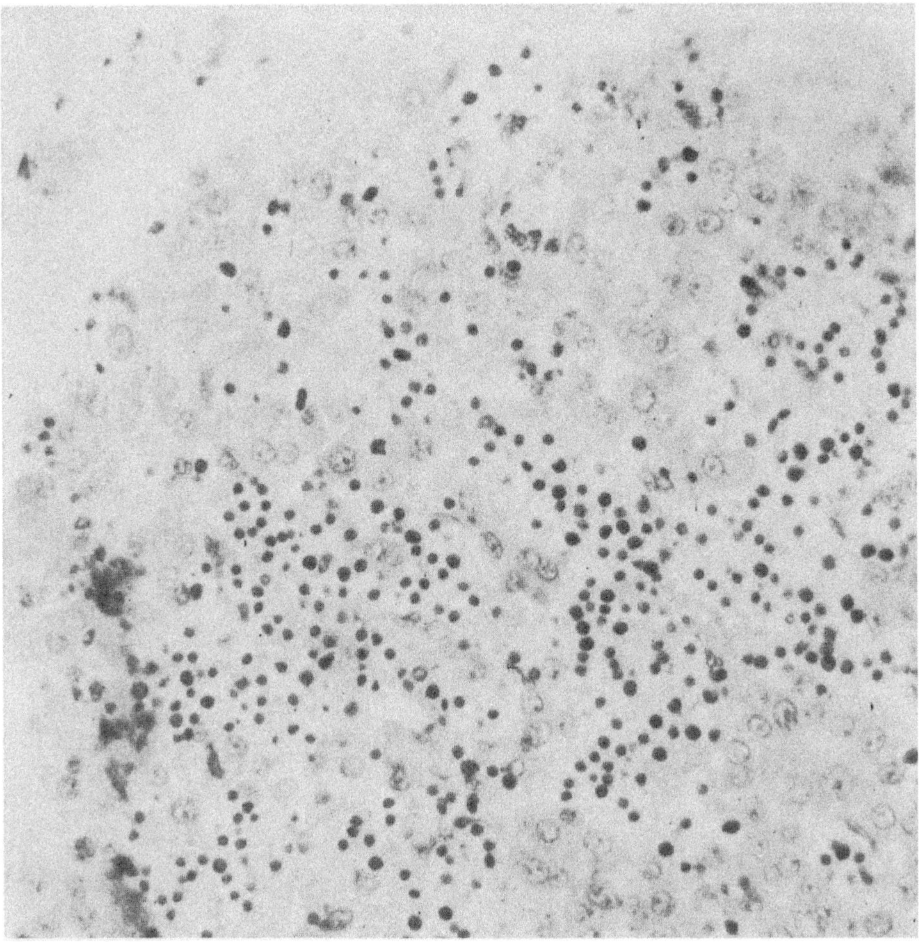

Fig. 5.

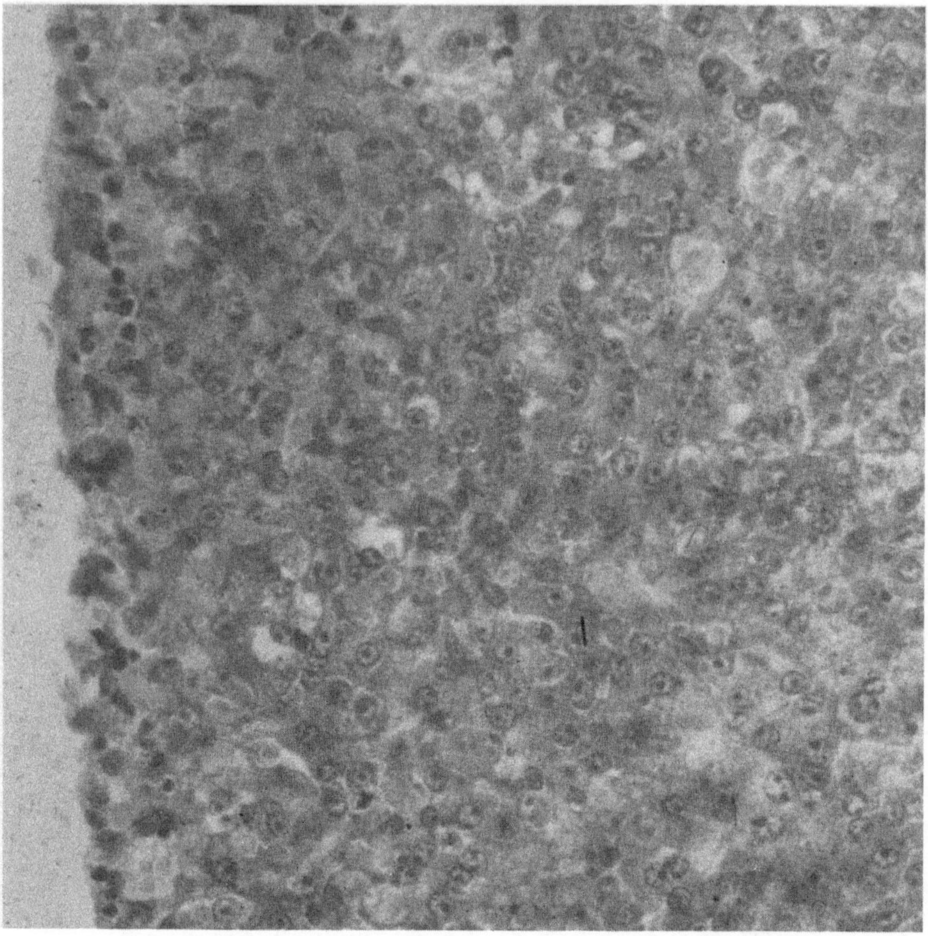

Fig. 6.

Table 2. *Development of transsulfuration in human liver.*

Gestation	Birth weight (grams)	Time death (hours)	Cystathionase (mμ moles/mg protein/hr.)	Cystathionine (μ moles/100g.)
Controls (9)			126 ± 12	0
Fetal (24)			0	14 ± 2
Premature	830	11	0	13.7
Premature	1000	8	0	16.2
Premature	1060	14	0	20.1
Premature	1260	3	0	6.5
Premature (35 wks)	1500	96	49	4.0
Full-term	3450	7	9	31.9
Full-term	4250	72	85	2.3

Table 3. *Development of transsulfuration in human liver*

Gestation	Birth weight (grams)	Time death (hours)	Methionine activating enzyme (mμ/moles/mg protein/hr.)	Cystathionine synthase (mμ/moles/mg protein/hr.)
Controls (9)			86 ± 16	98 ± 19
Fetal (24)			26 ± 3	21 ± 4
Premature	830	11	29.1	3.2
Premature	1000	8	13.1	21.5
Premature	1060	14	36.2	30.7
Premature	1260	3	29.4	18.2
Premature (35 wks)	1500	96	16.7	20.7
Full-term	3450	7	9.5	32.1
Full-term	4250	72	15.0	25.1

to its absence in mature human liver (10) supports the enzymatic results.

The activities of methionine activating enzyme and cystathionine synthase in the liver of the fetuses studied was about one-quarter to one-third of those found in mature human liver (tables 2 and 3).

In contrast to the human, cystathionase activity was present in the liver of fetal rats as early as day 12 of gestation.

Thus, in the human cystathionase activity does not appear until after birth. This means that cyst(e)ine is an essential aminoacid especially to the immature human who may require a diet supplemented with this aminoacid in order to grow and be able to adapt properly to extrauterine life. These results also point out the great species differences which may be found with respect to specific patterns of biochemical development. Results obtained using experimental animals cannot always be projected to the human.

REFERENCES

1. Sereni F., F. T. Kenney and N. Kretchmer, (1959) *J. Biol. Chem.* 234: 609.
2. Wicks W. D., (1968) *J. Biol. Chem.* 243: 900.
3. Rutter W. J., (1969) *Foetal Autonomy.* ed. Wolstenholme and O'Connor (Ciba Foundation) J. A. Churchill Ltd, London p. 59.
4. Kretchmer N., (1959) *Pediatrics* 23: 638.
5. Snyderman S. E., A. Boyer, E. Roitman, L. E. Holt and P. H. Prose, (1963) *Pediatrics* 31:786.
6. Sturman J. A., G. Gaull and N. C. R. Räihä, (1970) *Science* 169: 74.
7. Diamondstone T. I., (1966) *Anal. Biochem.* 16: 395.
8. Greengard O., (1969) *Science* 163: 891.
9. Gaull G. E., D. K. Rassin and J. A. Sturman, (1969) *Neuropädiatrie* 1: 199.
10. Brenton D. P., D. C. Cusworth and G. E. Gaull, (1965) *Pediatrics* 35: 50.
11. These studies have been supported by the Association for the Aid of Crippled Children and the Lalor Foundation.

DISCUSSION

Dr. Papadatos: Does anybody have any data about the activity of those enzymes in the placenta and whether the activities are changing with advancing gestational age?

Another question. You mentioned that corticosteroids induced tyrosine transaminase. Is this induction permanent or as soon as you stops the steroids the enzyme activity falls again.

Dr. Räihä: We did not study the activity of tyrosine transaminase in the placenta. We studied the transsulfuration enzymes in the placenta of the foetuses and there was no measurable activity of any of the transsulfuration enzymes. In the organ culture studies we kept our explants only for 72 hours. We don't know how long the effect of corticosteroids is lasting in our *in vitro* studies. In adults it is well known that the effect of corticosteroids is not permanent. The activity of tyrosine transaminase goes up for a while and goes down again. KERR, G. R., (1968) *Pediat. Res.* 2:493.

Dr. Nicoloponlos: I would like to report briefly on some studies of liver enzymes, done at the Pediatric Clinic of Athens University in collaboration with Drs. N. CONSTANTSAS and A. AGATHOPOULOS and Professor N. MATSANIOTIS: In one project were studied the phenylpyruvate tautomerase, the hydroxyphenyl pyruvate hydroxylase and the tyrosine aminotransferase, and in a second one the biochemical changes of catechol-O-methyltransferase (COMT) during development of human liver. In table 1 the variations of tautomerase, hydroxylase and tyrosine aminotransferase in the maturing liver can be seen.

COMT is the enzyme of the methylation, the main catabolic way to the inactivation of catecholamines and its study seemed indicated when we found significant differences of catecholamine metabolite (metacatecholamines, VMA, phenolic acids) exretion among premature and fullterm infants and adults.

Liver specimens were taken at autopsy within 12 hours after death. Twenty liver specimens were taken from individuals of 1 to 75 years

Table 1. *Phenylpyruvate tautomerase, p-Hydroxyphenylpyruvate hydroxylase and tyrosine aminotransferase in maturing liver*

	Phenylpyruvate tautomerase (K-units)	p-Hydroxyphenylpyruvate hydroxylase (μ moles/h)	Tyrosine aminotransferase (μ moles/h)
41–90-year-old adults (14)	2.5±0.04	23.7±0.73	5.3±0.25*
>1–5 kg newborn (13)	1.9±0.03	4.1±0.10	3.3±0.20
<1 kg newborns (7)	2.6±0.07	3.7±0.20	2.5±0.24
Stilborns (3)	1.6±0.01	2.9±0.33	0.8±0.03

* One high value (34 units) from a subject treated with glucocorticoids (tyrosine aminotransferase induction) was discarded.

of age and divided in 3 groups of age (table 2). In addition nine livers of infants aged 1 to 9 months and nine of newborns, of a few hours to 12 days of age as well as 6 livers from stillborn infants, were studied.

Our results are shown in table 2, with COMT activity expressed in nmol of formed methylepinephrine per g of liver tissue per hour.

It can be seen that enzyme activity increases with age: the average value for stillborn infants is 3 nmol/g liver per hour, for newborn 23,0 nmol/g liver per hour, during the first year of age 38,0, for children 58,0, for adults 233,0 and for older adults 71,0. It is interesting to note that the values of all five individuals above 59 years of age were as low as or lower than the lowest value of any younger adult. Another interesting observation was the low value (19 nmol/g liver per hour)

Table 2. *Activity of COMT in human liver at different ages – n mol/g of liver tissue per hour*

	Stillborn (6)	Newborn (9)	Infants (9)	Children (5)	Adults (10)	Older (5)
Mean value	3,0	23,0	38,0	58,0	233,0	71,0
Range	2,0–5,4	11,5–36,4	22,3–54,0	17,0–79,0	90–449	56–90

in the liver of an 18 year old girl, who died of self-induced barbiturate poisoning. This observation suggests inhibition by barbiturate upon COMT and some further investigations on the inhibitors of COMT are under way. (table 3).

Table 3. *Inhibitory effect of some substances on COMT'S activity. The concentration in the assay mixture is 10 moles*

Substance	Relative % activity
Calomel	5
Pyrogallol	20
Sodium diethylbarbital	30
Iron chloride (+++)	10
Iron chloride (++)	20

The enzyme from neonatal liver was found to have greater activity in pH 7.1, while that from the liver of adults was greatest at pH 7.7 (fig. 1). This suggests that intramolecular transformations probably take place.

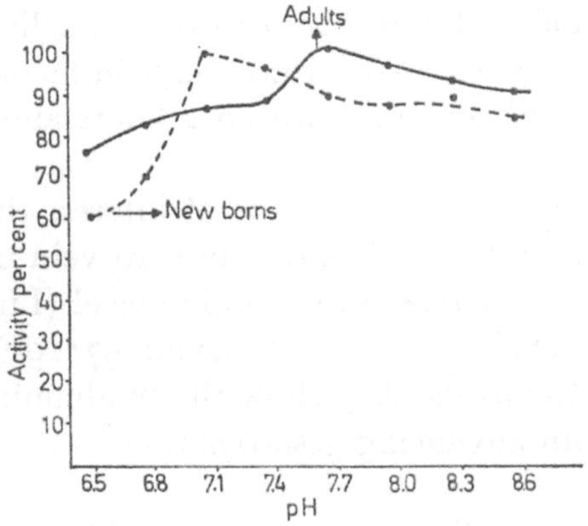

Fig. 1

The liver and kidney, which have a high concentration of catechol-O-methyltransferase and which receive a large portion of the cardiac output, are probably the organs mainly responsible for the destruction of circulating catecholamines. Oxidative deamination by monoamine oxidase plays a minor role in norepinephrine inactivation.

COMT is found in human liver before birth and its activity increases with age until the sixth decade. There is also evidence of change in properties of the enzyme within adult age. The increased amounts of metacatecholamines and VMA excreted during the first day of life in the urine of fullterm versus prematures and, still more, in the urine of adults, if compared to newborn, could be attributed to the increased COMT activity with advancing age.

Dr. Räihä: Why did you study the enzyme activities in the stillborn? How do you know how long they have been dead?

Dr. Nicolopoulos: That is a difficult question to answer. To obtain the whole range we took as many stillborns as we could. According to the information given by the obstetricians they were not dead many hours before delivery. In one or two cases we could take the liver almost immediately after the foetal death. We did not find great differences within the stillborns group.

Dr. Räihä: We take our liver samples immediately after therapeutic abortion. In the older children we can obtain a liver sample within two hours after death. All analyses are made in foetuses a few minutes after death and in the olde ones within 2 hours after death.

Dr. Lindblad: In this connection, it is of interest that the only consistant abnormality of the aminogram of cord vein plasma of a short-gestation group is an increased methionine level (Lindblad, B. S. and Zetterström, R., (1968) Acta Paediat. Scand. 57:195). It has also been demonstrated in Rhesus monkeys, how the methionine level decreases in cord plasma with advancing gestational age.

Dr. Räihä: Praemature-babies have high methionine levels.

Prof. De Meyer: You have mentioned that hydrocortisone does act on the induction only when there is yet a certain amount of transaminase activity present and not before. I would ask whether there is an explanation for this fact.

Dr. Räihä: Our results showed that if we took the liver explants from foetal rats less than 14 days (that means 9 days before birth), then we were not able to find an effect of hydrocortisone. But when we took the explants from foetal rats that were older, then we were able to get the effect.

It may be that the liver cells need to reach a certain stage of differentiation before they can respond to this stimulus.

FACTORS CONTROLLING BIOCHEMICAL DEVELOPMENT OF FOETAL AND NEWBORN LIVER

F. SERENI* AND L. P. SERENI*

INTRODUCTION

A great number of papers were published during the last years on biochemical development of the liver in mammals. It can be stated that a rather extensive knowledge was reached on variations of the most important enzyme activities during foetal and neonatal life, and that in many instances their physiological significance was clarified (1, 2).

Only very recently, however, the research work was focused on endogenous and exogenous factors which play an important role in regulating liver enzyme activities in various stages of development. This paper is mainly devoted to discuss some of the most important informations we have in this regard. The experimental approach which was used to investigate this aspect of liver developmental problems was obviously very different time by time, according with both the stage of maturity and the specific problem which had to be investigated. On table 1 a summary is reported of the most important approaches and of some of the conclusions which were reached.

No efforts will be made in this report to make a comprehensive review of all the important data which were published recently. The discussion will only be focused on the importance of hormonal and tissue factors on regulation of some liver enzyme activities in mammals.

IN VIVO EXPERIMENTS ON THE ROLE OF HORMONES ON LIVER ENZYME DEVELOPMENT

It is still questionable if certain hormones do in effect play an important role in determining the physiological great variations of activity of

* Pediatric Department of the Milano University. Supported by a research grant from Consiglio Nazionale delle Richerche n. 70.01184.04.115.4019.

Table 1. *Outline of the main experimental approaches used to investigate factors controlling mammalian liver development.*

General experimental approaches	Some examples of experiments performed	Type of conclusion reached
Administration or witdraw of hormones to fetus and newborn animals	Adrenalectomy of the newborn and lack of development of enzyme activity (3, 4, 5)	Adrenal cortex has a permissive role on some specific enzyme development
	Administration of hormones to fetus and newborn animals and different reply in comparison to adults. For example lack of reply to hydrocortisone (3, 6, 7)	In immature liver the hormonal regulation of enzyme activity should be different than in mature tissue
Changes in the quality and quantity of food intake during suckling period	Premature weaning and glucose feeding influence tissue carbohydrate metabolism (8, 9)	The adaptation of immature liver to metabolic requirements is good
Modification of the length of gestation	Premature delivery induces an increase of the activity of some liver enzyme systems (10, 11, 12)	Birth 'per se' has a great importance on enzyme development
In vitro cultures	Cells or explants cultures and control of factors necessary for specific enzyme development (3, 14, 15)	In some instances tissue factors play an important role in liver biochemical development

Table 2. *Permissive role of adrenal cortex on liver enzyme development*

Authors	Enzyme activity	Animal and age
JOST and JACQUOT (16) JACQUOT and KRETCHMER (17)	Many enzyme systems involved in glycogen synthesis	Rabbit and rat fetuses
SERENI et al. (3)	Tyrosine aminotransferase	Newborn rats
RÄIHÄ and SUIHKONEN (4)	Arginine synthetase	Newborn rats
HERTZFELD and GREENGARD (5)	Ornithine aminotransferase	Newborn rats
SERENI and BARNABEI (6)	Nuclear RNA synthesis	Newborn rats

Table 3. *Different response of immature versus mature liver to hormones*

Authors	Enzyme activity	Peculiarities of immature liver response
SERENI et al. (3)	Tyrosine aminotransferase	Lack of response of fetal liver to hydrocortisone – Normal reply only after birth when enzyme activity has reached adult levels.
GREENGARD (7)	Glucose-6-phosphatase Tyrosine aminotransferase Serine dehydratase Phosphoenolpyruvate-carboxylase	In fetuses 4–3 days before term only the injection of a cyclic AMP derivative (BcAMP) enhances enzyme activities In fetuses 2–1 days before term BcAMP, adrenaline and glucagon are all effective, but not hydrocortisone After birth only hydrocortisone is effective
SERENI and BARNABEI (6)	DNA dependent RNA polymerase	No corticosteroid activation in newborn rats in the first ten days of life

some enzyme systems during development. In this regard three series of data can be discussed. The first one concerns the so called 'permissive' role of adrenal cortex. In at least five instances it was well proved that adrenalectomy of fetus and newborn animals prevents the development of specific enzyme systems of the liver. These data are summarized on table 2.

It seems however important to remember that the permissive role of adrenal cortex is not a general phenomenon, but should be considered rather a very specific one. It was not demonstrated, for example, either for glucose-6 phosphatase (18) or for tryptophan pyrrolase (19) despite the fact that the developmental curve of these two enzyme activities is to a certain extent similar to that of tyrosine aminotransferase and arginine synthetase, and despite the fact that they can easily be induced by corticosteroids in the adult animal.

The second series of data which must be discussed are those supporting the evidence that at a certain stage of development the reply of liver tissue to hormonal stimuli may be different from that usually observed in adult life.

Some of the most significant experiments are listed on table 3.

Both series of data we have mentioned above on hormonal regulation of enzyme activities, i.e. those concerning the permissive role of adrenal cortex and those demonstrating a different reply of immature versus mature liver tissue to hormonal stimuli, are without any doubt relevant for a better understanding of regulation of enzyme activity during growth. It should however be stressed that in most of the cases we still miss the essential information of the extent during foetal and neonatal life of the endogenous secretion of those hormones which are supposed to play a critical role in regulating liver enzyme activities.

The third series of data which has to be discussed are those concerning the so called detoxicating enzyme systems. Since a long time we know that the activity of these microsomal enzymes is low in fetus and newborn animals (20). RANE and coworkers (21) have recently proved that this deficiency is to be related to a lack of NADP reductase activity, rather than to a low concentration of cytochrome-C. In the past it was stated that the low activity in early periods of life of these enzyme systems could be explained by the lack of endoplasmic reticulum in immature liver parenchymal cells (22).

However it is now well established that the activity of the mixed function oxidase systems usually remains low through the whole suckling period of the newborn animal, even after tissue liver cells have reached histologic maturity (23). It is therefore a reasonable hypothesis that inhibitor substances keep reduced these enzyme activities in newborn animals. On table 4 are reported some important data suggesting that these inhibitors may be hormones, either steroids, which are present in high concentration in serum and in milk, or growth hormones.

IN VITRO CULTURES OF FETAL LIVER CELLS. THEIR IMPORTANCE FOR A BETTER COMPREHENSION OF FACTOR CONTROLLING LIVER DEVELOPMENT

If the activity of a specific enzyme system increases abruptly from fetal to neonatal life (as it is for example for tyrosine aminotransferase or for glucose-6-phosphatase) two main hypotheses may be put forward to explain the mechanism of these variations. It may be that during fetal life the enzyme system is inhibited by the 'intrauterine milieu' or it is possible that a specific activation occurs as soon as the extrauterine life starts. To solve this problem the best experimental model is the evaluation of enzyme activity in 'in vitro' cultures, where the immediate environment of the cells could be easily defined and controlled.

To our knowledge NEMETH and coworkers were the first authors using the in vitro approach to evaluate factors controlling the development of enzyme activities of the immature liver (27, 14). They studied the UDP-glucuronyl-transferase activity in cultures of chick embryo liver and observed a sharp spontaneous in vitro development, as soon as the tissue was removed from embryonic milieu. The development of this enzyme activity was associated with a very active synthesis of rough endoplasmic reticulum.

The first data published by these authors (27) indicate an extrahepatic control of this enzyme activity, since fetal serum added to the medium inhibits the spontaneous development of this enzyme activity, while adult serum stimulated this process. This control mechanism needs however to be further investigated, since in a subsequent paper (14) the same authors have reported that the spontaneous activation of liver UDP-glucuronyltransferase activity may occur even in absence of adult serum.

Table 4. *Some known examples of hormone regulation of liver microsomal enzyme activities during development.*

Authors	Enzymes studied	Results
Arias et al. (24)	Glucuronyl-transferase	High amount of pregnane-3 (alpha)–20 (beta) diol in human milk significantly inhibits glucuronyl-transferase
Feuer and Liscio (25)	4-methyl-coumarin-3-hydroxylase UDPG-o-aminophenol-transglucuronylase	Low enzyme activities in pregnant animals. Increase after weaning. (Presumptive inhibitory effect of steroids)
Wilson (26)	Many hepatic microsomal drug metabolizing enzyme activities	High STH levels prevent normal postnatal development of enzyme activities
Soyka and Gyermek (23)	Aniline hydroxylation; p-Nitroanisole demethylation	In vitro inhibition of enzyme activities by pregnanolone

Table 5. *Comparison between developmental regulation of tyrosine aminotransferase and glucose-6-phosphatase in liver of mammals*

	Tyrosine aminotransferase	Glucose-6-phosphatase
Developmental curve	From very low values sharp rise after birth (3)	Slow rise during last period of intrauterine life – Sharp rise after birth (11)
Premature delivery	Sharp increase (10)	Increase as in the last period of gestation (11)
Glucose administration at birth	Inhibition of postnatal increase (?) (28, 10)	Inhibition of postnatal increase (18)
Effect of corticosteroids	Increase of activity in adult animals (de novo synthesis) No effect in fetal animals (3)	The same (28)
Permissive role of adrenal cortex (adrenalectomy at birth)	Yes (3)	No (18)
Intrauterine effect of glucagon	Activation (7)	Activation (7, 29)
Intrauterine effect of thyroxine	No effect (30)	Activation (30)

Important differences between tyrosine aminotransferase and glucose-6-phosphatase are printed in italics

These investigations in chick embryo liver have prompted us to use the in vitro technique to investigate some of the mechanisms controlling the postnatal development of enzyme activities of mammalian liver (15).

Our observations were focused on tyrosine aminotransferase and on glucose-6-phosphatase, two enzyme systems whose activity is low during fetal life but rises very sharply after birth.

On the basis of in vivo experiments the hypothesis was made (7) that these two enzymes may be controlled during the perinatal period of life by similar hormonal factors. However from an analysis of the literature on developmental peculiarities of these enzyme activities, we can draw the conclusion that besides many similarities, also important discrepancies exist, as is reported on table 5.

A different mechanism of regulation of these enzyme activities during fetal life is also indicated by our in vitro studies.

As a matter of fact when fetal liver tissue at different stages of maturity is taken from its maternal milieu and is cultured in vitro, a remarkable spontaneous activation of tyrosine aminotransferase activity is noticed (Fig. 1). This activation occurs very soon after the starting of the in vitro cultures when liver explants were obtained from fetuses close to term, but some time had to elapse when liver explants derived from very immature fetuses were used.

The in vitro development of tyrosine aminotransferase activity mimics therefore very well the postnatal increase of the same enzyme system.

Contrary to what was found for tyrosine aminotransferase, the glucose-6-phosphatase activity of fetal liver explants increases very slightly during in vitro cultures (fig. 2, left).

This increase is very comparable to what is usually observed in vivo during the last part of fetal life (fig. 2, right), and it is by no means comparable to the sharp postnatal activation of this enzyme activity.

From these data the conclusion was reached that tyrosine aminotransferase activity is inhibited during intrauterine life. This is primarily suggested by the observation that the simple removal of liver tissue from the foetal milieu is sufficient to induce a sharp activation of the enzyme activity. This seems not to be true for fetal glucose-6-phosphatase activity, which increases 'in vitro' at the same rate as 'in vivo'.

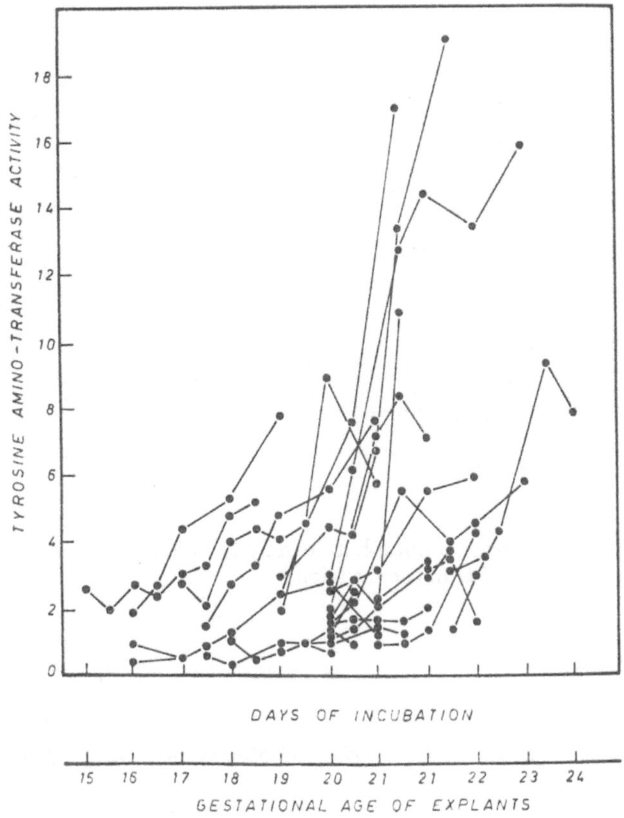

Fig. 1. Spontaneous changes in tyrosine aminotransferase activity in explants of fetal liver cultures (15).

This statement is further supported by some data we have collected on the different 'in vitro' responses to hydrocortisone of these two enzyme activities in fetal liver cultures. It is well known that the 'in vivo' injection of glucocorticoids enhances both enzyme activities in adult animals, but is not effective during fetal life (see table 5).

We have found that by adding hydrocortisone to the medium of the in vitro fetal liver cultures it was possible to obtain a sharp activation of tyrosine aminotransferase activity (15) whereas no significant effect on glucose-6-phosphatase activity was observed (31) (Table 6).

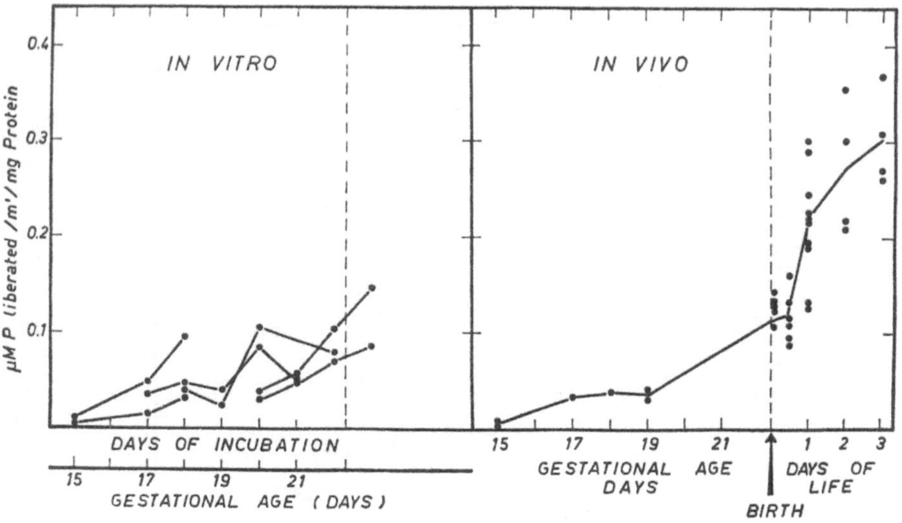

Fig. 2. Variations of glucose-6-phosphatase activity in fetal liver culture (left) and during fetal and neonatal life in the rat (right) (31)

Table 6. *Influence of hydrocortisone on glucose-6-phosphatase activity of fetal rat liver explants* (31)

Experiment N.	Gestational age (days)	Incubation time (hours)	Glucose-6-phosphatase activity (μM P/m^1/mg Protein $\times 10^{-2}$) Control	Hydrocortisone
1	15	48	4.83	15.73
			9.40	1.19
2	15	48	1.41	8.32
		72	3.22	2.82
3	17	24	4.71	2.92
		48	3.84	2.65
		72	8.50	11.70
4	20	24	5.05	6.33
		48	6.91	6.37
		72	8.45	1.22

CONCLUSIONS AND SUMMARY

Many experiments were performed during recent years with the main aim to clarify the factors which are involved in controlling liver enzyme activities during development. The experimental approaches were multiple, but only a relatively small number of enzyme activities was studied. A large part of the investigations concerns the perinatal period of life, since in this period some of the most striking variations of liver enzyme activities occur.

Our discussion was mainly focused, for pragmatic reasons, on tyrosine aminotransferase and on glucose-6-phosphatase, i.e. on two enzyme systems very extensively studied in adult animal and also very much investigated in foetal and neonatal tissue.

The relative value of in vivo and of in vitro studies was discussed and the conclusion was reached that while tyrosine aminotransferase is inhibited during foetal life, this is not true for glucose-6-phosphatase.

Additional studies in this field are needed for a more comprehensive understanding of these important problems on biochemical development of mammals.

REFERENCES

1. SERENI F. and B. LUPPIS, (1968) In: *Aspects of Prematurity and Dysmaturity*, Jonxis J. H. P., H. K. A. Visser and J. A. Troelstra eds., H. E. Stenfert Kroese N.V., Leiden, p. 68
2. SERENI F. and N. PRINCIPI, (1971) In: *Developmental Biochemistry*, P. Benson ed., Spastic International Medical Publications, London (in press)
3. SERENI F., F. T. KENNEY, N. KRETCHMER, (1959) *J. Biol. Chem.* 234, 609
4. RÄIHÄ N. C. R. and J. SUIHKONEN, (1966) *Proc. 36th Ann. Meet. Soc. Ped. Res.*, Atlantic City, Paper N. 6
5. HERTZFELD A. and O. GREENGARD, (1969) *J. Biol. Chem.* 244:4394
6. SERENI F. and O. BARNABEI, (1967) In: *Advances in Enzyme Regulation*, G. Weber ed., Pergamon Press 5:165
7. GREENGARD O., (1969) *Biochem. J.* 115:19
8. WALKER D. G. and S. W. EATON, (1967) *Biochem. J.* 105:771
9. VERNON R. G. and D. G. WALKER, (1968) *Biochem. J.* 106:331
10. HOLT P. G. and I. T. OLIVER, (1968) *Biochem. J.* 108:333
11. DAWKINS M. J. R., (1961) *Nature* 191:72
12. NEMETH A. M., (1959) *J. Biol. Chem.* 234:2921
13. LE DOUARIN N., (1968) *Develop. Biol.* 17:101
14. SKEA B. R. and A. M. NEMETH, (1969) *Proc. Nat. Acad. Sci* 69:795

15. Sereni F. and L. Piceni Sereni, (1970) In: *Advances in Enzyme Regulation*, G. Weber ed., Pergamon Press, 8:253
16. Jost A. and R. Jacquot, (1958) *Compt. Rend.* 247:2459
17. Jaquot R. and N. Kretchmer, (1964) *J. Biol. Chem.* 239:1301
18. Dawkins M. J. R., (1963) *Ann. N. Y. Acad. Sci.* 111:203
19. Nemeth A. M., (1963) *Ann. N. Y. Acad. Sci.* 111:199
20. Fouts J. R. and R. H. Adamson, (1959) *Science* 129:897
21. Rane A., S. Yaffe and S. Orrenius ,(1970) *Acta Paediat. Scand.* 59:596
22. Peters U. B., G. W. Kelly and H. M. Dembitzer, (1963) *Ann. N. Y. Acad. Sci.* 111:87
23. Soyka L. F. and L. Gyermek, (1970) *Ped. Res.* 4:471
24. Arias I. M., L. M. Gartner, S. Seifter and M. Furman, (1964) *J. Clin. Invest* 43:2037
25. Feuer G. and A. Liscio, (1969) *Nature* 223:68
26. Wilson J. T., (1970) *Nature* 225:861
27. Ko V., G. J. Dutton and A. M. Nemeth, (1967) *Biochem. J.* 104:991
28. Greengard O. and H. K. Dewvey, (1967) *J. Biol. Chem.* 242:2986
29. Holt P. G. and I. T. Oliver, (1969) *Biochemistry* 8:1429
30. Greengard O. and H. K. Dewvey, (1968) *J. Biol. Chem.* 243:2745
31. Sereni F. and L. Piceni Sereni, Unpublished data

DISCUSSION

Prof. Villee: You haves hown that there is no response before a certain age of gestation. You used the word immaturity to define the stage during which the tissue does not respond. Could you speculate on the meaning of this immaturity?

Dr. Sereni: One possible way to define tissue immaturity from a biochemical point of view is to evaluate the response to physiologic stimuli. We may consider a tissue to be immature if it does not reply as the adult one. You should however always remember that the development of various tissue functions is not synchronous. This is particularly true for the liver. Consequently it is very possible that at a certain stage of development a tissue could be considered mature for some respect, but still immature for others.

Prof. Villee: One of my co-workers Dr. RHODA MAKOFF carried out experiments very much like yours on the appearance of tyrosine-aminotransferase. She found the same remarkable peak 16 hours after birth, where it is much higher than it is subsequently for a long time. We had no real explanation as to why is got so high. Do you have an explanation?

She also carried out an adrenalectomy in the newborn, and she managed to get the mother to take back the adrenalectomized young and to feed them again. When those adrenalectomised babies were refed, the tyrosine aminotransferase came up just as if corticosteroids had been given. It seemed therefore that the important thing was the nutrition, the refeeding. The nutrition could act as an alternative stimulator rather than giving the hydrocortisone. Perhaps hydrocortisone has some permissive effect in the system.

Dr. Sereni: I am surprised by the possibility to increase the activity of tyrosine aminotransferase in adrenalectomized newborn rat by mother feeding. I may recall two different sets of experiments. OLIVER has shown that it is possible to inhibit tyrosine aminotransferase development by early feeding of glucose and other authors have demonstrated that suckling mother milk has an inhibitory influence on development of microsomal enzyme systems. Your interesting data are just the reverse, since they suggest a permissive role of milk feeding.

For some microsomal enzymes there is some evidence that corticosteroids could have some suppressive action. In pregnant animals and in the newborn animal till weaning time there is a low activity of some microsomal and metabolising enzymes. As soon as you remove the animal from the mother and if you get an early weaning you have a rise of those enzyme activities. Maybe the newborn is ingesting with the milk of the mother some substance which suppress those enzyme activity. But with tyrosine transaminase it is just the reverse.

Prof. Villee: I think there is some difference between giving a great deal of a single compound such as glucose, which is clearly inhibitory and giving a much more balanced nutritional substrate as mothermilk.

Dr. Sereni: Few years ago we artificially fed newborn rabbits and we have shown that the protein intake in the first 36 hours of life is very critical for liver plasma protein synthesis in the newborn. These experiments are in some way in agreement with yours.

EFFECT OF HORMONES ON THE DEVELOPMENT OF ENZYME SYSTEMS

C. A. VILLEE*

The nature of the biochemical mechanisms underlying the appearance of a specific enzyme in a specific tissue of the fetus at a specific time in development is among the most challenging of current biological problems. Advances in molecular biology have greatly increased our

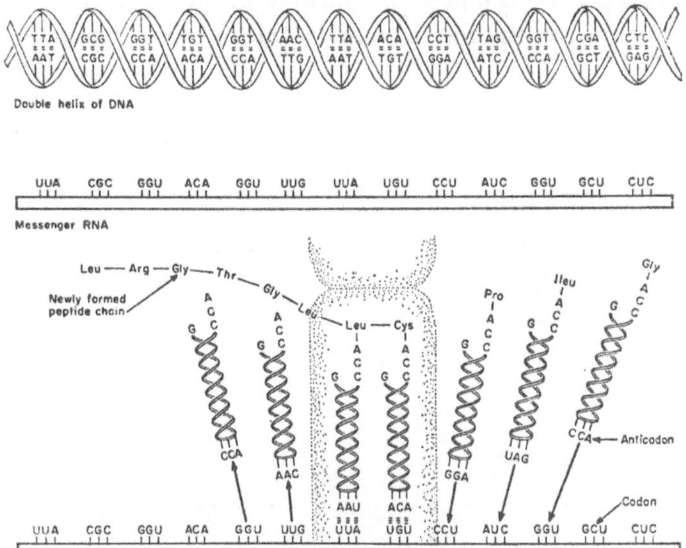

Fig. 1. A diagram of the relations between the codons of DNA and messenger RNA and the anticodons of transfer RNA which lead to the synthesis of specific peptide chains. From Villee C. A., *Biology*, 5th ed., W. B. Saunders Co., 1967.

* Department of Biological Chemistry and Laboratory of Human Reproduction and Reproductive Biology, Harvard Medical School, Boston, Massachusetts.
This research was aided by a grant from the Association for the Aid of Crippled Children and by grants HD 00006 and HD 1232 of the National Institute of Child Health and Human Development.

understanding of the means by which biological information is transferred from one generation of cells to the next and transcribed in each cell to produce its constituent proteins. It is not yet possible, within the framework of this hypothesis to explain either how a gene may determine the quantity of an enzyme produced, what determines the time in development at which the enzyme appears, or how certain cells of a multicellular organism may have a given enzyme or protein when other cells of the same organism with the same genome do not.

Each gene, composed of a specific sequence of deoxynucleotides, has two primary functions: to undergo replication so that one of the two replicates can be transmitted to each daughter cell, and to undergo one or more transcriptions so that its information can be used to direct the synthesis of a specific protein within that cell. The product of the transcription process is RNA with information coded in triplet sequences of purine and pyrimidine ribonucleotides termed codons (fig. 1).

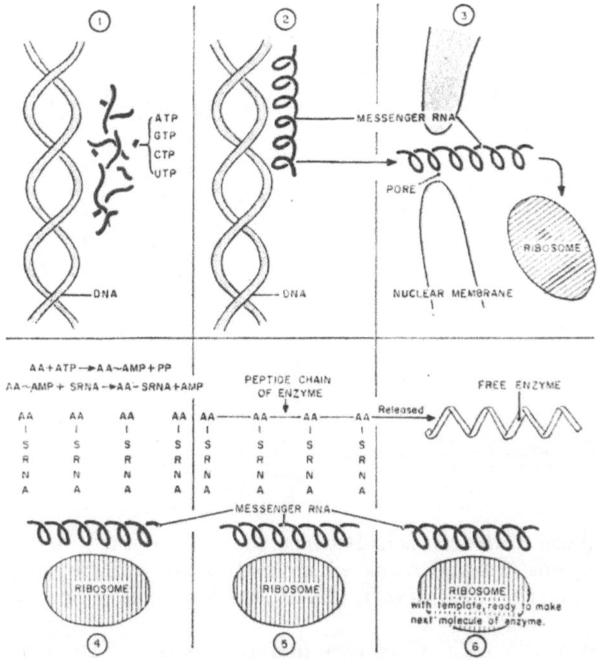

Fig. 2. Diagram of the assembly of messenger RNA on a DNA template inside the nucleus and its passage to the ribosome where it serves as a template for the assembly of a peptide chain. From VILLEE C. A., *Biology*, 5th ed., W. B. Saunders Co., 1967.

The sequence of ribonucleotides in the RNA codons is determined by the sequence of deoxynucleotides in genic DNA. The three major types of RNA – messenger, ribosomal and transfer – are formed in the nucleus and pass through the nuclear membrane to the cytoplasm (fig. 2). Messenger RNA combines with the ribosomes and provides a template for the synthesis of the specific protein. Thus the sequence of amino acids in the peptide chain, which dictates the molecular conformation of the protein and its enzymatic and other properties, is determined by the sequence of nucleotides in messenger RNA and ultimately by the sequence of nucleotides in genic DNA.

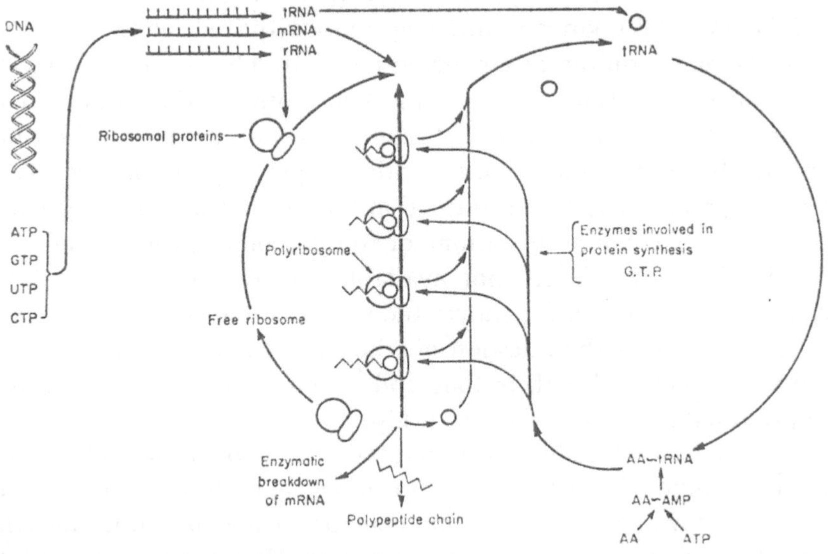

Fig. 3. Diagram of the activation of amino acids and their assembly on a messenger RNA by polyribosomes. VILLEE C. A., *Biology*, 5th ed., W. B. Saunders Co., 1967.

Each kind of amino acid is activated by a reaction with ATP and then forms a complex with a specific kind of transfer RNA (fig. 3). The transfer RNA contains on one of its loops a specific sequence of three nucleotides, the anticodon, which determines where the amino acid-transfer RNA molecule will fit onto the codon of the messenger RNA. The complementarity between the nucleotides in codon and anticodon serves to line up the amino acids in a specific order so that synthesis of the specific protein may proceed.

It is apparent that differentiation does not involve any assortment of genes into the daughter cells during mitosis; each cell in a multicellular organism has the same complement of genes, the same quota of biological information, as every other cell. Cellular differentiation then must result in some way from the differential activity of a common set of genes in different cells.

How a cell can contain all the various kinds of DNA represented by its entire genic complement and not produce the entire spectrum of corresponding messenger RNAs is a vexing problem. It would clearly be advantageous to the cell if its ribosomes were not encumbered with nonfunctional molecules of messenger RNA, and if it were able to produce only those kinds of messenger RNA required for the synthesis of the proteins required at any given moment. The control of enzyme formation could occur either in the gene, during the formation of messenger RNA, during the translation process occurring on the ribosome, or during the folding of the ultimate polypeptide product. One currently popular hypothesis states that the DNA in the genes of eukaryotic organisms is bound to histone or to some other protein, and that the bound DNA is 'silent', not available for transcription (1). This hypothesis however simply moves the problem of differentiation back one step and raises the question of what determines which molecules of DNA are combined with histone and which are free – what controls this presumably reversible relationship.

The processes of cellular differentiation and of hormonal control may have much in common at the molecular level, for each may involve the turning on of a specific gene or set of genes to initiate the production of one or more specific enzymes. Hormones may regulate metabolic processes within a cell by altering the permeability of the cell membrane or of the membrane surrounding the mitochondrion or other subcellular organelle. By increasing or decreasing the uptake of a specific substrate or cofactor the hormone may alter the pattern of metabolism within the cell. Secondly, a hormone may activate a preexisting protein, perhaps by changing its conformation, so that it acquires enzymatic properties not previously apparent. Each of these mechanisms has been documented for the action of one or another hormone in adult tissues and each provides for the rapid response of a tissue to the hormone.

A third currently popular mechanism suggests that a hormone may act by initiating the readout of a portion of the genome, by interacting either with the DNA or with the histone to initiate the transcription of a specific gene or genes. There is now a substantial body of evidence supporting the hypothesis that most steroid hormones and some peptide hormones produce their specific effects in the adult by this mechanism. This is also a reasonable hypothesis regarding the means by which the hormone might affect the appearance of a specific enzyme during development.

Thus, a hormone may act by initiating for a brief time the readout of a portion of the genome. Differentiation appears to involve the long term activation of certain genes in certain cells. Each must involve some mechanism for selecting one portion but not another of the genic DNA for transcription.

Hormones may act in the adult by transferring information from one cell to another. Secretin tells the acinar cells of the pancreas to secrete their enzymes but its message is unintelligible to other cells in the body. Hormones may act jointly to set limits on the concentration of some metabolite. The concentration of glucose in the plasma is maintained reasonably constant by the combined action of insulin and glucagon. More complex interrelations of hormones are evident in feedback controls such as the reciprocal control of pituitary and adrenal cortex by ACTH and cortisol, or the complex regulation of estrous and menstrual cycles by pituitary and ovarian hormones. Only the first of these mechanisms, the transfer of information, appears to be important in controlling the development of enzymes.

Prenatal development proceeds largely without hormonal control; the fetus does not require growth hormone for its growth, its somatic growth will proceed essentially normally even in the complete absence of the fetal pituitary (2).

The experiments of Price (3) and others have shown that the differentiation of the fetal male reproductive tract and accessory sex glands does require testosterone. The metamorphosis of amphibians under the control of thyroxine is accompanied by the synthesis of a variety of proteins and by changes in many enzyme systems. Thyroxine increases the amounts of hydrolytic enzymes that degrade proteins, nucleic acids and polysaccharides, causing resorption of the tadpole's tail. As Tata (4) has shown, the resorption of the tail can be inhibited by substances such as actinomycin which prevent the transcription of

RNA; thus the resorbtion of the tail in response to thyroxine is an active process which requires the synthesis of new enzymes.

The regulation of molting in insects by ecdysone provides a classic example of the hormonally controlled appearance of new enzymes during development. Under the stimulus of a tropic hormone produced in the neurosecretory cells of the intercerebral gland of the brain and released in the corpus cardiacum, the insect's prothoracic gland synthesizes ecdysone, a 27 carbon steroid. Certain tissues of dipteran insects have giant chromosomes, composed of many chromatids, which permit the cytologist to recognize specific bands and loci in the chromosome. Injecting minute amounts of ecdysone into the larva of the midge *Chironomus* causes the puffing or swelling of a specific region of a particular chromosome (5) (fig. 4). Puffing has been shown to

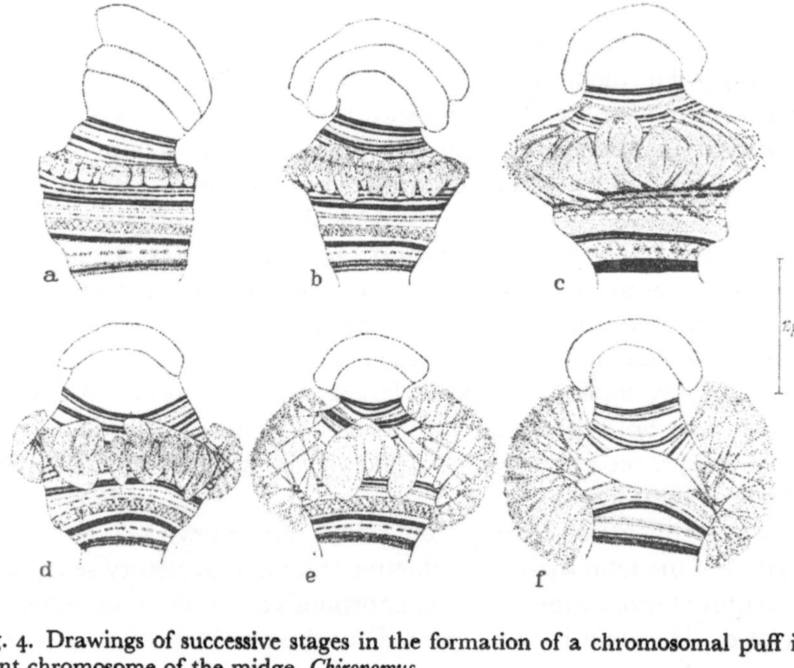

Fig. 4. Drawings of successive stages in the formation of a chromosomal puff in a giant chromosome of the midge, *Chironomus*.

represent the synthesis of RNA. Injecting ecdysone into a larva causes puffing at a specific band and the subsequent production in epidermal cells of the enzyme dopa decarboxylase. This enzyme catalyzes the conversion of dihydroxyphenylalanine (DOPA) to N-acetyl dihydroxyphenylethylamine, a compound involved in the hardening of the cuticle which follows molting.

Among the more striking phenomena of perinatal enzymology is the appearance at or shortly after birth in man and other mammals of enzymes such as liver tyrosine transaminase, tryptophan pyrrolase (6) histidase (7) and fructose 1, 6-diphosphatase (8). The enzymes increase within a few days or a week from essentially zero activity to the adult level of activity. The increase does not appear to be initiated by a hormone, but may represent the induction of the enzyme by its substrate or some not yet understood response of the protein synthesizing system to a biological clock that goes off at a particular time in development.

The clearest examples of hormonal control of enzymic development in mammals appear later in development. Androgens, for example, increase the activities of many enzymes in the seminal vesicle and the prostate (9). Estrogens increase certain enzymic activities in the uterus and vagina (10). Estrogens together with other hormones regulate enzymic activity in the mammary gland during growth, pregnancy and lactation (11).

Evidence is accumulating that the tissues that respond to a given hormone are characterized by the presence of a specific binding protein ('receptor') which reacts with the specific steroid hormone. The estrogen binding protein of the uterus (12, 13), the anterior pituitary (14) and anterior hypothalamus (15) has been characterized and purified (16). A specific androgen binding protein has been described in prostatic nuclei (17), and a progesterone binding protein has been found in the chick oviduct (18). In seeking an explanation for the production of an enzyme in response to a hormone during development we must consider the possibility that this results from the appearance of a specific receptor protein in the target tissue and not simply from the initiation of secretion of that hormone by its endocrine gland.

Let us examine the hypothesis that a hormone interacts with the genome and frees a certain part of the DNA so that it can be transcribed, producing an RNA which codes for the synthesis of certain proteins (fig. 5). The hypothesis predicts that we should be able to detect some sort of interaction of the steroid either with the DNA or with one of the

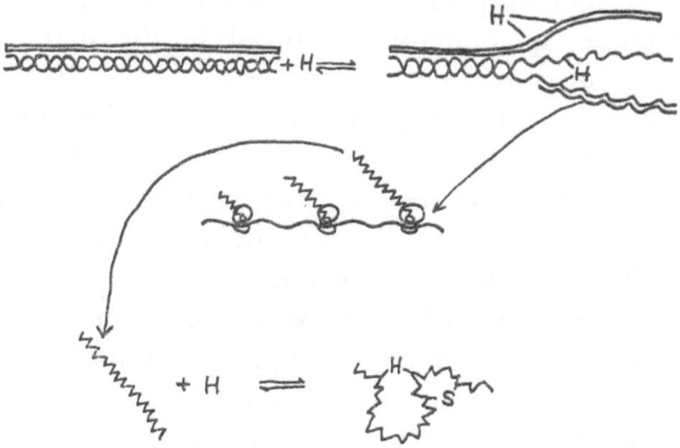

Fig. 5. A diagram illustrating the several ways in which a hormone (H) might interact with the DNA (double helix) or the histone (indicated by the open bar) bound to the DNA to initiate transcription of the genome.

nuclear proteins such as histone. It predicts that the hormone should lead to a rapid increase in the synthesis of RNA and it predicts that this RNA, when isolated and reintroduced into the target cell, should increase protein synthesis and the activity of those enzymes known to respond to the application of the steroid *in vivo*. Interactions between testosterone and a histone present in the nuclei of the ventral prostate and between cortisol and a histone present in the liver were demonstrated by SLUYSER (19). GOLDBERG and ATCHLEY (20) provided evidence of interactions between hormones and DNA prepared from the nuclei of human placental cells. The DNA was incubated with a hormone and the combination of hormone and DNA was measured by changes in the melting profile of the DNA. In this way interactions of DNA with estradiol, cortisol, insulin, growth hormone and epinephrine were demonstrated. The altered melting profile of the DNA which resulted was interpreted as a weakening of the bonds between the DNA strands produced by interaction with the hormone. The biologically inactive isomer, 17a estradiol, was ineffective in changing the melting profile.

In a different approach to this problem DR. MICHAEL MITCHELL working in my laboratory (21) took advantage of the fact that actinomycin D binds specifically with non-complexed, double helical DNA. Mitchell compared the amount of DNA in the chromatin that is free and ready to be transcribed in control and in the steroid treated state by measuring the binding of tritium labelled actinomycin D to the DNA (table 1). He prepared chromatin from the livers of normal

Table 1. *Effect of steroids on the binding of actinomycin D to chromatin from the livers of adrenalectomized rats.*

Steroid added	^{3}H-AMD bound, cpm/μg DNA		Percent change
	Control	Steroid	
None	398	405	1.8
Cortisol, 30 μg	311	356	14.5
Cortisol, 30 μg	229	273	19.1
Corticosterone, 37 μg	528	622	17.8

Chromatin isolated from the livers of adrenalectomized rats was complexed with an excess (0.1 μM) of unlabeled actinomycin (AMD) to bind all available sites on the chromatin. The unbound AMD was removed by a Sephadex G50 column. The chromatin was then reacted with ^{3}H-AMD with or without the steroid at 5° for 18 hours. The unbound ^{3}H-AMD was then removed by passing the mixture through a second column of Sephadex G50. The chromatin samples with and without steroid were passed through parallel columns of Sephadex.

and adrenalectomized rats and mixed portions of the chromatin with steroids; other portions were kept as control. Labelled actinomycin D was added, the mixture was incubated at 37° for ten minutes, then rapidly chilled. Free actinomycin was separated from the bound, either by passing the mixture through a Sephadex column or by equilibrium dialysis (table 2). By either method MITCHELL found that cortisol or corticosterone at 10^{-6} molar increased the binding of tritium labelled actinomycin D to the chromatin. This was interpreted as reflecting a hormone-induced increase in the amount of DNA free to bind with actinomycin D.

Nuclei isolated from rat liver responded to cortisol added in vitro with an increase in the template activity of RNA as measured in an amino acid incorporating system (22). Other experiments of SEKERIS suggested that a primary action of cortisol is to increase the activity of RNA polymerase. The stimulation of RNA polymerase in the nuclei of cells in the rat uterus by estradiol was reported by GORSKI and NELSON

Table 2. *Effect of steroids on the binding of actinomycin D to rat liver chromatin.*

Steroid added	DNA-bound AMD/free AMD
None	38 ± 2
Corticosterone, 1.9 μg	38 ± 2a
Corticosterone, 9.4 μg	51 ± 3b
Cortisol, 1.5 μg	43 ± 1c
Cortisol, 30 μg	44 ± 2c
Androstenediol, 10 μg	37 ± 1a
None*	27 ± 1
Corticosterone*, 7.5 μg	32 ± 1b

To a solution of chromatin, 20 μg/4 ml reaction mixture, was added ^{3}H-AMD, 3.5×10^{-2} μM, and the mixture was incubated at 37° for 10 minutes. It was then cooled rapidly and duplicate aliquots were placed in dialysis bags for equilibrium dialysis.

* Chromatin from livers of normal rats; all other chromatin from livers of adrenalectomized rats.

a not significantly different from control
b significantly different, $p < 0.1\%$
c significantly different, $p < 5\%$

(23). Experiments in many laboratories have shown a marked increase in RNA synthesis occurring in the uterus within a short time of the administration of estradiol, and in the seminal vesicle or prostate following testosterone.

The question of whether RNA produced in a target tissue in response to a steroid could be applied to another target tissue and mimic the effects of the steroid was first investigated by MANSOUR and NIU (24) and by SEGAL ET AL. (25). MANSOUR and NIU instilled RNA from the uterus of estradiol treated mice into the uterus of adult castrate mice and found it increased the uterine content of alkaline phosphatase, a phenomenon which usually occurs in response to estradiol administered *in vivo*. SEGAL demonstrated that RNA from the uterus of estradiol treated rats perfused into the lumen of the uterus of a castrate adult rat produced cytologic changes similar to those seen when estradiol is injected.

Investigations in our laboratory have shown that an increased synthesis of RNA, measured by the incorporation of ^{3}H-cytidine into RNA, is an early response in the seminal vesicle to testosterone administered to either adult castrate rats (26) or to immature rats (27) (fig. 6). Analysis of the RNA on sucrose density gradients showed that

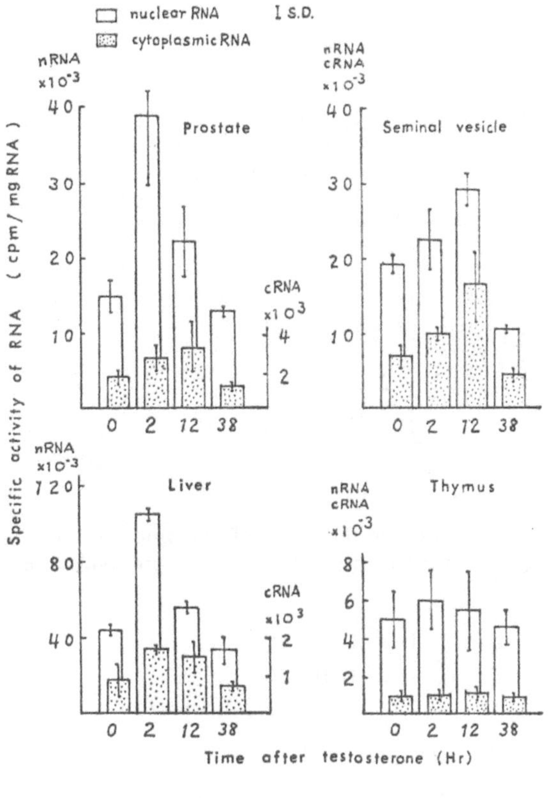

Fig. 6. Effect of testosterone on the synthesis of nuclear and cytoplasmic RNA in the prostate, seminal vesicle, liver and thymus.

the steroid increased the specific activities of RNAs with the sedimentation constants of transfer, messenger and ribosomal RNA (fig. 7). In continuing this investigation we found (28) that RNA isolated from the seminal vesicle of androgen treated rats and instilled into the lumen of the seminal vesicle of another immature rat brought about an increase in weight and increased protein synthesis (fig. 8). RNA extracted from any of the tissues of immature rats not treated with testosterone was without effect. Of several tissues tested from immature rats treated with testosterone only RNA from the seminal vesicle caused growth

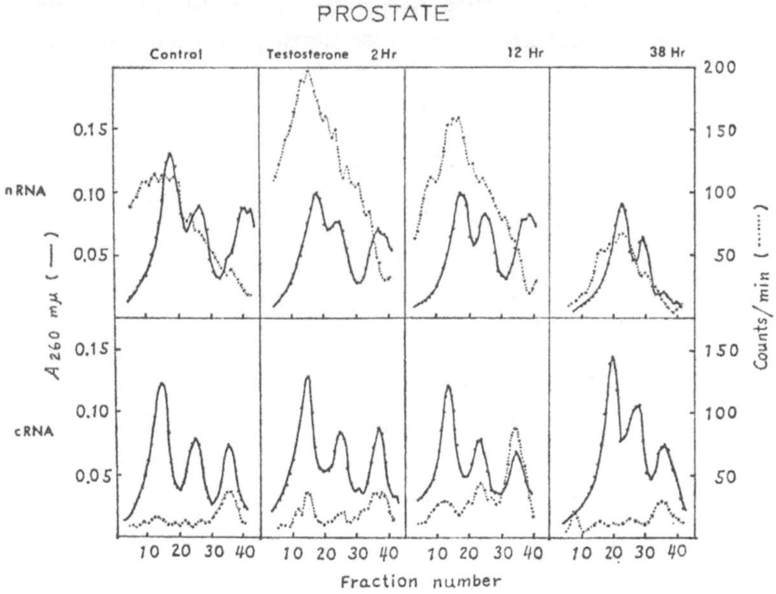

Fig. 7. Sucrose density gradient analyses of the nuclear and cytoplasmic RNAS present in the prostate at zero time and at varying intervals after the injection of testosterone.

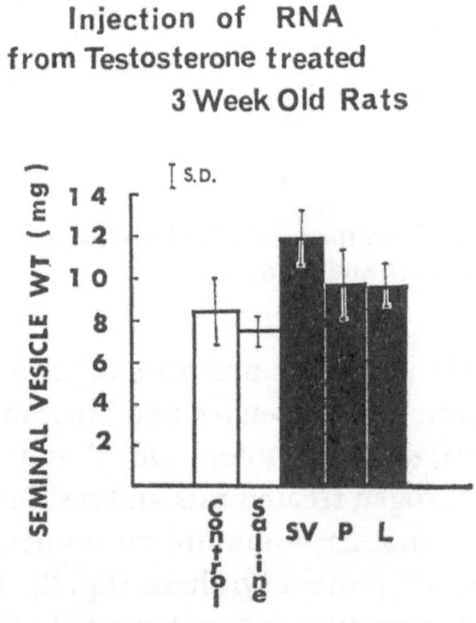

Fig. 8. Growth promoting effect of the injection of RNA from testosterone treated three week old rats into the seminal vesicles of control three week old rats. SV, RNA from the seminal vesicle; P, RNA from the prostate; L. RNA from the liver.

when instilled. RNA from the prostate, liver or kidney as well as from the seminal vesicle of adult male rats was effective in stimulating growth and protein synthesis when instilled into the seminal vesicle of three week old rats (fig. 9). Treating the RNA with ribonuclease or

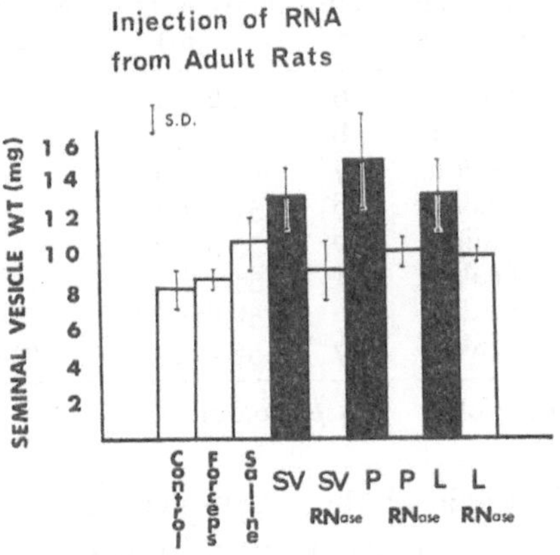

Fig. 9. The growth promoting effect of RNAs from the tissues of adult rats instilled into the seminal vesicles of three week old rats. SV, seminal vesicle; P, prostate; L, liver. RNAse indicates the effects of RNA that was treated with ribonuclease before being instilled.

boiling it for 15 minutes before instillation destroyed the growth promoting effect and showed that it was due to the RNA and not to a possible contaminating androgen. RNA extracted from the tissues of rats injected with ^{14}C-testosterone contained no detectable ^{14}C.

When the synthetic polynucleotide, polyuridylic acid (poly U) was instilled into the seminal vesicle it did not lead to increased weight or increased protein synthesis but it did increase the incorporation of labeled phenylalanine into protein (29). This suggests that the poly U entered the cells and directed the synthesis of polyphenylalanine on their ribosomes.

Fractionating the RNA on sucrose density gradients revealed that only the central one of the three peaks is biologically active in stimulating protein synthesis and growth when instilled into the seminal vesicle (table 3). It is this peak which becomes labeled most rapidly when an animal is injected with testosterone and labeled cytidine.

The seminal vesicle of the three week old rat responded equally well to RNA from seminal vesicle, prostate, liver or kidney of the adult male

Table 3. *Effects of RNA fractions from the liver on the growth of the seminal vesicles of three week old rats. The RNA was extracted from livers and fractionated by sucrose density gradient centrifugation into three peaks which were then separately instilled into the seminal vesicles. Only peak two, the middle peak representing 16s to 18s RNA, was effective in stimulating growth.*

Source of RNA	Material instilled	Rats (no.)	Body weight (gm)	Seminal vesicle weight (mg)	Per cent increase
	Saline	6	53.8 ± 2.4	11.6 ± 0.4	
Control liver	Peak 1	8	52.5 ± 1.4	12.6 ± 0.6	
	Peak 2	7	54.1 ± 1.3	14.0 ± 1.0*	22
	Peak 3	6	54.0 ± 1.5	11.5 ± 0.6	
	Saline	10	55.5 ± 5.0	11.5 ± 0.6	
DOC-treated liver	Peak 1	11	54.1 ± 2.2	11.7 ± 0.6	
	Peak 2	10	56.6 ± 2.0	15.5 ± 0.7†	32
	Peak 3	7	54.4 ± 1.5	12.9 ± 0.9	

* $p < 0.025$ vs. saline controls. † $p < 0.001$.

(28). The seminal vesicle of the seven-week old rat showed a three-fold greater growth in response to RNA from the seminal vesicle than to RNA from prostate or liver (29) (fig. 10). Finally, the seminal vesicle

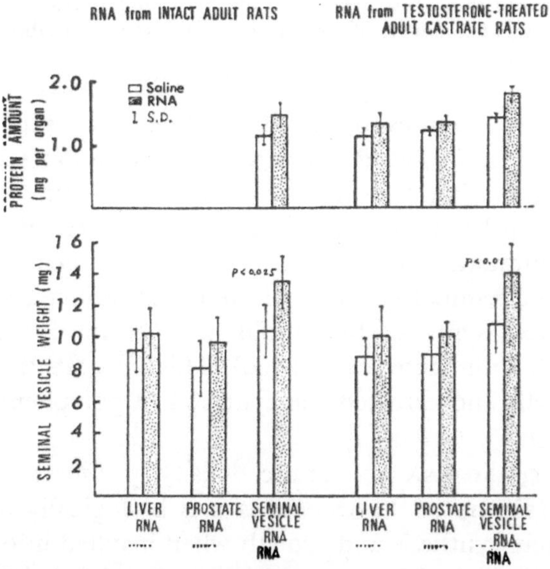

Fig. 10. The effects of RNA derived from the liver, prostate and seminal vesicle of intact adult rats or testosterone treated castrate rats on the growth of the seminal vesicle of seven weeks old rats. The open column represents the weight or protein content of the control seminal vesicles. The dotted column indicates the weight or protein content of the contralateral seminal vesicle which received the RNA.

of the 12 week old rat responded only to RNA from the seminal vesicle (30) (table 4). During the course of development the seminal vesicle

Table 4. *Effects of* RNA *from various tissues and given a variety of treatments on the weight and protein content of the seminal vesicles of castrate twelve week old rats.*

Material Instilled	No. of Animals	Seminal vesicle		Protein content	
		Wt. (mg)	Mg/g body wt.	µg/mg S.V.	Mg/gland
Saline	5	104 ± 3	3.2	44.6 ± 0.4	4.6
Native RNA from:					
Seminal Vesicle	7	141 ± 13	4.0	47.4 ± 1.4	6.3
Prostate	5	108 ± 7	2.9	44.5 ± 0.9	4.8
Liver	6	112 ± 8	3.3	41.7 ± 0.9	4.6
Heated RNA from:					
Seminal Vesicle	5	87 ± 7	2.8	41.9 ± 0.9	3.6
Prostate	4	110 ± 11	3.4	38.4 ± 1.0	4.2
Liver	3	101 ± 2	3.1	41.1 ± 0.3	4.2
Ribonuclease treated RNA from:					
Seminal Vesicle	5	81 ± 4	2.4	45.2 ± 0.8	3.7
Prostate	5	75 ± 9	2.3	45.4 ± 0.2	3.5
Liver	3	82 ± 8	2.3	42.2 ± 1.5	3.4
Uterine RNA from normal adult	5	105 ± 4	3.1	43.4 ± 0.5	4.6

Rats were castrated when 10 weeks old. RNA was instilled (80 µg/lobe) into the seminal vesicles when the rats were 12 weeks old. The rats were killed 48 hours after instillation of RNA and the seminal vesicle was dissected free of the coagulating gland, weighed, and analyzed for protein content (Lowry).
The RNA was isolated from the tissues of normal adult (10 week old) male rats. Uterine RNA was isolated from normal adult female rats.

gradually becomes more specific in the kind of RNA that can enter it and be effective in stimulating proteins synthesis. It is of interest to recall that MANSOUR and NIU (24) found only uterine RNA from adult mice to be effective in stimulating the appearance of alkaline phosphatase in the uteri of castrate adult mice. Only uterine RNA from estrogen treated castrate rats initiated the cytologic changes in the endometrium of adult castrate rats characteristic of estrogen (25). Thus all three experiments suggest that well differentiated tissues respond only to organ specific RNA whereas the less fully differentiated tissue of immature animals may respond to certain kinds of heterologous RNA.

Perhaps there are receptor sites of some kind for RNA that become established in cells after sexual maturation or after the cells have been exposed to a certain level of androgens for a suitable period.

In a comparable series of experiments RNA has been shown to mediate the effects of estradiol on the rat uterus (31). RNA extracted with cold phenol and sodium dodecyl sulfate from uteri of three-week old rats treated with estradiol, or from the uteri of intact adult rats, and instilled into the lumen of the uterus of a three-week old rat, increased protein synthesis. This was measured by the incorporation of uniformly ^{14}C-labeled amino acids into proteins (table 5). Compared

Table 5. *Protein synthesis in the uterus following intraluminal application of* RNA.

Series	Control horn cpm/mg protein	RNA-treated horn cpm/mg protein	Exp/Control	Significance
A (11)	1359	1798	1.34	$p < 0.05$
B (8)	1630	2040	1.28	$p < 0.02$
C (5)	678	1230	1.73	$p < 0.05$

Numbers in parenthesis indicate number of rats injected with RNA. The control horn was injected with saline (series A), with RNA from untreated immature rats (series B), or with RNA from estradiol-treated rats inactivated by ribonuclease (series C). RNA was prepared from uteri of three week old rats injected with 5 μg 17β estradiol 12 hours before death. Approximately 60 μg of RNA was instilled into the lumen of one uterine horn. The rats were injected with 2 μc of ^{14}C-labelled amino acid mixture 2 hours before death.

with any of four types of controls, the RNA increased significantly the incorporation of amino acids into protein. This increased uptake was decreased when 7.5 μg of actinomycin D was injected into the uterus along with the 70–75 μg of RNA.

The uterus of the three-week old rat responded to liver RNA as well as to uterine RNA but RNA from any of the other tissues tested – kidney, adrenal, skeletal muscle, lung and thymus – was ineffective (table 6.) Uterine RNA was ineffective when instilled into the seminal vesicle and seminal vesicle RNA was without effect when instilled into the uterine lumen.

We have carried out two series of experiments with explants of seminal vesicle and of uterus grown in organ culture. The explants were

Table 6. *Protein synthesis in the uterus following intraluminal application of* RNA *from various tissues of immature (three-week old) female rats.*

Source of RNA		Experimental/Control cpm/mg protein	Significance
Uterus	(8)	1.28	$p < 0.02$
Liver	(7)	1.29	$p < 0.05$
Kidney	(6)	1.01	--
Adrenals	(5)	1.16	$p > 0.50$
Skeletal muscle	(4)	0.92	--
Lung	(5)	0.86	--
Thymus	(5)	0.78	--

Numbers in parenthesis indicate number of rats injected with RNA.

RNA was prepared using phenol-sodium dodecylsulfate from tissues of three week old rats injected with 5 μg 17β estradiol 12 hours before death. Approximately 60 μg of RNA was instilled into the lumen of one uterine horn. The rats were injected with 2 μC of ^{14}C-labeled amino acid mixture 2 hours before death.

cultured 24 hours in medium 1066 with or without RNA extracted from the appropriate target organ of the hormone. RNA extracted from the seminal vesicle was added to organ cultures containing seminal vesicle and RNA extracted from the uteri of adult rats was added to explants of uteri from three-week old rats. The rate of protein synthesis in the tissue in organ culture was measured by adding a pulse of uniformly labeled ^{14}C-amino acids one or two hours before the culture was terminated. In the experiments to date we have found no consistent difference in the rate of protein synthesis in experimental versus control cultures. This is in marked contrast to the clear response to exogenous RNA of certain enzymatic activities in the adrenal and ovary in organ culture (32, 33).

Experiments in several laboratories have described specific enzymes in target tissues which increase markedly in activity in response to androgen (9) or estrogen (10). Dr. RISTO SANTTI working in my laboratory has demonstrated increased activity of hexokinase in the prostate following testosterone administration. We plan to use this as a reference enzyme to determine whether its activity is increased when RNA is instilled as well as when testosterone is injected. If this does occur it would suggest that the RNA instilled does contain some sort of biological information. Our experiments to date in these systems have shown that RNA increases protein synthesis but the experiments were not designed to detect the synthesis of a specific protein. The increased protein synthesis found consistently in the experiments could have been brought about by the RNA acting in any of several different ways.

There are now several experimental systems which provide strong presumptive evidence that a hormone may lead to the production of a new species of RNA and that at least some of this RNA is template RNA which provides biological information for the synthesis of specific enzymes. The mechanism by which this result is achieved remains unknown. Is the action of the hormone on the genetic mechanism direct or indirect? With which component of the gene system does the hormone interact? Or, if the effect of the hormone is indirect, with which component of the cell does the hormone interact initially and how does this secondarily affect the readout of the genes? When satisfactory answers to these basic questions have been found, we will be closer to an understanding of the effect of hormones on the development of enzyme systems.

REFERENCES

1. BONNER J., (1965) *Molecular biology of development*, Oxford Univ. Press, New York and Oxford.
2. JOST A., (1957) In: *Gestation: transactions of the third conference*, VILLEE C. A. ed., JOSIAH MACY, Jr. Foundation, New York, p. 129.
3. PRICE D., In: *Gestation: transactions of the third conference*, VILLEE, C. A. ed., JOSIAH MACY, Jr. Foundation, New York, p. 173.
4. TATA J. R., (1966) *Developmental Biol.* 13: 77.
5. CLEVER U. and P. KARLSON, (1960) *Exper. Cell Research* 20: 263.
6. NEMETH A., (1960) *Science* 132: 1497.
7. CORNELL N. and C. A. VILLEE, (1968) *Comp. Biochem. Physiol.* 27: 603.
8. VILLEE C. A., (1966) *Federation Proc.* 25: 874.
9. SINGHAL R. L. and G. M. LING, (1969) *Canad. J. Physiol. Pharmacol.* 47: 233.
10. NOACK I. and H. SCHMIDT, (1968) *Endokrinologie* 53: 291.
11. TURKINGTON R. (1970) In: *The sex steroids: molecular mechanisms*, McKERNS, K. W. ed., Appleton-Century-Crofts, New York.
12. JENSEN E. V., H. I. JACOBSON, J. W. FLESHER, N. N. SAHA, G. N. GUPTA, S. SMITH, V. COLUCCI, D. SHIPLACOFF, H. G. NEUMANN, E. R. DESOMBRE, and P. W. JUNGBLUT, (1966) In: *Steroid dynamics, proc of the symposium on the dynamics of steroid hormones*, PINCUS G., T. NAKAO, J. F. TAIT, eds., Academic Press, New York, p. 133.
13. TOFT D. and J. GORSKI, (1966) *Proc. Nat. Acad. Sci.* U.S. 44: 15.

14. EISENFELD A. J. and J. AXELROD, (1965) *J. Pharmacol. Exper. Ther.* 150: 469.
15. KATO J. and C. A. VILLEE, (1967) *Endrocrinology* 80: 567.
16. JENSEN E. V., T. SUZUKI, M. NUMATA, S. SMITH and E. R. DESOMBRE, (1969) *Steroids* 13:417.
17. ANDERSON K. M. and S. LIAO, (1968) *Nature* 219: 277.
18. O'MALLEY B., (1970) In: *The sex steroids: molecular mechanisms*, MCKERNS, K. W. ed., Appleton-Century-Crofts, New York.
19. SLUYSER M., (1966) *J. Molec. Biol.* 22: 411.
20. GOLDBERG M. L. and W. A. ATCHLEY, (1966) *Proc. Nat. Acad. Sci. U.S.* 55: 989.
21. MITCHELL M., (1969) *The interaction of rat liver chromatin with steroid hormones as measured by ^{3}H-actinomycin D binding*. Thesis, Harvard University.
22. SEKERIS C. E. and N. LANG, (1964) *Life Sciences* 3: 169.
23. GORSKI J. and N. J. NELSON, (1965) *Arch. Biochem. Biophys.* 110: 284.
24. MANSOUR A. M. and M. C. NIU, (1965) *Proc. Nat. Acad. Sci. U.S.* 53: 764.
25. SEGAL S. J., O. W. DAVIDSON and K. WADA, (1965) *Proc. Nat. Acad. Sci. U.S.* 54: 782.
26. WICKS W. D. and C. A. VILLEE, (1964) *Arch. Biochem. Biophys.* 106: 353.
27. FUJII T. and C. A. VILLEE, (1968) *Endocrinology* 82: 463.
28. FUJII T. and C. A. VILLEE, (1967) *Proc. Nat. Acad. Sci. U.S.* 57: 1468.
29. FUJII T. and C. A. VILLEE, (1969) *Proc. Nat. Acad. Sci. U.S.* 62: 829.
30. ITO Y. and C. A. VILLEE, (1970).
31. FENCL M. and C. A. VILLEE, (1971) *Endocrinology*, 88: 279.
32. VILLEE D. B., (1967) *Science* 158: 652.
33. VILLEE D. B., L. GREENOUGH and J. RETTIG, (1968) *Science* 159: 1365.

DISCUSSION

Prof. Sereni: About three years ago you published some data on template activity of chromatin in the mammalian liver during perinatal period of life. There was an increase in activity just after birth. Could you speculate a little bit on those very important findings?

Prof. Villee: In a series of experiments, I did not allude for here, we did find an increase of template activity in isolated chromatin just after birth. We also reported that there is an increase template activity of chromatin isolated from regenerating liver. When you remove 70% of the liver and then follow the properties of the chromatin in the remaining 30% of the liver over the next 24–48 hours there is a demonstrable increase in template activity. It appeared that the increased template activity must reflect some change in the binding of DNA by histones. In bacterial systems there are no histones and the control of gene-acivity must depend in one way or another on the interaction of repressors and redrepressors. It appears that genic control is basically different in several respects in mammalian systems as compared to bacterial systems. Mammalian system does have histones. There is good evidence that the histones play some role in determining which genes are active and which genes are not active. I do believe that when we have a better idea of the nature of these mechanisms we will be closer to a full understanding of the mechanism of cell differentiation and of hormone action. I believe the two have many similarities.

DRUG SUSCEPTIBILITY AND THE DEVELOPMENT OF ERYTHROCYTE ENZYME SYSTEMS

WERNER SCHRÖTER*

INTRODUCTION

Some peculiarities of the erythrocytes of newborn infants are now well documented. The best known are their high hemoglobin F concentration and their shortened life span of about 80 days (1, 2). Clinically most important is the susceptibility of newborn infants, especially of prematures, to develop hemolytic anemia, characterized by Heinz bodies within the red cells, or methemoglobinemia on exposure to a variety of agents (Reviews see 3, 4). The mechanism of this high susceptibilty, mainly, against oxidizing drugs, has been the subject of numerous studies in the past 20 years. The examination of the erythrocytes of newborn infants has been stimulated especially by the introduction of enzymology. Due to the relative homogeneity and availability of erythrocyte suspensions and their comparatively small number of metabolic pathways, the biochemical characterization of the human erythrocyte is more accomplished than that of most other human tissues. The developmental variations of the erythrocyte enzyme activities are well known too. But all these more descriptive studies do not definitely explain why the erythrocytes of newborn infants live only 80 instead of 120 days and why these cells are highly vulnerable to oxidizing agents.

HETEROGENEITY OF THE ERYTHROCYTE POPULATION OF NEWBORN INFANTS

The homogeneity of an erythrocyte population is more apparent than

* Department of Pediatrics, University of Hamburg, Hamburg, Germany. This work was supported by research grants (Schr 86/6, Schr 86/7) of the Deutsche Forschungsgemeinschaft, Bad Godesberg, Germany.

real. BEUTLER has stressed this problem in 1966 especially with regard to the evaluation of gene action in hereditary disorders of the red cell (5). In the newborn infant the heterogeneity of the erythrocyte population is much more marked than in adults (6). Although we are used to express the size and the hemoglobin content in terms of mean corpuscular volume, mean corpuscular hemoglobin and mean corpuscular hemoglobin concentration, we have to recognize that we only describe hypothetical average values, in spite of the present anisocytosis. Similarly, when we measure erythrocyte enzymes, we express enzyme activity in terms of a unit of red cells or of hemoglobin; we also have to recognize that young and old cells contain different levels of enzyme activity. The variability in red cells may be due to the effect of any random factors or to aging.

Table 1. *Corresponding metabolic characteristics of red cells of newborns and young red cells of adults.*

High rate of glycolysis
High rate of the pentose phosphate pathway
Increased adenosine triphosphate content
Slightly increased levels of reduced glutathione
Diminished stability of 2, 3-DI-phosphoglycerate during incubation

From SCHRÖTER (13)

The erythrocyte population of newborn infants contains a high portion of immature cells. The reticulocyte counts are relatively high in the first days of life with an average of 5 per cent. Biochemical equivalents of the young cell age are the high rates of the glucose metabolism with concomitantly increased activities of the corresponding enzymes, the slightly increased concentrations of ATP and GSH and the instability of 2,3-diphosphoglycerate as summarized in table 1 (7–12). Despite their high metabolic activities the erythrocytes of newborn infants seem to consume less glucose than would be expected from their mean age (14).

The metabolic differences between the red cells of newborn infants and young red cells of adults shown in table 2 clearly demonstrate that the two populations consist of principally different cell types. This is evident from the low levels of some enzymes in the red cells of newborn infants compared with the elevated levels of the corresponding enzymes in young red cells of adults. One further bit of evidence to the fact of the erythrocytes of newborn infants being different to those of normal adults is the decreased membrane ATPase activity with resultant decrease in the active transport and leak of potassium demonstrable during the incubation of the cells *in vitro* (15, 16).

Table 2. *Different metabolic characteristics of red cells of newborns and young red cells of adults compared to normal red cells of adults*

	Red cells of newborns	Young red cells of adults
Activities of the enzymes Cholinesterase Carbonic anhydrase Catalase Glutathione peroxidase Glyoxalase NADH-dependent methemoglobin reductase Membrane ATPase	Decreased	Increased
ATP stability during incubation	Decreased	Increased
Potassium efflux during storage	Increased	Decreased

From Schröter (13)

Whether these 'minus deviations' of the red cells of newborn infants render them more liable to hemolysis or not is not yet clearly understood. From the theoretical point of view this assumption is more hypothetical, since most of the deviations are only small with regard to the corresponding adult parameters. We have to recognize that even the decrease of an enzyme activity of 30 to 50 per cent generally is not rate limiting under normal conditions.

The heterogeneity of the newborn erythrocyte population has been further confirmed by the biophysical studies of DANON et al. (17). The bimodality of the osmotic fragility curve shown in fig. 1 suggests that a small portion of the erythrocytes hemolyzes later, i.e. at lower salt

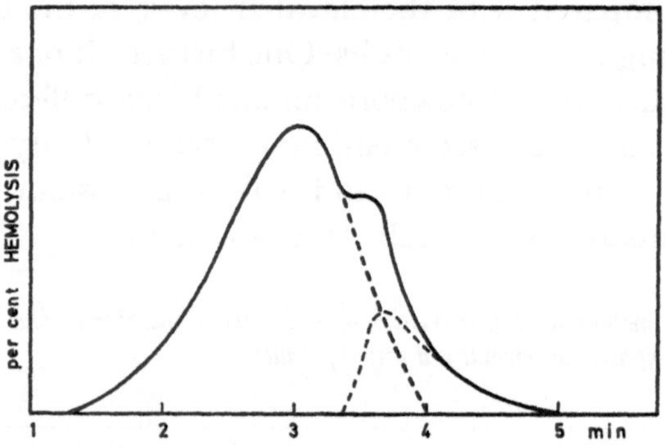

Fig. 1. Bimodality of the fragility curve obtained from umbilical cord blood. ----- Hypothetic cell population with low fragility (modified from DANON et al., 17).

concentrations than the most resistent cells from adults as has been pointed out earlier by SJÖLIN (18). This even more resistent portion seems to be higher than 10 per cent.

The density distribution curve of the cord blood red cells is also bimodal (fig. 2). Most of the cells are of lower specific gravity than

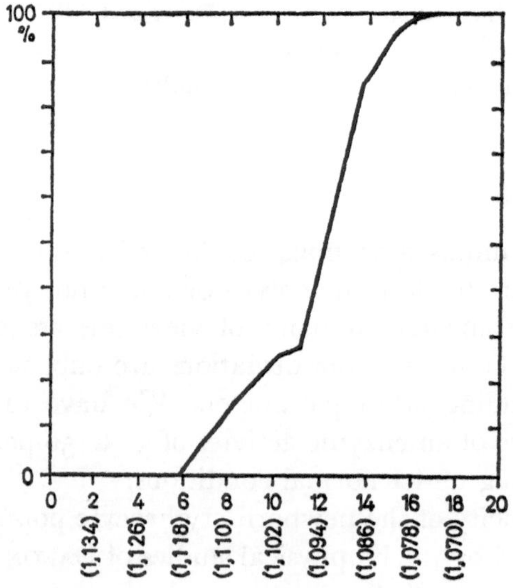

Fig. 2. Bimodal density distribution of the red cells of umbilical cord blood (from DANON et al., 17).

adult cells, indicating mainly higher hydration; but there appears to be a considerable number of cells with a high specific gravity, similar to the densest cells of adult blood. Also this portion, which corresponds to senescent fetal-type red cells may occasionally account for up to 10 per cent.

Apart from the biochemical and biophysical examination, the existence of two different cell populations can be demonstrated morphologically by the alkali elution of adult hemoglobin from the fetal cells according to BETKE and KLEIHAUER (19). A marked tendency for concentration of fetal hemoglobin in some cells and adult hemoglobin in others has been found.

MECHANISM OF DRUG SUSCEPTIBILITY OF THE ERYTHROCYTES OF NEWBORN INFANTS

Most of the drugs which injure the red cells of newborn infants are directly or indirectly acting oxidants (table 3). They produce de-

Table 3. *Some drugs causing Heinz body formation in the erythrocytes of newborn infants*

Directly acting oxidants	
Nitrite	
Chlorate	
Acide	
Indirectly acting oxidants (in the presence of oxygen, in part via the formation o peroxides)	
Nitrogen-containing	*Nitrogen-free*
Acetylphenylhydrazine	Naphthalene
Anilin derivatives	Menadione
Acetanilide	Resorcin
Aminophenol	Acetophenetidin
Dinitrophenol	(Phenacetin)
Nitrobenzene	Dichlorophenol
Dinitroglycol	
Erythroltetranitrate	
Sulfonamides	
Sulfanilamide	
Sulfathiazole	
Sulfapyridine	

Many, but not all of these drugs also produce methemoglobinemia.

naturation of the hemoglobin associated with Heinz body anemia. Many, but not all of them also produce methemoglobinemia. As a logical consequence defect mechanisms normally protecting the cells against oxidation or a more facilitated oxidation of intracellular components have been postulated.

Virtually, some enzymatic reactions involved in the detoxification of oxidants are less active in cord blood red cells than in red cells of adults. The activity of the NADH-dependent methemoglobin diaphorase, which mainly catalyzes the reduction of methemoglobin to oxyhemoglobin is reduced to approximately 60 per cent of that in the erythrocytes of adults (20). Moreover, there is an increased susceptibility of fetal hemoglobin to oxidizing agents (21). These two abnormalities may explain the tendency of newborn infants to develop methemoglobinemia. Compared with the methemoglobin formation the denaturation of hemoglobin with concomitant formation of Heinz bodies and premature destruction of the cells is a more complex process. A central role in the protection of hemoglobin from oxidative hemolysis play the thiols of the red cell (22). Fig. 3 shows schematically that the SH-groups of the hemoglobin by far outnumber the thiols located in or at the membrane, the SH-groups of GSH and those of the enzymes. Glutathione provides a primary defense against intracellular oxidation.

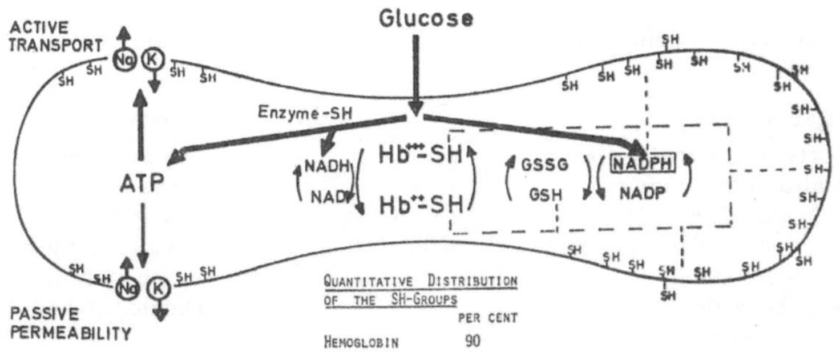

QUANTITATIVE DISTRIBUTION OF THE SH-GROUPS	PER CENT
HEMOGLOBIN	90
MEMBRANE	5
INSIDE	4,95
OUTSIDE	0,05
GSH AND ENZYMES	5

Fig. 3. Schematic graphs of the erythrocyte SH-groups and their relationship to the intracellular metabolism. Their stability depends on the formation of NADPH in the hexosemonophosphate-shunt. Quantitative data from WEED et al. (23) and VANSTEVENINCK et al. (24).

It is supported in this function by active reducing systems via the hexosemonophosphate shunt. The addition of glucose to the suspensions of erythrocytes likewise slow down the oxidative changes whereas hereditary enzyme defects of the hexosemonophosphate shunt accelerate them.

Glutathione is rapidly oxidized by some indirect oxidants in the presence of oxygen. From acetylphenylhydrazine the active agent phenyldiimide is formed (fig. 4) reacting with oxyhemoglobin and

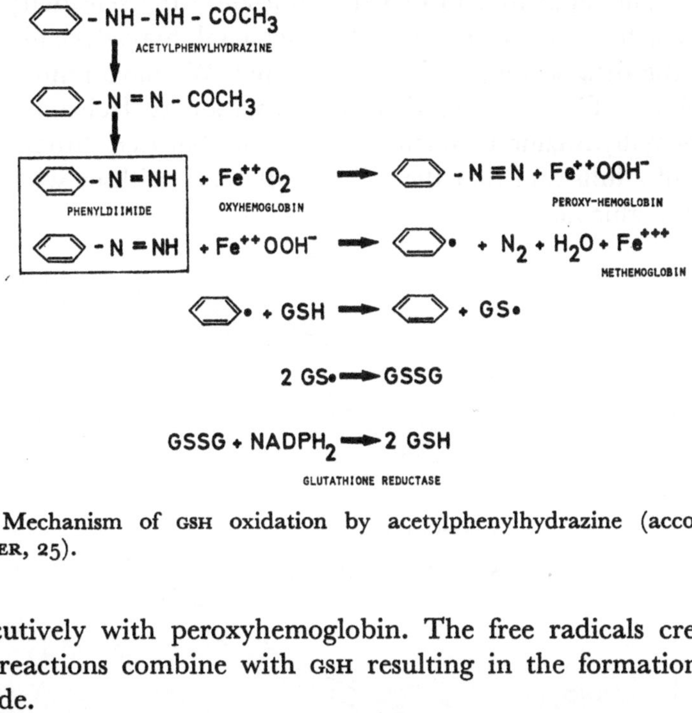

Fig. 4. Mechanism of GSH oxidation by acetylphenylhydrazine (according to KOSOWER, 25).

consecutively with peroxyhemoglobin. The free radicals created in these reactions combine with GSH resulting in the formation of the disulfide.

Other agents, for example menadione and ascorbic acid, act by the formation of hydrogen peroxide. Glutathione peroxidase (fig. 5) efficiently detoxifies low levels of H_2O_2. It is assumed that catalase is important only when the erythrocytes are exposed to high concentrations of peroxide (26).

The erythrocytes of newborn infants are highly sensitive to both acetylphenylhydrazine and peroxides, agents which oxidize glutathione within the cell. Therefore, the in vitro observation of ZINKHAM (27) in 1959, that GSH is more instable in erythrocytes of newborn infants

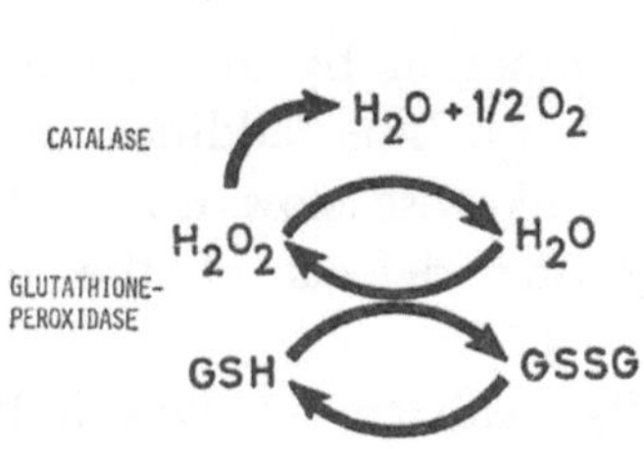

Fig. 5. Peroxide detoxification in human erythrocytes.

than in adults appeared to explain sufficiently the sensitivity of the fetal red cells. The hypothesis, that neonatal hypoglycemia might support the drug sensitivity has been stated. We have reinvestigated this problem. Fig. 6 shows that the formation of Heinz bodies by acetylphenylhydrazine is much higher in newborn erythrocytes than in those of adults and that there is no difference with or without the addition of glucose.

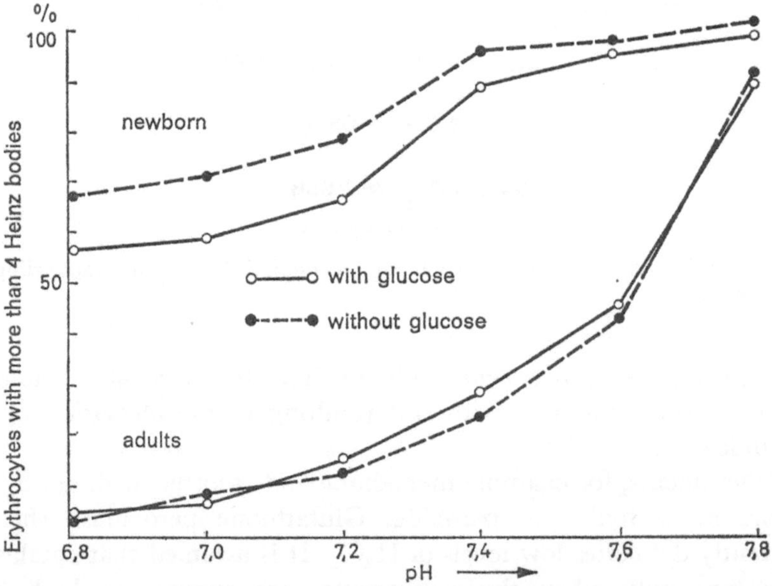

Fig. 6. The effect of pH and glucose concentration on Heinz body formation in neonatal and adult erythrocytes exposed to acetylphenylhydrazine. Twice washed erythrocytes were incubated in a mixture of 9 parts isotonic NaCl solution and 1 part 0,1 M phosphate buffer. Glucose concentration: 200 mg/100 ml, acetylphenylhydrazine concentration: 80 mg/100 ml, temperature 37 °C, duration of incubation: 2 hours. Demonstration of inclusion bodies by Nile-blue sulphate. The points on the curve represent mean values of 10 individual tests (from SCHRÖTER, 28).

Furthermore, the figure shows that the formation of Heinz bodies becomes less as pH falls, both in newborn infants and adults. From these data we conclude that there probably is no relationship between neonatal hypoglycemia and drug sensitivity. Also the postulated relation between acidosis and the tendency to hemolysis is apparently the same as in adults (4).

The significance of the low glutathione peroxidase activity for the sensitivity of neonatal red cells against oxidizing agents is not yet clearly understood. The reduction of the enzyme activity for about 15 per cent in full-term infants and 25 per cent in prematures (29–31) does not necessarily indicate that the relative enzyme deficiency is the cause of the drug sensitivity of the erythrocytes. In vivo the relative

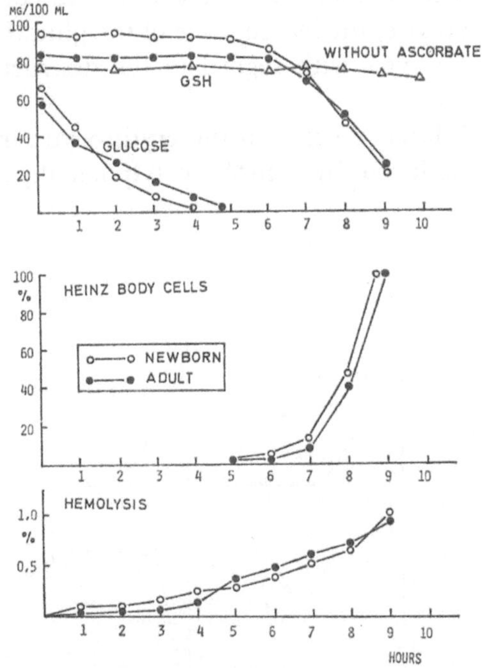

Fig. 7. The effect of 0,015 M ascorbic acid on glucose and GSH concentration, Heinz body formation and hemolysis of erythrocytes of adults and newborn infants. Twice washed erythrocytes were incubated at 37 °C in an isotonic mixture containing 3,5 mMol K^+, 160 mMol Na^+, 30 mMol HPO_4^{--}, 25 mMol HCO_3^- and 109,4 mMol Cl^- per liter. pH 7,4. Hematocrit 30%. Determination of GSH according to BEUTLER et al. (34).

glutathione peroxidase deficiency alone does not appear to result in neonatal hyperbilirubinemia (31).

In vitro hydrogen peroxide is formed in red cells through the coupled oxidation of ascorbate with oxyhemoglobin (32, 33). We have studied the effect of 15 mM ascorbate on both erythrocytes of newborn infants and adults (fig. 7).

The concentration of GSH decreases – after a lag period of 1 hour – when glucose has been consumed. Simultaneously Heinz bodies are formed. Hemolysis is only minimal. It is noteworthy that in this case there is no significant difference between the erythrocytes of newborns and adults. If the glutathione peroxidase activity would be the rate limiting step for the detoxification of peroxide, we would have to expect a slower decrease of the GSH concentration in the erythrocytes of newborns, due to their lower enzyme activity, as compared to adult erythrocytes. Therefore, the leading role of the glutathione peroxidase in newborn erythrocytes with regard to the destruction of peroxide seems very unlikely.

A significant difference between the erythrocytes of newborns and adults can be produced by 5 mM acetylphenylhydrazine (fig. 8).

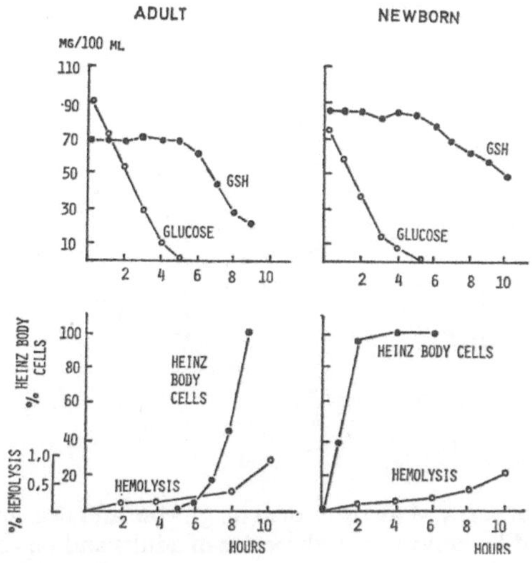

Fig. 8. The effect of 0,005 M acetylphenylhydrazine on glucose and GSH concentration, Heinz body formation and hemolysis of erythrocytes of adults and newborn infants. Experimental conditions as in fig. 7.

In the erythrocytes of newborns Heinz bodies are formed in the first hour of incubation despite active glycolysis and high GSH concentrations.

In contrast, in adult cells Heinz bodies appear only when glucose disappears and when the concentration of GSH begins to decrease. These experiments clearly demonstrate that the formation of Heinz bodies by acetylphenylhydrazine in the erythrocytes of newborn infants neither depends on the concentration of GSH nor on glucose metabolism as well. This assumption is further supported by experiments with other sulfhydryl reagents such as N-ethylmaleimide and iodoacetate, which inhibit glycolysis by alkylating protein and nonprotein SH-groups, but no Heinz bodies appear despite of the complete blocking of intracellular glutathione.

If we summarize the reported experiments, we may conclude that the discussed intracellular metabolic deviations of the erythrocytes of newborn infants do not sufficiently explain their high susceptibility to oxidizing agents. We will now consider the role of the erythrocyte membrane.

THE ROLE OF THE ERYTHROCYTE MEMBRANE WITH REGARD TO DRUG SUSCEPTIBILITY IN NEWBORN INFANTS

The composition of the erythrocyte membrane is now well documented. Essential structural components are the lipids, membrane proteins, ions and water (35). There are reported differences between the erythrocytes of newborns and adults with regard to the total and individual phospholipids (6, 36, 37) as well as to the membrane structure (38–40). Among the essential functional ligands of the red cell membrane protein, the membrane SH-groups are most important for the protection of the red cell against oxidative injury. The membrane SH-groups bind lipid peroxides, a mechanism which is greatly enhanced in vitamin E deficiency (33, 41, 42).

In the erythrocytes of newborn infants the number or the stability of the membrane SH-groups may be decreased as suggested by SCHRÖTER and BITTER (43). This assumption is based on the following experiments. If we incubate erythrocytes with the indirect oxidant menadione in a concentration of 2,5 mM the cells of newborn infants hemolyze totally within 6 hours, whereas the hemolysis of adult cells is only minimal (fig. 9).

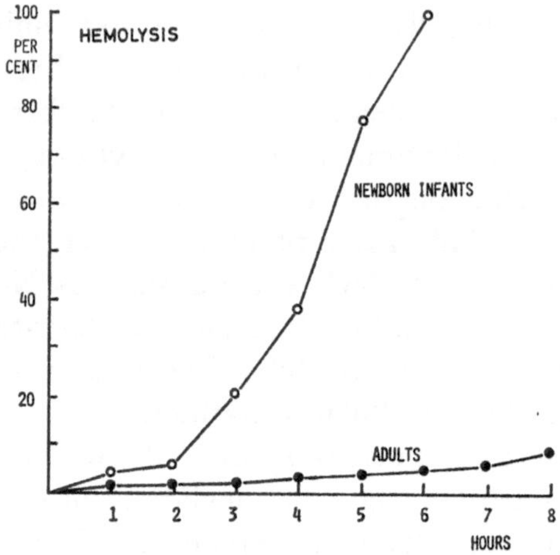

Fig. 9. The effect of 0,025 M menadione on hemolysis of erythrocytes of adults and newborn infants. Experimental conditions as in fig. 7.

This difference is not due to differences in the intracellular metabolism, since glucose consumption, decrease of GSH and the formation of Heinz bodies are identical in both cell types under the conditions of the experiment.

The functional state of the membrane SH-groups also influences the cation permeability of the red cells (44). In an attempt to define any increased susceptibility to membrane injury of the erythrocytes of newborns, we studied the effect of iodoacetate plus ferricyanide on the passive cation permeability and on hemolysis (fig. 10). In adult cells we found both an increase of the potassium efflux and the sodium influx, followed by osmotic hemolysis. In the red cells of newborn infants the kinetics of the cation fluxes and of hemolysis differ markedly from those seen in adults. It is remarkable that the rate of hemolysis is higher than in suspensions of adult cells though the cation fluxes are much less affected. Therefore, we assume that the suspensions of fetal red cells consist of two different populations which exhibit a different susceptibility to iodoacetate plus ferricyanide. The one population, probably the older one, is more sensitive to the membrane injury than the other. In the older population the membrane injuring agents

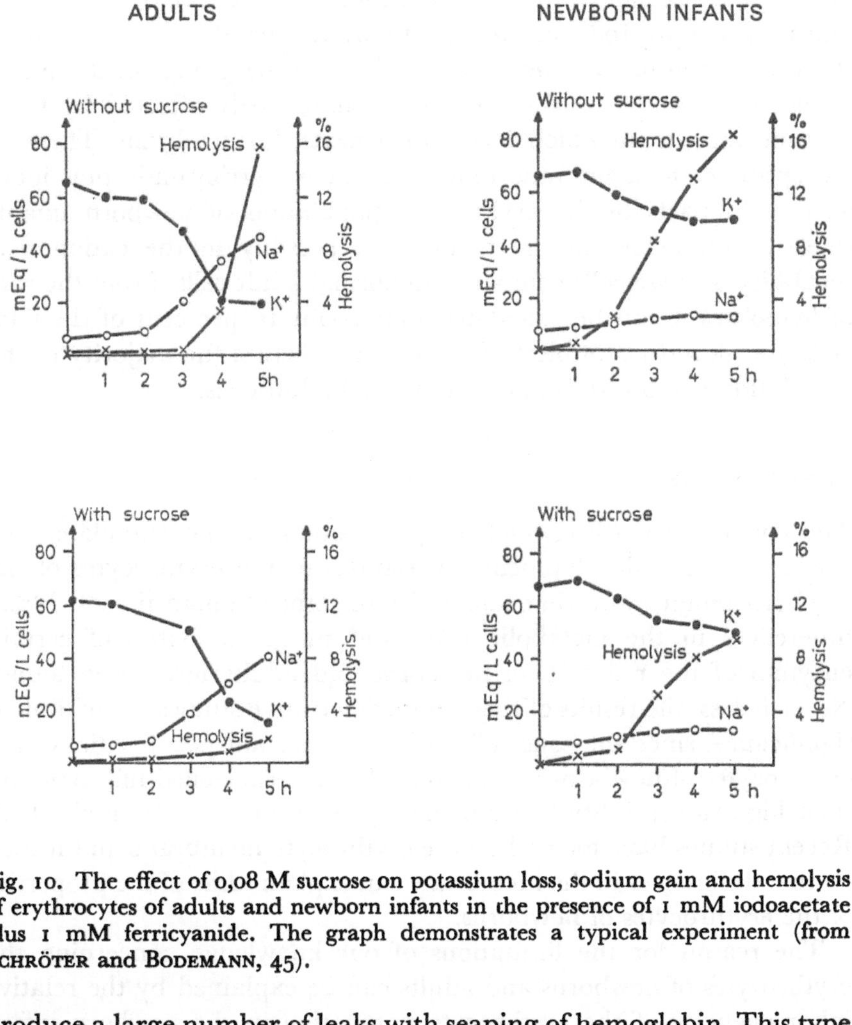

Fig. 10. The effect of 0,08 M sucrose on potassium loss, sodium gain and hemolysis of erythrocytes of adults and newborn infants in the presence of 1 mM iodoacetate plus 1 mM ferricyanide. The graph demonstrates a typical experiment (from SCHRÖTER and BODEMANN, 45).

produce a large number of leaks with seaping of hemoglobin. This type of hemolysis is not due to osmosis, because the non-penetrating sucrose, which abolishes the osmotic hemolysis of adult cells nearly completely, has only little effect on the red cells of newborn infants. On the other hand, the red cells of the younger population must be more resistant against iodoacetate plus ferricyanide than red cells of adults, because the cation fluxes are less affected in the remaining non-hemolyzed cells than in the red cells of adults.

The mechanism of the combined effect of iodoacetate plus ferricyanide may be explained by the 'conditioning hypothesis' of LINDEMANN and PASSOW (46). Iodoacetate 'conditions' the membrane by inhibiting the production of ATP and by alkylating the SH-groups of the membrane, thus rendering the membrane more easily affected by ferricyanide, an oxidant which does not permeate the membrane. The high susceptibility to membrane injury caused by ferricyanide plus iodoacetate in parts of the erythrocyte population of newborn infants suggests differences in the membrane, possibly in the cation permeability of these cells compared to normal adult cells. From the rate of hemolysis it can be calculated that about 10 per cent of the fetal cells are more susceptible to ferricyanide whereas the majority of the population is more resistant than normal adult cells.

CONCLUSIONS

The convenience with which they are obtained has stimulated the research on the developmental variations of the erythrocytes of the newborn infant more than those of most other human tissues. Many differences in the metabolic rates and in the activities of certain enzymes of the red cells of newborns and adults have been found. Nevertheless, the results of these more descriptive studies are of limited significance, since the cause of the most important peculiarities of the erythrocytes of newborn infants, namely their shortened life span and their high susceptiblity to oxidizing agents has not yet been clarified. Recent studies have focused on the erythrocyte membrane and it may be that differences in the membrane can explain some of the properties of the erythrocytes of newborns.

The reason for the limitations of our knowledge concerning the erythrocytes of newborns and adults can be explained by the relative inhomogeneity of the erythrocyte population in the newborn infant due to biochemical and biophysical properties. About 10 per cent of the cells of the newborn infant are younger than the youngest cells of adults. On the other hand, a second portion, which as well may exceed 10 per cent, may be senescent fetal-type cells which are older than the oldest cells of adults. We have to consider this complex situation when we determine the activities of enzymes or other parameters in the erythrocyte population of newborn infants.

Which conclusions might be drawn from these considerations? First of all, we have to establish that the 'red cell of the newborn infant' does not exist. If we determine the difference between the red cells of adults and newborns, we do not know whether this difference is valid for the whole population or not. It may be that the demonstrated deviation is only valid for a small portion of cells, for example the very old or the very young cells. Secondly, we have to delineate the perspectives for further research in this field. Here we can only postulate that we have to find out new methods which make possible the separation of the different cell types of which the erythrocyte population consists.

A last point should be mentioned, which has been neglected hitherto. This is the possible influence of the surrounding plasma on the red cells. It is well documented that the phospholipids of the red cell's membrane reflect the composition of the phospholipids of the plasma (6) and that the vitamin E concentration of the plasma may determine the susceptibility of the erythrocytes to peroxides (47).

REFERENCES

1. Garby L., S. Sjölin and J. Vuille, (1964) *Acta paediat.* (Uppsala) 53: 165.
2. Pearson H. A., (1967) *J. Pediat.* 70: 166.
3. Kleihauer E., (1966) *Fetales Hämoglobin und fetale Erythrocyten*, Ferdinand Enke Verlag, Stuttgart.
4. Oski F. A. and J. L. Naiman, (1966) *Hematologic problems in the newborn*, W. B. Saunders, Philadelphia and London.
5. Beutler E., (1966) *Amer. J. Med.* 41: 724.
6. Hürter P., W. Schröter, I. Schedel and G. Gercken, (1970) *Pediatrics* 46: 259.
7. Oski F. A., (1967) *Pediatrics* 39: 689.
8. Oski F. A. and J. L. Naiman, (1965) *Pediatrics* 36: 103.
9. Schröter W. and H. von Heyden, (1965) *Z. Kinderheilk.* 94: 263.
10. Schröter W. and P. Winter, (1967) *Klin. Wschr.* 45: 255.
11. Witt I., H. Müller and W. Künzer, (1967) *Klin. Wschr.* 45: 262.
12. Witt I., M. Herdan and W. Künzer, (1968) *Klin. Wschr.* 46: 149.
13. Schröter W., (1969) In: *Enzymopenic Anaemias, Lysosomes and Other papers*, Allan J. D., K. S. Holt, J. T. Ireland and R. J. Pollitt, eds., Livingstone, Edinburgh and London, p. 19.
14. Oski F. A. and Ch. Smith, (1968) *Pediatrics* 41: 473.
15. Whaun J. M. and F. A. Oski, (1969) *Pediat. Res.* 3: 105.
16. Blum S. F. and F. A. Oski, (1969) *Pediatrics* 43: 396.
17. Danon Y., A. Kleimann and D. Danon, (1970) *Acta haemat.* 43: 242.
18. Sjölin S., (1954) *Acta paediat.* (Uppsala), Suppl. 98, 43: 390.
19. Betke K. and E. Kleihauer, (1958) *Blut* 4: 241.
20. Ross J. D., (1963) *Blood* 21: 51.

21. BETKE K., (1953) *Naturwissenschaften* 40: 60.
22. ALLEN D. W. and J. H. JANDL, (1961) *J. clin. Invest.* 40: 454.
23. WEED R., J. EBER and A. ROTHSTEIN, (1961) *J. gen. Physiol.* 45: 395.
24. VANSTEVENINCK J., R. I. WEED and A. ROTHSTEIN, (1965) *J. gen. Physiol.* 45: 617.
25. KOSOWER N. S., (1968) In: *Hereditary disorders of erythrocyte metabolism*, E. Beutler ed., Grune & Stratton, New York and London, p. 176.
26. JACOB H. S., S. H. INGBAR and J. H. JANDL, (1965) *J. clin. Invest.* 44: 1187.
27. ZINKHAM W. H., (1959) *Pediatrics* 23: 18.
28. SCHRÖTER W., (1968) *Dtsch. med. Wschr.* 93: 1202.
29. GROSS R. T., R. BRACCI, N. RUDOLPH, E. SCHROEDER and J. A. KOCHEN, (1967) *Blood* 29: 481.
30. VETRELLA M., W. BARTHELMAI and J. RIETKÖTTER, (1970) *Klin. Wschr.* 48: 85.
31. WHAUN J. and F. A. OSKI, (1970) *J. Pediat.* 76: 555.
32. HILL A. S., A. HAUT, G. E. CARTWRIGHT and M. M. WINTROBE, (1964) *J. clin. Invest.* 43: 17.
33. JACOB H. S. and S. E. LUX, IV, (1968) *Blood* 32: 549.
34. BEUTLER E., O. DURON and M. KELLY, (1963) *J. Lab. clin. Med.* 61: 882.
35. WEED R. I. and C. F. REED, (1966) *Am. J. Med.* 41: 681.
36. CROWLEY J., P. WAYS and J. W. JONES, (1965) *J. clin. Invest.* 44: 989.
37. NEERHOUT R. C., (1968) *Pediat. Res.* 2: 172.
38. DERVICHIAN D., C. FOURNET, A. GUINIER and E. PONDER, (1952) *Rev. Hémat.* 7: 567.
39. SACHTLEBEN V. P., H. LEHMANN and G. RUHENSTROTH-BAUER (1961) *Blut* 7: 369.
40. HOLLAN S. R., J. G. SZELENYI, J. H. BREUER, V. MEDGYESI and G. N. SÖTER (1968) *Folia haemat.* (Lpzg.) 90: 125.
41. CENTURY B. and M. K. HORWITT, (1960) *J. Nutrition* 72: 357.
42. LEWIS S. E. and E. D. WILLS, (1962) *Biochem. Pharmacol.* 11: 60.
43. SCHRÖTER W. and K. BITTER, (1969) *Klin. Wschr.* 47: 727.
44. JACOB H. S. and J. H. JANDL, (1962) *J. clin. Invest.* 41: 779.
45. SCHRÖTER W. and H. BODEMANN, (1970) *Biol. Neonat.* 15: 291.
46. LINDEMANN B. and H. PASSOW, (1960) *Pflügers Arch. ges. Physiol.* 271: 497.
47. OSKI F. A. and L. A. BARNES, (1967) *J. Pediat.* 70: 211.

DISCUSSION

Prof. Jonxis: We can confirm your results working along quite other lines. We are interested in haemoglobin synthesis. We have found two types of reticulocytes in the newborn. One type is more or less the adult type, with a low rate of synthesis of foetal haemoglobin. The other type of reticulocytes, whose occurrence is stimulated by severe bleeding of the newborn animal, can be found in newborn babies with severe erythroblastosis foetalis synthesizing a high rate of foetal haemoglobin.

Dr. Schröter: This is a very important comment. Have you found also a clone of cells which synthesizes foetal haemoglobin and adult haemoglobin in similar amounts as well?

Dr. Papadatos: Do you think that the heterogeneity of the red blood cell population, that you mentioned, is the same in the fullterm baby as compared to the praemature baby or the small-for-date baby?

Dr. Schröter: We didn't determine that. In the praemature baby the proportion of immature cells is much larger than in the full term baby.

GENERAL DISCUSSION

SESSION I

Dr. Meeuwisse: I'm not quite satisfied about the question of oxygen consumption of liver slices and what we heard of Dr. HOMMES on enzyme activities in foetal rat livers. I wonder if these studies you mentioned and also the studies by Dr. Young are on another species. It may be that the foetal rat liver is much more immature than the species where whole oxygen consumption was measured.

Prof. Villee: The studies I referred to were done in the human.

Dr. Young: The studies of oxygen consumption in the intact foetus were made during the last 2/3 gestation by DAWES in the sheep and by ASSAN in the human subject. The oxygen consumption of a perfused placenta is about twice that for the foetus per kg body weight in the sheep.

Prof. Villee: Maybe your figures are peculiar for the sheep placenta. Some years ago we measured oxygen consumption in human placental slices. More recently a study was published on oxygen consumption in perfused human term placentas. The placentas were perfused both at the maternal and at the foetal side. Those results were quite comparable, within 10% of each other.

There was also agreement when you calculated for the foetal consumption of oxygen. They are quite consistent with the calculated value for oxygen consumption of the placenta in situ when you subtract how much the foetus uses from the total oxygen delivered by the arteries to the uterus. These studies don't indicate a great difference in oxygen consumption between slices and perfused organs.

Of course Dr. YOUNG referred to different species and different experimental circumstances, so that may account for. I simply say that I don't think it is necessarily true that tissue slices experiments give you figures 1/10th compared to experiments with perfused organs.

Prof. Villee: There was a difficult question this morning. What does one mean by tissue immaturity. Is there anyone who would like to pick up that question again?

Dr. Hommes: I don't know if you can speak of immaturity, but rather of dysmaturity which is one aspect of it. Sometimes you find under-developed embryos in the pregnant rat. Table 1, column 1, first line gives the weight of the liver in mg, that is the average value for the normal littermates. Column 2 gives the value for the dysmature embryos: the value is 2/3rd of normal.

Table 1.* *Activities of glycolytic anzymes –μ moles per min per gram soluble protein of embryonic rat liver* 0,5 *days before birth.*
I: Well developed embryo's,
II: Dysmatures.

	I	II
Weight of liver (mg)	323	228
Hexokinase	13,7	8,8
Glucose-6-phosphate dehydrogenase	42,6	60,9
6-phosphogluconate dehydrogenase	69,5	39,9
Phosphoglucomutase	51,1	36,5
Phosphoglucoisomerase	625	669
Phosphofructokinase	13,7	10,3
Fructokinase	14,7	15,2
Aldolase	185	45,1
α-Glycerophosphate dehydrogenase	91,4	52,4
Triosephosphate isomerase	2083	1568
Glyceraldehyde phosphate dehydrogenase	587	262
Phospholycerate kinase	824	657
Phosphoglycerate mutase	597	457
Enolase	341	152
Pyruvate kinase	99,4	105
Lactate dehydrogenase	4374	3470

* From: F. A. Hommes and C. W. Wilmink, *Biol. Neonat.* 13, 181 (1968) Reprinted with permission of the copyright owners.

All the enzymes are about the same, but there are a few important differences. For instance aldolase, 185 in the normal one and 45 in the dysmature embryo. The values for alpha-glycero-phosphate-dehydrogenase are significantly different. The same is true for glyceral aldehyde-phosphate dehydrogenase. All the other enzymes have about the same activity. You have indeed very specific decreased activities of enzymes in dysmature tissue or animal.

Prof. Villee: All these enzyme activities are stated in μ mol per min per g. These are all turnover numbers of the enzymes. When you have enzymes that act in sequence it is only least active enzyme, that is the rate limiting one, which determines the overall activity. Then it is even more curious, that there are such wide differences in the ones that are not rate limiting. What do you think about that?

Dr. Hommes: I just don't know. It may be a different susceptibility.

Prof. Villee: It would appear that aldolase would even not be rate limiting in group 2 and yet it is 1/4 of the activity.

Dr. Hommes: This is certainly true. I don't say that the decreased activity results in dysmaturity, but I observe that it just goes together. Any further conclusion cannot be drawn.

Dr. Räihä: Dr. HOMMES, do you have any values for enzymes of gluconeogenesis in normal embroys or in dysmature embryos.

Dr. Hommes: You can see that those measurements are made in embryos half a day before birth. This is indeed the period that the gluconeogenetic enzymes are increasing. We just happened to be interested at that time in glycolysis and didn't have a single look at gluconeogenesis, so I can't answer your question.

Dr. Schröter: If we find an increase of enzyme activity short before or after birth then we have to ask is this a new synthesis of enzyme protein or is this due to an increase of cell organelles. The glucose-6-phosphatase is located in the endoplasmatic reticulum. I would like to ask Dr. Sereni what he thinks about the suggestion that the increase of glucose-6-phosphate activity is due to an increase of endoplasmatic reticulum or to a de novo synthesis of protein.

Dr. Sereni: It seems likely that in the postnatal increase of glucose-6-phosphatase a de novo enzyme synthesis occurs. But I have no specific data on that.

Dr. Räihä: When we measure any enzyme activity in fetal tissue as compared to adult we should always try to use different substrate concentrations to see whether the foetal enzyme has a different km for the substrate or any of the co-factors.

Prof. Teller: I was surprised that we did not embark on the question of enzyme inductions by phenobarbital. We are faced with the problem to treat infants with phenobarbital in order to avoid hyperbilirubinaemia. Nobody really understands what is going on. The fact is there that hyperbilirubinaemia is less striking in the infants treated with phenobarbital. Are there any experiments available to show that phenobarbital does increase enzyme activity.

Dr. Räihä: I don't know if there are any in vitro studies. We should do much more in vitro studies on the effect of phenobarbital on enzyme and protein synthesis before we do clinical trials. Phenobarbital may have a lot of other effects. The effect on the microsomal enzyme systems is probably very unspecific.

Dr. Sereni: Few years ago we made some experiments on isolated and perfused newborn rabbit liver.

We were then studying glucuronyl-transferase activity. Adding to the perfusion medium phenobarbital, no increase of enzyme activity could be demonstrated. This is not surprising, since 'in vivo' a delay of many hours is necessary before activation occurs.

SESSION II

AMINO ACID METABOLISM

PLACENTAL TRANSPORT OF FREE AMINO ACIDS

MAUREEN YOUNG*

Measurement of the rate of accumulation of nitrogen in the foetus during gestation is difficult and has not been made in many species. The difficulties have been clearly described by Dr. Elsie Widdowson (1) who provided the first figures for the human infant, which contains about 15 g protein at 20 weeks gestation and 500 g. at term. These values give an indication of the net transfer of amino nitrogen from the mother to the foetus across the placental membrane throughout gestation (2, 3). Our knowledge of some of the mechanisms of this transport is already twenty years old. Christensen first suggested, and his colleagues subsequently proved, that the qualitative aspects of amino acid transfer across the placental membrane were very similar to the transfer of amino acids across the other cells in the body (4, 5). Active transport was demonstrated by the selective transfer of the natural L-isomer of histidine (6, 7); competitive inhibition between members of the same transport group and saturation of the transport mechanisms were also observed. Finally, transport occurs against a concentration gradient; the foetal plasma levels of amino acids are usually about twice that found in the maternal blood stream but may be as much as five times the maternal concentration in the guinea pig, (4, 8).

Clinically, Dent and his colleagues found that the maternal plasma levels of α amino nitrogen were reduced in pregnant women (9) and it has subsequently been shown that this reduction occurs early in pregnancy before the demands of the conceptus are large (10, 11). Page (12) was swift to use Stein and Moore's method for the separation of the plasma amino acids by ion exchange chromatogrophy, and his description of some of the maternal-foetal plasma interrelationships

* **Department of Gynecology, St. Thomas Hospital, Medical School, London, U.K.**

for the individual amino acids has been frequently confirmed (8). The pattern of the individual amino acids in plasma is subject to a diurnal rhythm (13), it is known to alter during the menstrual cycle (14); and the changes seen during pregnancy can be reproduced in males by the administration of a combination of oestrogen and progesterone (15).

Our own work has been concerned with a further exploration of the maternal-foetal plasma amino acid relationships, in the human subject at delivery, in the sheep, during her last trimester, and in the guinea pig with the foetal placenta, perfused 'in situ' through the umbilical vessels. The experimental results are described first and applied to the clinical observations.

PLACENTAL TRANSFER OF AMINO ACIDS IN THE SHEEP

In sheep, the placental transfer of amino acids was investigated in the chronic preparation with indwelling catheters in the umbilical and maternal uterine vessels first described by Barron and his colleagues (16). The maternal plasma amino acids were raised within

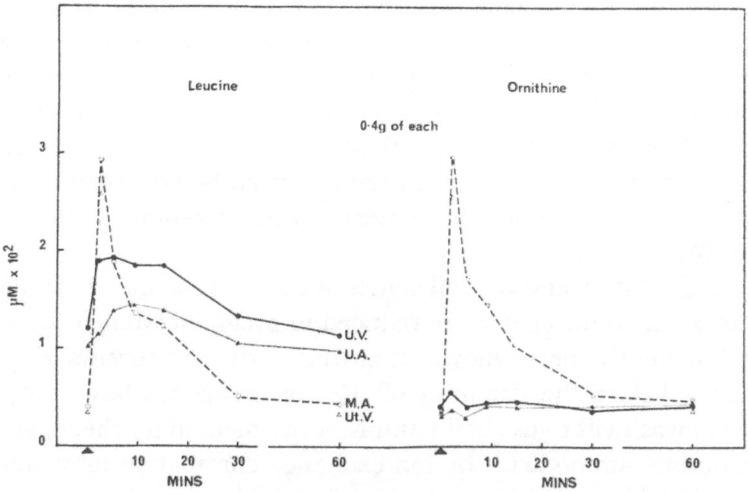

Fig. 1. The relation of maternal and foetal free amino acid levels following the intravenous injection of 0.4 g. leucine and ornithine into the maternal blood stream of the pregnant ewe. (Young and McFadyen (1971), *J. Physiol.* (in press)).

physiological limits by a single intravenous injection of a mixture of six amino acids (17). Figure 1 shows the influence on the foetal plasma levels and foetal uptake for leucine, belonging to the 'L preferring' group of neutral, branched chain, amino acids and for ornithine, a basic amino acid. Note that the foetal levels are higher than the maternal and also that the A-V differences for each amino acid on both sides of the placenta are small. Leucine was transferred readily across the membrane raising the foetal levels; the umbilical V-A difference, and therefore, foetal uptake was also increased. The broad shape of the foetal curve is due to the accumulation of the amino acids within the placenta prior to release into the foetal plasma which has been demonstrated using isotopes (18). A raised level of ornithine in the maternal plasma barely influenced the level in the foetal blood and similarily, raised levels of glycine, alanine or citrulline in the maternal plasma did not alter the foetal values. These results were characteristic for each of the other members of all three transport groups, the 'A preferring' neutral group, the 'L preferring' neutral group and the basic group; the observations were readily predictable from the characteristics of the transport of amino acids across the epithelium of the gut, reabsorption by the proximal renal tubule and uptake by muscle cells (19, 20). The majority of the amino acids essential for growth in the young animal are, therefore, the most readily accessible to the foetus, during the last trimester of gestation at least. The concept of essentialness of amino acids probably has to be modified for the foetus. Early in gestation all the amino acids must be important to supplement those already present in the fertilized ovum. Later, the development of enzymes necessary for the conversion of one amino acid to another in the foetus will also be important as RAIHA has shown for methionine and cystine; moreover he has also found that there are likely to be species differences for the time of development of these enzymes 'in utero'. (21).

PLACENTAL TRANSFER OF AMINO ACIDS IN THE GUINEA PIG

The relative influence of the maternal and foetal blood flows and the activity of the parenchyma on the transfer of α amino nitrogen was studied with the foetal guinea pig placenta perfused 'in situ' through the umbilical vessels with an artificial fluid (22). The arrangement of

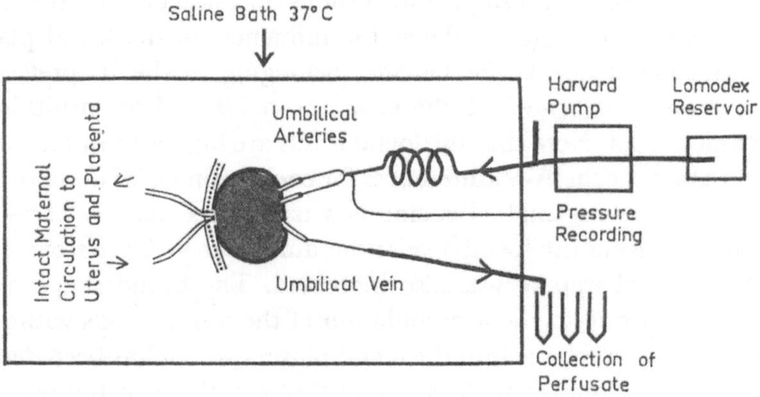

Fig. 2. Arrangement for perfusion of the guinea pig foetal placenta 'in situ'. (REYNOLDS and YOUNG (1971). *J. Physiol.* 214).

the open perfusion circuit, is shown in Fig. 2. A low molecular weight dextran, containing physiological salts but no amino acids, was perfused at a pressure of 30–40 mm Hg. Antipyrine, a readily diffusible substance, was infused at a constant rate into the maternal blood stream and changes in maternal placental blood flow were followed by measuring its transfer into the perfusate.

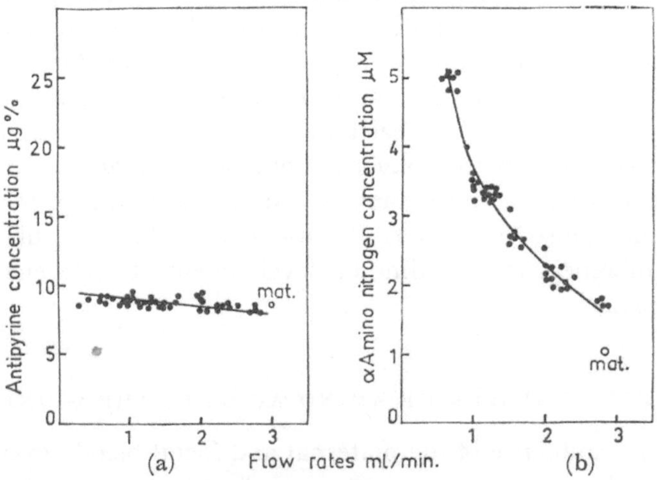

Fig. 3. Foetal placental perfusate concentration-flow relationships for a) antipyrine, b) amino nitrogen. Transfer from maternal blood to foetal perfusate/min. for c) antipyrine d) amino nitrogen. (REYNOLDS and YOUNG (1971) *J. Physiol.* 214).

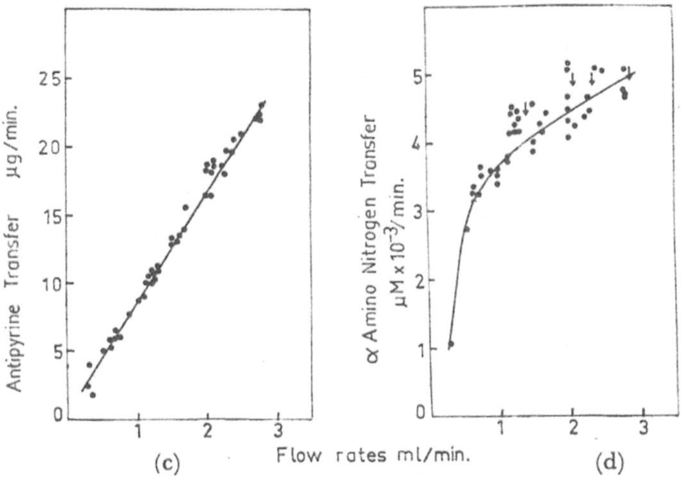

Fig. 3a) and b) show that the concentration of *a* amino nitrogen in the perfusate was high at low flow rates on the foetal side of the placenta, decreasing as the flow increases, while that of antipyrine decreases only slightly. Transfer of the latter is therefore completely flow dependent, as expected, while that of amino nitrogen is relatively little altered by flow within the physiological limits of 1–3 ml/min (fig. 3c) and d). In contrast, fig. 4 shows that as the maternal placental blood flow was reduced by bleeding the progressive fall in transfer of antipyrine was accompanied by a decreased transfer of amino nitrogen. However, a decrease below 50% was never observed, unless the acid base balance of the mother was impaired.

High foetal: maternal plasma concentration ratios of *a* amino nitrogen are maintained in all species in spite of a reduction of the maternal plasma level during pregnancy; this suggests that the active process at the placental membrane together with the provision of an adequate supply of amino nitrogen, are the more important factors than maternal plasma concentration in the foetal accumulation of nitrogen. The experimental results in the guinea pig provide some confirmation of this hypothesis; the inverse relationship between the flow and amino nitrogen concentration of the perfusate, on the foetal side of the placenta, is evidence for a secretion from the maternal circulation and at least half of the transfer has been shown to depend upon the maternal blood flow.

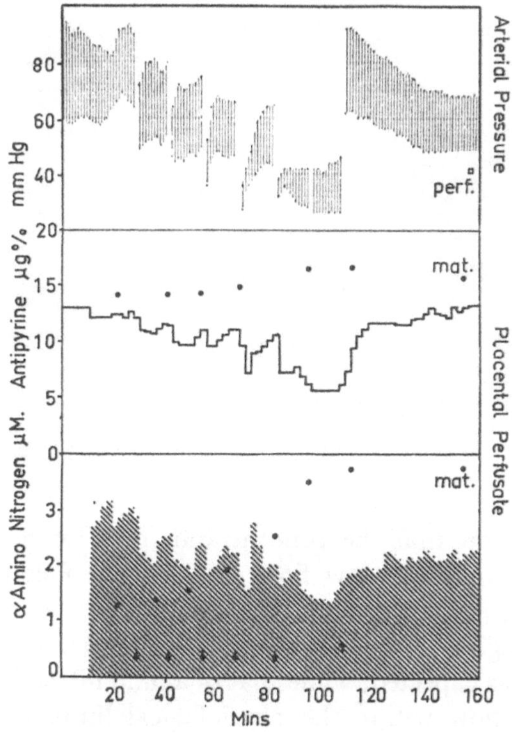

Fig. 4. Influence of changes in maternal placental blood flow on amino nitrogen, 7 ml blood withdrawn at each arrow ↓. Return of blood to maternal circulation ↑ restores the maternal placental blood flow to the control levels; restoration of *a* amino nitrogen output is incomplete. Note the rise in maternal plasma levels of both following bleeding.
Perfusion rate 1.1 ml/min. (Reynolds and Young (1971) *J. Physiol.* 214).

THE RELATIONSHIP OF THE AMINO ACIDS TRANSFERRED ACROSS THE PLACENTAL MEMBRANE TO THE MATERNAL AND FOETAL PLASMA LEVELS OF AMINO ACIDS

The perfused guinea pig's placenta also gave us the opportunity of observing the part played by placental transfer relative to foetal metabolism in determining the foetal plasma levels of amino acids. Fig. 5 shows an aminogram of the maternal and foetal plasmas and foetal placental perfusate: the maternal levels are arranged in order of

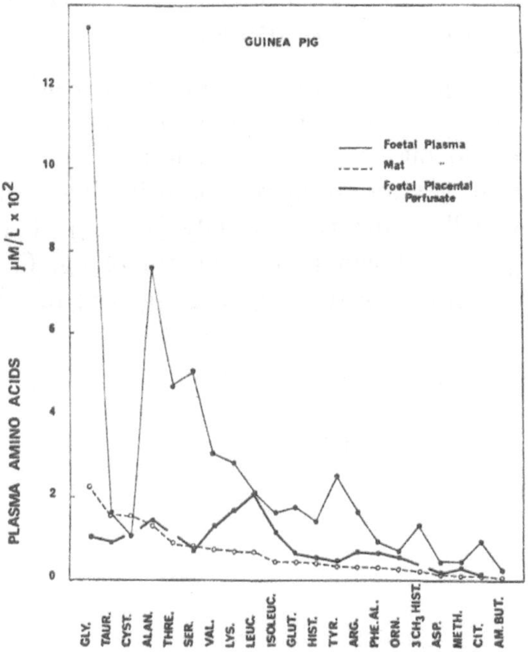

Fig. 5. Aminograms of maternal and foetal guinea pig plasma and foetal placental perfusate. With the exception of the relatively high lysine and branched chain amino acid concentration the perfusate resembles the maternal plasma. The difference between the foetal and perfusate aminogram represents the contribution of foetal metabolism to the foetal plasma levels.

magnitude of their concentration in the conventional way. The levels of amino acids in the foetal plasma are much higher than in the maternal plasma. Those in the perfusate are similar to the maternal plasma, with the exception of lysine and the branched chain amino acids belonging to the 'L preferring' neutral transport group; the latter are present in higher concentration demonstrating once more their ready passage across the placental membrane. The difference between the amino acid levels in the perfusate and in the foetal plasma will represent the contribution of the foetal metabolism to the high foetal plasma concentration of amino acids.

MATERNAL-FOETAL PLASMA AMINO ACID RELATIONSHIPS IN THE HUMAN SUBJECT AT DELIVERY

Our clinical colleagues were interested to know whether conditions in which there may be placental dysfunction were associated with impaired maternal-foetal plasma amino acid relationships such as in the 'light for dates' infant and in the postmaturity. The results are already published and will be described briefly (11, 23). The patients were divided into groups shown at the bottom of fig. 6. The ranges of gestational age, and of birth weights are given; the first five groups

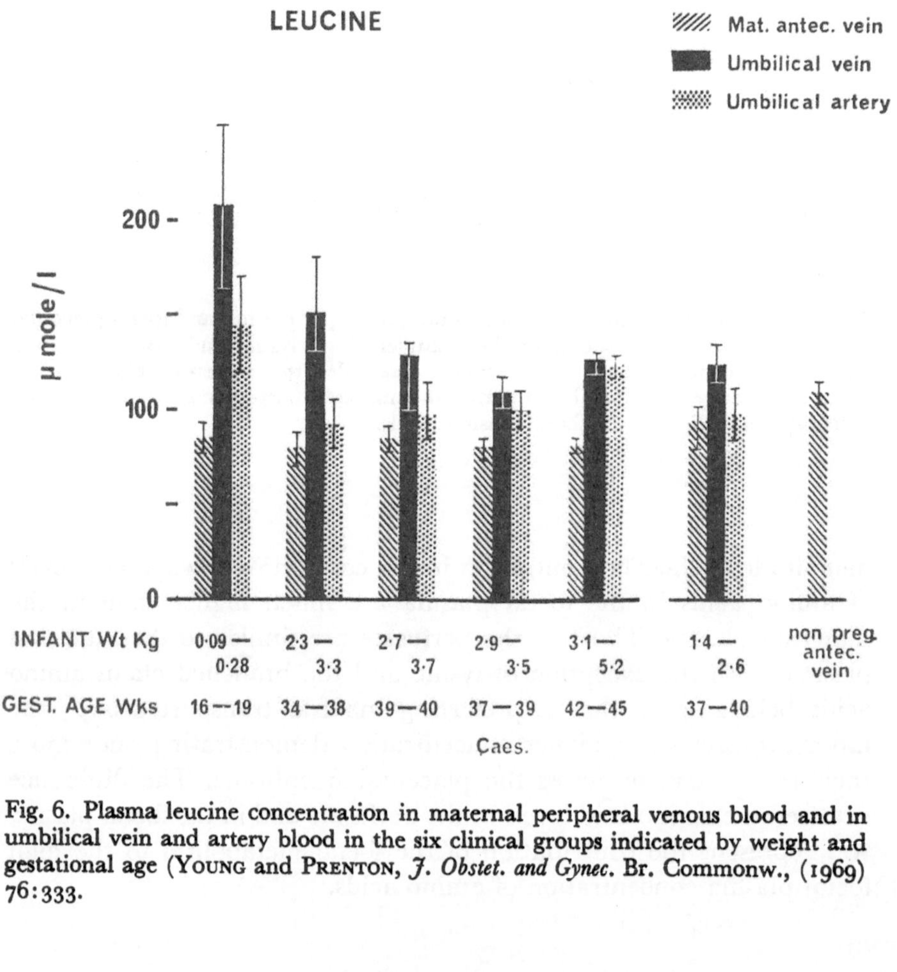

Fig. 6. Plasma leucine concentration in maternal peripheral venous blood and in umbilical vein and artery blood in the six clinical groups indicated by weight and gestational age (Young and Prenton, *J. Obstet. and Gynec.* Br. Commonw., (1969) 76:333.

are arranged in order of gestational age of the infant. The last group consists of infants whose birthweights were low: the average weight was about two-thirds of that expected for the gestational age, and the daily pregnandiol excretion of the mothers prior to delivery was also low; they were all delivered by Caesarian Section. The pattern of results is shown using leucine as an example. The maternal levels of this amino acid are lower than in the nonpregnant state but no differences were found between any of the groups. Both umbilical vein and artery levels are higher than in the maternal plasma and again no differences could be demonstrated between the groups: the mean umbilical vein and artery values are highest in the 16–19 week group but not significantly so. There was a large scatter of values on each side of the placenta and the data was analysed for maternal foetal interrelationships. Fig. 7 shows the ten out of a possible nineteen

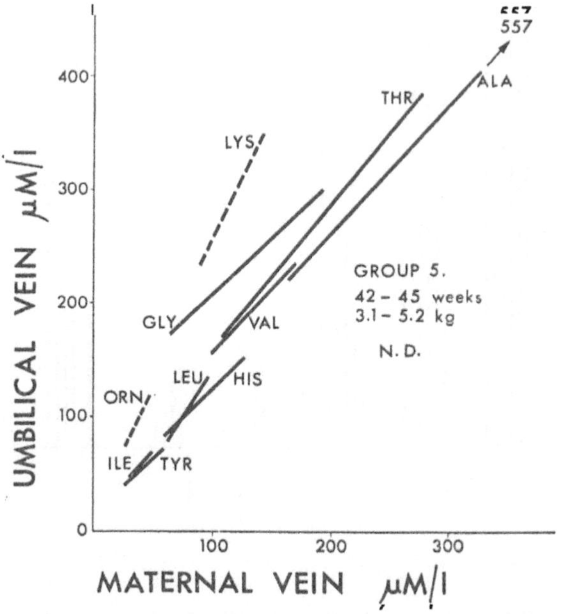

Fig. 7. Significant correlations between umbilical venous and maternal venous plasma amino acid concentrations in post-term deliveries. ALA, Alanine; GLY, Glycine; HIS, Histidine; ILE, Isoleucine; LEU, Leucine; LYS, Lysine; ORN, Ornithine, THR, Threonine; TYR, Tyrosine; VAL, Valine. (YOUNG and PRENTON, *J. Obstet. and Gynec.* Br. Commonw. (1969) 76:333.

amino acids in the post-term group which gave significant correlations between umbilical venous and maternal venous levels. The lines are drawn over the range of values observed and the slopes fall roughly into two groups; the majority of amino acids, consisting of the neutral amino acids, both 'L preferring' and 'A preferring' have slopes of 1–1.3, while the basic amino acids have slopes of 2.7. This suggestion of a direct maternal: foetal relationship for the 'A preferring' neutral group and the basic group is in contrast with the short term observations following a single injection just described.

The umbilical V-A differences in the clinical material are shown in fig. 8. The very small V-A differences in the Caesarian Section group correspond to the low umbilical V-A differences in the lamb, 'in

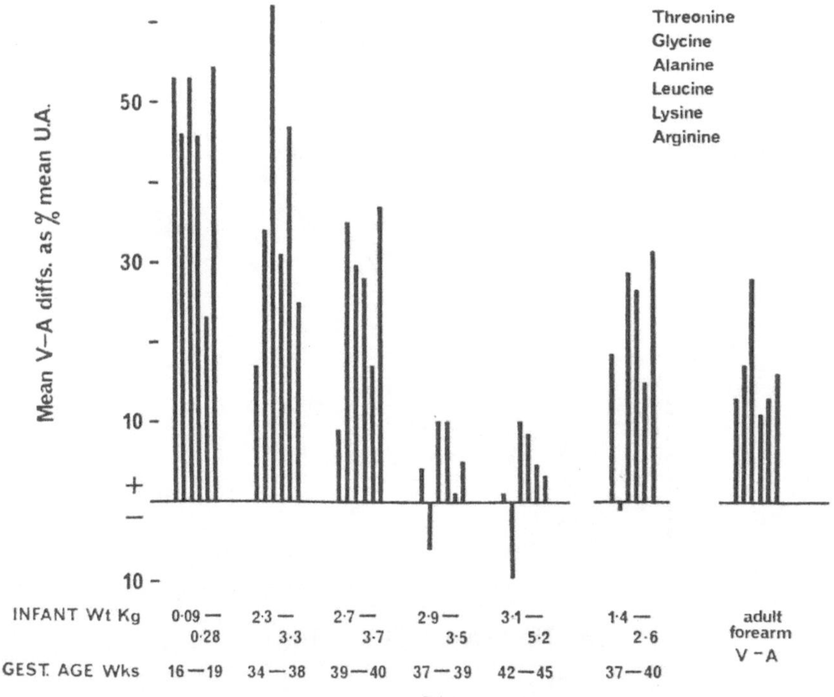

Fig. 8. Mean umbilical V-A differences for six amino acids, expressed as a percentage of the mean umbilical artery value during ges ation, in different types of delivery and 'small for dates' infants. (From 'Foetus and Placenta', ed. by A. KLOPPER, E. DICZFALUSY (1969) p. 145).

utero' with good acid base conditions and, presumably, no impairment of blood flow, and suggest that the placental circulations were less influenced by Caesarian section than by vaginal delivery. The umbilical V-A differences are also elevated in the 'light for dates' group which would suggest that the circulations are readily impaired, in spite of the Caesarian Section delivery. Since it is difficult to obtain blood quickly from the cord of infants at termination, the high values and large V-A differences observed are probably due to the impairment of blood flow and correspond to the high values for total and α amino nitrogen found in the perfusate at low flow rates in the guinea pig placenta perfused 'in situ'. Finally because plasma amino acids levels change readily with alterations in placental and foetal blood flow their pattern is likely to be changed by delivery and, therefore, influence the baseline from which subsequent changes occur in the early post natal period (24, 25, 26).

In conclusion, the experimental evidence suggests a secretion of amino acids from the maternal to the foetal circulation. On the maternal side of the placenta this transfer is dependent upon the blood flow and to a lesser extent upon the concentration of amino acids in the maternal plasma. On the foetal side of the placenta the flow is relatively unimportant within physiological limits. Finally, the placental transfer of amino acids is related to the transport groups, the 'A preferring' neutral group and the basic group were transferred slowly in comparison with the branched chain amino acids. The majority of the amino acids essential for growth in the newborn belong to this group of neutral amino acids, and because of their ready accessibility to, and uptake by the foetus, the possibility of supplying them by mouth, therapeutically, to the mother carrying a suspected 'light for dates' infant may be considered.

ACKNOWLEDGEMENTS

This work would have been impossible without good colleagues, Mrs. Margaret Reynolds, Mr. Iain McFadyen and Miss Lynda Hopkins.

REFERENCES

1. WIDDOWSON E. M., (1965) In: *Human Body Composition* p. 31 Brozek, J. ed. Pergamon Press Ltd., Oxford.
2. WIDDOWSON E. M. and C. M. SPRAY, (1951) *Arch. Dis. Childh.* 26: 205.
3. KELLY H. J., R. E. SLOAN, W. HOFFMANN, and C. SAUNDERS, (1951) *Human Biol.* 23: 61.
4. CHRISTENSEN H. N. and J. A. STREICHER, (1948) *J. Biol. Chem.* 175: 95.
5. DANCIS J., G. OLSEN and G. FOLKART, (1958) *Am. J. Physiol.* 194: 44.
6. PAGE E. W., M. B. GLENDENNING, A. J. MARGOLIS and H. A. HARPER, (1957) *Am. J. Obstet. Gynec.* 74: 705.
7. MISCHEL W., (1963) *Arch. Gynäk.* 198: 181.
8. YOUNG M., (1969) In: *Foetus and Placenta* p. 139. Klopper A. and E. Diczfalusy eds. Blackwell, Oxford.
9. CLEMETSON C. A. B. and J. CHURCHMAN, (1954) *J. Obstet. Gynec. Br. Commonw.* 61: 364.
10. GHADIMI H. and P. PECORA, (1964) *Pediatrics* 33: 500.
11. YOUNG M. and M. A. PRENTON, (1969) *J. Obstet. and Gynec. Br. Commonw.* 76: 333.
12. GLENDENNING M. B., A. J. MARGOLIS and E. W. PAGE (1961) *Am. J. Obstet. and Gynec.* 81: 591.
13. FEIGIN R. D., A. S. KLAINER, W. R. BEISEL, (1967) *Nature* (Lond.) 215: 512.
14. SOUPART P., (1960) *Clin. Chim. Acta.* 5: 235.
15. ZINNEMAN H. H., A. S. SEAL and R. DOE, (1967) *J. Clin. Endocr.* 27: 397.
16. MESCHIA G., J. R. COTTER, C. S. BREATHNACH and D. H. BARRON, (1965) *Quart. J. exp. Physiol.* 50: 185.
17. YOUNG M. and I. R. MCFADYEN, (1971) (in press.).
18. HAYTER C. J., E. A. HUTCHINSON, M. J. KARVONEN and M. YOUNG, (1964) *J. Physiol. Lond.* 175: 11.P.
19. MILNE M. D., (1964) *Brit. Med. J.* (1) 327.
20. OXENDEN D. L. and H. N. CHRISTENSEN, (1963) *J. Biol. Chem.* 238: 3687.
21. GAULL G., J. STURMAN, N. RAIHA, (1970) *Proc. Soc. Ped. Res.* p. 31.
22. REYNOLDS M. L. and M. YOUNG, (1969) *J. Physiol. Lond.* 207: 13.P.
23. PRENTON M. A. and M. YOUNG, (1969) *J. Obstet. Gynec. Br. Commonw.* 76: 404.
24. LINDBLAD B. S. and A. BALDESTAN, (1969) *Acta. Paediat. Scand.* 58: 252.
25. MESTYAN J., M. FEKETE, GY. SOLTESZ, L. LAJOS, I. GATI, J. PREISZ and J. DOSZPOD, (1969) *Biol. Neonat.* 14: 153.
26. MESTYAN J., M. FEKETE, I. JARAI, S. IMHOF and GY. SOLTESZ, (1969) *Biol. Neonat.* 14: 164.

DISCUSSION

Dr. Wiseman: I wonder which cells in the placenta are actually doing the work. It seems there are two possibilities: either the amino acids are pushed by cells directly into the foetal circulation or cells are doing their work by raising an extracellular pool of amino acids and the amino acids are leaking into the foetal circulation. A second question is quite different. I wonder if there is a possibility of peptide, going from the maternal to the foetal circulation, being hydrolysed there and thus giving a higher content of amino acids in the foetal blood than in the maternal blood.

Dr. Young: By analogy with transport across other cells, one can assume that there is an active membrane on one side of the cell. As far as the placenta is concerned say it must undoubtedly be on the maternal side. Following the injection of isotopes into the maternal blood stream we could show that there is a considerable concentration of amino acids in the placenta probably in the syncytial trophoblast. Then we assume there is simple diffusion down the gradient from the syncytial trophoblast into the foetal blood. Such concentration in the trophoblast did not occur following injection into the foetal blood stream.

I think there is active transport of amino acids. To prove this experimentally you have to perfuse the placenta on both sides, then to give inhibitors on the maternal side and secondly on the foetal side. But we have not yet been able to perfuse the placenta succesfully on both sides.

In regard to the placental transport of polypeptides I do know nothing at all about that.

Prof. McCance: Is it not true that the intestinal mucosa cells can transport some simple peptides as fast as amino acids?

Dr. Wiseman: It has been demonstrated recently that peptide disappears from the intestinal lumen more rapidly than an equivalent amount of free amino acids. The uptake of peptides by cells in the intestine has now been well documented. The same phenomenon might occur in the placenta.

Dr. Young: Do you have to postulate this for the placenta? Are there polypeptides in the plasma?

Prof. Teller: Did you find any changes in transfer of amino acids in relation to gestational age. In regard to your last slide were the gestational ages of those animals and human individuals comparable?

Prof. Young: I don't have any observation on the effect of gestational age. We have studied guinea pigs and sheep in their last trimester. The human individuals were studied at term. Some of them were studied after therapeutic abortion. The high values we found in the plasma of 12–14th week infants was most probably an artefact due to the fact that it is difficult to get into the vessels at this age. While you are doing this you impair the circulation and there will be more time for the amino acids to be transferred from the placenta to the foetal plasma.

KERR showed that the concentration of amino acids in the plasma decreases with gestational age in monkeys. I don't know if it is easy to sample from the vessels of the placenta in monkeys without impairing the circulation. I'm sure this study was very careful.

THE PLASMA AMINOGRAM IN 'SMALL FOR DATES' NEWBORN INFANTS

B. S. LINDBLAD*

Many newborn babies, who are unduly short and light for the period of gestation ('short and light for dates' or 'small for dates', SFD, by definition below the 10th percentile for gestational age) show certain clinical features indicating impairment of prenatal nutrition (1). In addition to growth retardation they may suffer from hypothermia and hypoglucosaemia, sometimes with symptoms from the CNS. The hypoglycaemic attacks occasionally seen in growth retarded newborn babies seem to be aggravated by a high protein intake (2). These problems are also well known to those dealing with the rehabilitation of postnatal undernutrition (3).

Are some SFD babies born undernourished? Theoretically, impaired foetal nutrition may be caused by 1) conditions affecting the nutrient content of maternal blood or the utero-placental circulation; 2) disturbed development, damage or abnormality of the placental membranes, and 3) impaired foeto-placental circulation. Some maternal diagnoses, like primiparity and hypertension and social circumstances, like low family income, are associated with an increased frequency of SFD newborn babies (4). This may be explained by one of the nutritional mechanisms already mentioned.

Recent animal experiments show that undernutrition of pregnant animals may produce growth retardation of the offspring (5, 6), and that undernutrition during the phase of intensive cell multiplication causes an irreparable deficit in cell population of organs (7). These results raise the old question of maternal undernutrition and its effect on the foetus with increased significance. Ignorance in this area

* The Department of Paediatrics of Karolinska Institutet at St Göran's Children's Hospital, Stockholm, Sweden. This work was supported by grants from AB Semper Fund for Nutritional Research, Expressen's Prenatal Fund and Grant No 2583 from the Swedish Medical Research Council.

is unfortunate as the nutritional situation of pre-pregnant and pregnant women seems to be growing worse. For example, it is evident from the Pakistan Medical Research Council pilot study in the urban areas of Khodadad Colony, Karachi, and Jurain Village, Dacca, and the first phase of the Nutritional Health Laboratories' study in the rural area of Lehtrar as well as the Nutrition Survey of East Pakistan (8) that: in contrast to the villagers, the wives of the factory workers of the bigger cities make no change in their diet during pregnancy and lactation. The villagers say they act upon the advice of the elders, while the city's group of women of low income often say that they depend only on their own or their husband's knowledge. This could mean that a growing tendency towards industrialization means a growing gulf between the nutritional habits of the modern pregnant and lactating woman and the old, perhaps wise, nutritional habits of the former generation. This should also be connected with the poverty and the lack of cheap milk and vegetables in the city areas.

In its recommendations for paediatric research of 1969 the WHO has stated: '...the developing countries should concentrate on the effect of maternal nutrition on birth weight and the survival and subsequent development of infants of low birth weight.' (9). Difference in birth weight between different races seems to be largely dependent on socio-economical differences (10). According to investigations in economically developing countries where an attempt has been made to measure the length of pregnancy, the birth weight is low even with regard to the gestational age of the newborn infant (11, 12). Our knowledge about the endocrinological and metabolic consequences of pre-maternal undernutrition is limited. The importance of maternal undernutrition to foetal development, to the adaptation of the newborn to extra-uterine life and the prognosis as regards physical and mental development should be investigated.

There is a lack of objective criteria for undernutrition in pregnant women and the newborn infant. We need such a basis for studies of the effects of foetal undernutrition in man. Can we apply any of the tests used in the assessment of subclinical postnatal undernutrition? The test must be of such a nature that it can be used on both the pregnant woman; healthy and sick; nervous and stable, educated and full of prejudice; and on the much loved newborn baby with the mother's consent, in the highly developed society as well as far away from sophisticated laboratories.

METHOD

In the assessment of postnatal undernutrition the tests most often combined are the hydroxyproline/creatinine concentrations of the urine and the urinary 24-hour excretion of urea (13, 14). The urinary concentrations are difficult to assess before commencement of postnatal nutrition, because of the great variability of kidney function of newborn infants. Assessment of protein nutrition in the pregnant woman by weight increase, and urea, creatinine and hydroxyproline excretion is complicated by pregnancy toxaemia. The use of serum albumin levels is not feasible as they are lowered during normal pregnancy.

In infants and adults a low dietary nitrogen intake leads to a characteristic pattern of the individual post-absorptive free amino acid concentrations of plasma, to what Dr. SNYDERMAN has called a characteristic 'plasma aminogram' (15). This change is also seen in the clinical syndrome of protein deficiency of children ('kwashiorkor') (fig. 1).

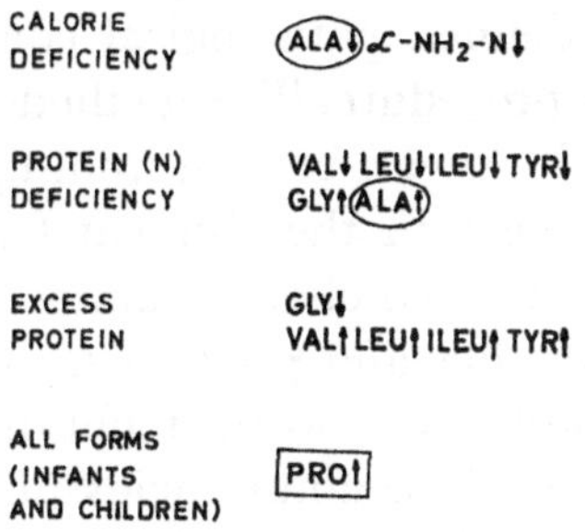

Fig. 1. 'Characteristics' of the postabsorptive plasma aminogram in different nutritional states according to the literature (15, 16, 17, 18, 19, 20, 21, 22, 23, 24). Arrow pointing upwards means increased plasma level, or a 'resistance' to a general decline. Arrow pointing downwards means decreased level.

Modern quantitative techniques have revealed a marked uniformity of the plasma amino acid concentrations of normal fasting human subjects (25). The numerous investigations on infant malnutrition in South America, Africa and Asia show the same range of the plasma amino acid levels in the normal or post-habilitation material as Western European or North American normal materials (for references see fig. 1). This speaks against any racial differences. However, the age differences are marked. Each age group seems to have its own characteristic normal fasting plasma levels and urinary concentrations of free amino acids (25).

The present day knowledge of the normal plasma aminogram of mother and child at birth is based on the results of the analyses, by different methods, of a limited number of samples, with a frequent lack of clinical correlation. The plasma amino acid pool can be influenced by liver and kidney disease, stress and hormonal disturbances. The age of the mother, the number of previous pregnancies, disease and anomaly of the placenta, umbilical blood flow interruption and asphyxia are factors which may well hypothetically influence the plasma amino acid levels of mother and child.

The automatic amino analyzer is such a familair tool, that many authors in their communications today give only the particular instrument used as reference to the method. This leads to scant information about collection, storage, and preparation of samples, special adaptations of the apparatus and the calculation method employed. As the present investigation aimed at providing a basis for studies of the plasma levels under well defined pathological conditions, emphasis was laid on a standardized procedure. The methods used have been given in detail before (26, 27). As can be seen from fig. 1, the plasma animo acid levels that are changed in the different forms of protein aminotrition are those of the branch-chained amino acids (valine, leucine, isoleucine), glycine, alanine and proline. A modified system of ion-exchange chromatography was worked out in order to give reproducible determinations of these amino acids on the small amounts of neonatal plasma (28). See fig. 2.

RESULTS. THE NORMAL AMINOGRAM

The normal venous plasma aminogram of fasting, non-pregnant women of fertile age is shown in fig. 3. (26). The venous plasma aminogram of pregnant women at term is quite different (26). See fig. 4. There is a general decrease, but the decrease is not uniform. There seems to be a relative hyperalaninaemia and hyperhistidinaemia in the pregnant woman at term. In cord vein plasma the aminogram shows yet another pattern. See fig. 5. There is a general increase, most marked in the levels of alanine, lysine and taurine. Mean, range and S.D. for 18 free amino acid levels in pregnant women at term and in

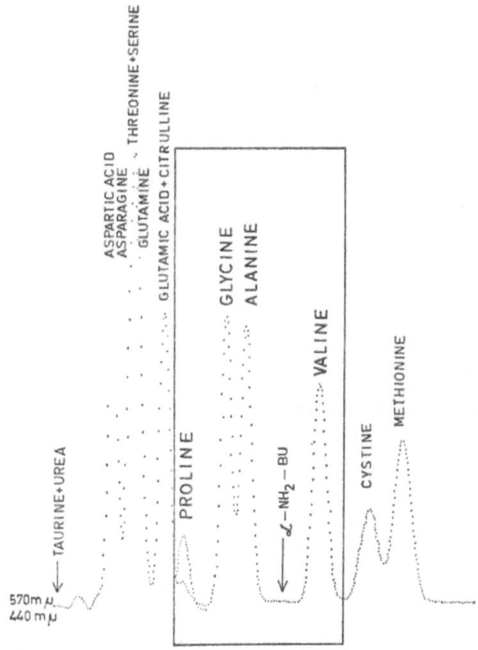

Fig. 2. Modified standard run of ion-exchange chromatography for determination of proline, glycine, alanine and valine concentrations. 50 μmoles of each amino acid were loaded on the column (28).

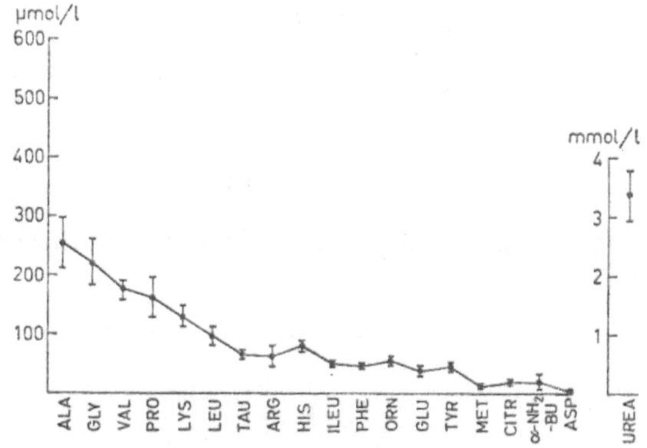

Fig. 3. The plasma aminogram of non-pregnant women of fertile age. Mean and double S. E. are given (26).

cord vein plasma are given in table 1. The pattern of the cord vein plasma agrees with that of the 8 cases of GHADIMI and PECORA (29).

Already during the first postnatal hours there is a fast decline in the levels of most free amino acids of plasma, most marked in the case of the branch-chained amino acids and of alanine and lysine, while the glycine level increases (28). See table 2. If fasting is prolonged till 48 hours of age, the isoleucine, alanine and lysine levels show a further

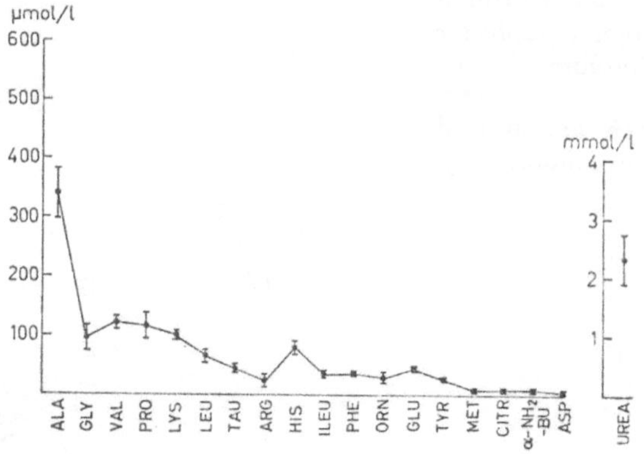

Fig. 4. The plasma aminogram of mothers during delivery. Mean and double S. E. are given. (26).

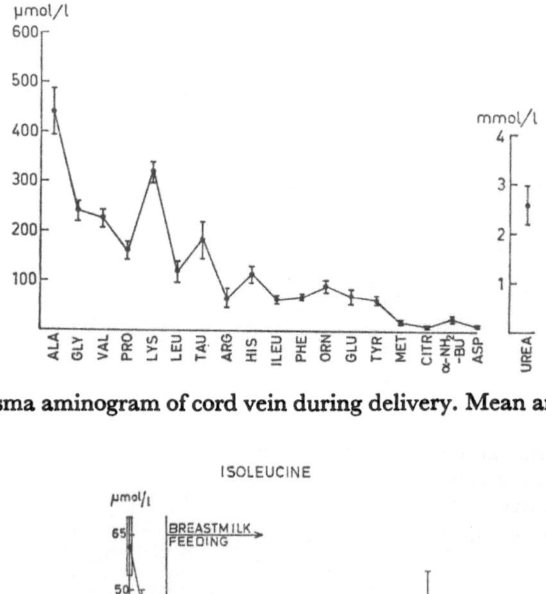

Fig. 5. The plasma aminogram of cord vein during delivery. Mean and double S. E. are given (26).

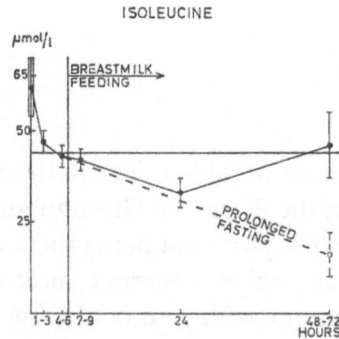

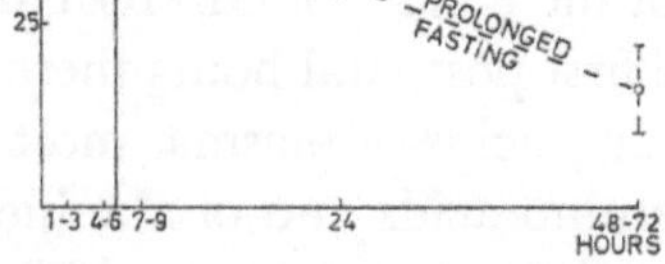

Fig. 6. Isoleucine levels of plasma during the first hours of life. The horizontal line is the level of infants (25). Mean and double S. E. are given (28).

decline. A fast decline of the taurine plasma level characterizes the second part of this observation period. See fig. 6. and 7. The aminogram during the rest of the neonatal period is markedly influenced by the feeding procedure (27). With the possible exception of lysine it was evident that the fast decline of the plasma amino acid levels was not due to urinary excretion. The immediate postnatal change of the plasma aminogram is the same as that found during experimental

Table 1. *Free amino acid levels in venous plasma from normal non-pregnant women, the mother during delivery and the cord during delivery with ratios between the cord vein level and that of the mother's cubital vein (26). Range, mean and standard deviation are expressed in μmol/l plasma. Mean is also given in mg/100 ml plasma (in brackets). n=number of cases where the amino acid was successfully determined. Compounds below dotted line are those which are better determined with other methods.*

	Non-pregnant women				Mothers			
Amino acid	Range	*n*	Mean	S.D.	Range	*n*	Mean	S.D.
α-Alanine	188–341	8	255 (2.3)	61	286–496	10	339 (3.0)	67
Glycine	161–322	8	222 (1.7)	55	64–160	10	94 (0.7)	35
Valine	153–211	7	174 (2.0)	21	81–149	10	121 (1.4)	18
Proline	94–240	8	162 (1.9)	48	58–168	10	115 (1.3)	32
Lysine	97–171	9	130 (1.9)	27	84–114	10	99 (1.5)	12
Leucine	77–111	8	96 (1.3)	22	40–83	10	64 (0.8)	17
Taurine	51–84	9	64 (0.8)	11	29–69	10	43 (0.5)	11
Arginine	29–101	8	62 (1.1)	26	15–33	4	23 (0.4)	8
Histidine	64–107	9	79 (1.2)	13	65–83	4	79 (1.2)	8
Isoleucine	41–63	8	49 (0.6)	8	23–46	10	34 (0.5)	8
Phenylalanine	41–54	8	46 (0.8)	5	23–44	10	36 (0.6)	7
Ornithine	41–70	9	55 (0.7)	11	19–47	6	29 (0.4)	11
Glutamic acid	21–52	8	38 (0.6)	11	34–54	10	44 (0.7)	7
Tyrosine	34–63	8	45 (0.8)	10	16–32	10	26 (0.5)	5
Methionine	6–19	8	13 (0.2)	5	4–12	9	8 (0.1)	3
Citrulline	12–31	8	20 (0.4)	7	5–16	9	8 (0.1)	4
α-NH_2-BU	11–39	4	21 (0.2)	13	6–11	3	9 (0.1)	3
Aspartic acid	1–7	9	4 (0.1)	2	2–7	10	5 (0.1)	2
Urea	2670–4610	9	3370 (20.4)	646	1290–3210	10	2320 (13.9)	670
- - - - -	- - -	-	- - -	- -	- - -	-	- - -	- -
Threonine	112–208	4	145 (1.7)	43	92–144	3	124 (1.5)	29
Serine	117–197	4	147 (1.5)	37	58–101	3	73 (0.8)	24
Cystine	27–46	6	37 (0.9)	7	29–40	4	36 (0.9)	10
Glutamine	555–792	4	716 (10.5)	115	284–376	3	331 (4.8)	47
Asparagine	53–94	4	74 (1.0)	17	38–68	3	51 (0.7)	16
Total amino acids			(22.6)				(17.0)	

calorie undernutrition of adults (16, 20). The assumption of a calorie deficiency agrees with the increased mobilization and utilization of fat observed during the neonatal period (30).

In the case of abnormally short, but otherwise normal pregnancy (31) the maternal levels were normal, but the cord vein plasma showed an increase of methionine and the levels of taurine and lysine were occasionally very high. The cord plasma methionine level has been found to decrease during the end of pregnancy in the Rhesus monkey (32), which is in accordance with the present findings. The plasma aminogram during the first hours of life of the early born infant was

Table 1. *(continued)*

	Cord-blood				Ratio cord/maternal plasma			
Amino acid	Range	*n*	Mean	S.D.	Range	*n*	Mean	S.D.
α-Alanine	324–591	10	441 (3.9)	75	1.0–1.5	10	1.3	0.2
Glycine	205–298	10	239 (1.8)	32	1.8–3.5	10	2.5	0.6
Valine	189–272	10	224 (2.6)	28	1.5–2.4	10	1.9	0.3
Proline	119–205	10	160 (1.8)	28	1.2–2.5	10	1.5	0.4
Lysine	277–368	10	318 (4.6)	33	2.5–4.1	10	3.3	0.7
Leucine	82–195	10	118 (1.6)	33	1.3–2.9	10	1.9	0.5
Taurine	97–272	10	181 (2.3)	58	3.0–5.7	10	4.3	1.0
Arginine	37–135	9	65 (1.1)	30	2.2–5.5	3	3.4	1.9
Histidine	93–135	4	112 (1.7)	17	1.2–1.8	4	1.5	0.3
Isoleucine	43–90	10	62 (0.8)	12	1.3–2.5	10	1.9	0.4
Phenylalanine	55–90	10	67 (1.1)	10	1.3–2.6	10	1.9	0.4
Ornithine	60–121	9	89 (1.2)	20	2.0–4.6	6	3.3	1.0
Glutamic acid	46–128	10	68 (1.0)	24	0.9–3.4	10	1.6	0.7
Tyrosine	43–83	10	61 (1.1)	14	1.7–3.4	10	2.4	0.6
Methionine	10–32	10	18 (0.3)	6	1.5–3.9	9	2.4	0.7
Citrulline	5–15	9	9 (0.2)	3	0.6–1.6	8	1.1	0.4
α-NH_2-BU	15–31	5	24 (0.3)	7	1.5–3.6	3	2.6	1.1
Aspartic acid	5–20	9	10 (0.1)	5	1.2–3.7	9	2.0	0.8
Urea	1530–3440	10	2590 (15.5)	610	0.9–1.4	10	1.1	0.1
Threonine	209–262	3	234 (2.8)	26	1.6–2.3	3	1.9	0.4
Serine	127–133	3	130 (1.4)	3	1.3–2.2	3	1.9	0.5
Cystine	33–43	5	38 (0.9)	5	1.0–1.2	3	1.1	0.1
Glutamine	492–590	3	550 (8.0)	58	1.5–2.0	3	1.7	0.3
Asparagine	53–66	3	59 (0.8)	4	1.0–1.5	3	1.2	0.2
Total amino acids			(32.8)				1.9	

Table 2. *Normal newborns (28). Cord vein plasma levels of free amino acids, CB are compared to those of the cubital vein plasma at 4 hours of age, CUB. Mean and S.D. are given in μmol/l plasma.*

Amino acid		*n*	Mean	S.D.	Significance of difference
Valine	CB	10	224	25	
	CUB	12	139	20	***
Leucine	CB	10	118	32	
	CUB	12	67	13	***
Isoleucine	CB	10	62	12	
	CUB	12	36	5	***
Lysine	CB	10	318	32	
	CUB	5	212	33	***
Alanine	CB	10	441	75	
	CUB	9	311	65	***
Glycine	CB	10	239	35	
	CUB	9	293	48	*

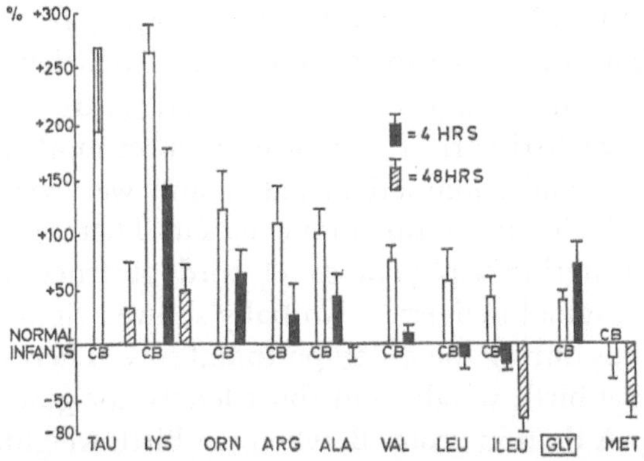

Fig. 7. Change of the free amino acid levels of plasma during the first hours of life of the fasting normal newborn (28). The 4 hour level is indicated if different from the cord vein level (26), the 48 hour level if different from the 4 hour level. The other 8 amino acid levels investigated showed a not significant decrease and urea a not significant increase during this period. The normal infant level is that of infants 9 months to 2 years of age (25).

characterized by an increase of tyrosine; higher levels of taurine than in the full term newborn, and a slower decline of the phenylalanine levels. The amino acid pattern of the urine was the same as that of term infants. The findings are in accordance with the known deficiency of the enzymes phenylalanine hydroxylase and p-hydroxy-phenylpyruvate oxidase in the liver of foetuses (33); with the decreased tolerance for phenylalanine demonstrated in early born infants (34), and with the high taurine and tyrosine levels found later during the neonatal period of early borns (27, 35).

RESULTS. LOW SOCIO-ECONOMIC GROUP

The plasma aminogram of mother and cord were determined in 10 cases of a low socio-economic group (A) and in 10 cases of a middle-class group (B) in Karachi, West Pakistan (36). The aminogram of the neonates was determined in 21 cases of group A (37). Group A was nutritionally characterized by maternal low consumption of vegetable protein during both the prematernal as well as maternal stage. Group B had a balanced diet with meat daily. There was no hypertension and no protein or glucose in the urine of the mothers at the time of delivery and a malaria smear was negative. Maternal care during pregnancy was negligible in both groups. Gross anaemia was present in one case of group A. The mothers showed no clinical deficiency symptoms, such as angular cheilosis, pre-tibial oedema, goitre, bone pains or signs suggestive of beri-beri (13). However, most mothers of group A showed weakness and conjunctival pallor and were thin with sometimes marked depletion of subcutaneous fat. There were no signs of intra- or extra-uterine asphyxia or of cord obstruction during the normal crown vaginal deliveries. No baby showed signs of malformations or infections during the 3-day postnatal stay. There was a greater frequency of low birth weight and short length for gestational age in the poor group A than in group B, when the birth weights and lengths were compared to an 'ideal' standard (38).

There was a significant increase in the maternal plasma levels of glycine and ornithine in the poorer group (A). Cord plasma was characterized by a general hyperaminoacidaemia with significantly increased glycine and proline levels. The plasma aminogram changed during the first hours of life to significantly increased levels of the non-essential amino acids alanine, proline, glycine and taurine. See fig. 8. The taurine level, which is increased in the plasma of the early born was excluded from the figure because of the difficulties of assessing

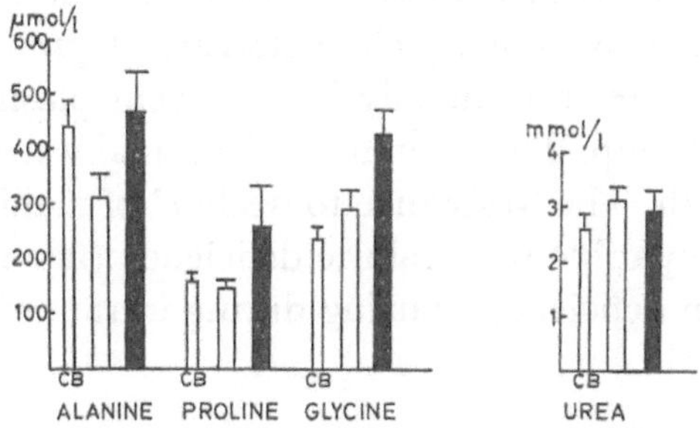

Fig. 8. Low socio-economic group. The normal cord vein levels (26) are indicated with CB. 2 S.E. are indicated. The unfilled columns represent the normal cubital vein levels at 4 hours of age (28). The filled columns represent the cubital vein levels of the low socio-economic group at 4 hours of age (37).

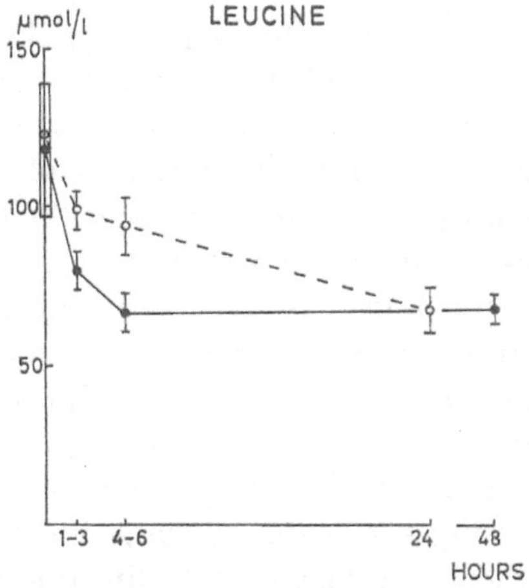

Fig. 9. Low socio-economic group. Leucine plasma levels during the immediate neonatal period. Filled circles indicate normal levels (26, 28). 2 S. E. are indicated. Unfilled circles indicate the levels of the low socio-economic group (37).

length of pregnancy with accuracy in this material. The branch-chained amino acids showed a delay in their normal decline. See fig. 9.

The increased plasma levels of alanine, proline and glycine found are characteristic of protein deficiency in infants and children, both after experimental protein restriction (15, 17) and in the clinical syndrome of kwashiorkor grade I (21). The increased levels of glycine, typical of the calorie deficiency of the first fasting period of the normal newborn (28), and of proline, characteristic of protein malnutrition of infants (15), were seen already in cord vein plasma of the lowest socio-economic group. The alanine level normally declines in plasma rapidly after birth. The 'resistance to decline' of alanine found in this group is not compatible with calorie deficiency (fig. 1.). The findings suggest a protein deficiency, starting during intrauterine life.

DISCUSSION

The use of the free amino acid levels of plasma for the early detection of malnutrition has been criticized (39). The criticism is based on the controversial results in the use of a rapid paper-chromatographic method intended for mass-screening (40, 41, 42). This method includes adding up several essential and non-essential amino acid levels and deals with a non-essential/essential amino acid ratio. The controversial results may depend on the sensitivity to storage of glutamine (43, 44), whose level makes up part of the numerator. It is also known that essentiality or non-essentiality of an amino acid is not necessarily relevant to the response of its plasma concentration to undernutrition. Histidine, lysine and phenylalanine, which are essential amino acids to the child, 'resist' the general decline in kwashiorkor, while all other essential amino acid levels of plasma decrease (fig. 1 with references).

If a ratio is to be used, which seems justified, as it will probably not be too sensitive to changes in plasma volume and to the catabolism of serious cases, then the use of the glycine/valine quotient is proposed. It seems to be a practical thing, as glycine increases and valine decreases in plasma very early both in experimental starvation (16, 20), and in experimental protein under-nutrition (15, 17). The same changes are seen in the clinical syndromes of kwashiorkor and marasmus (18, 19, 21, 22, 24). In the present investigation, the glycine/valine quotient was increased in the mothers of the low socio-economic group A, not significantly increased in the middle-class group B and increased in the newborn of group A at 4 hours of age. See fig. 10. Fig. 10 shows that the maternal glycine/valine quotient is not changed by hypertension as a complication during pregnancy (31, 36). The cord quotient, however, seems to be increased in hypertension of the mother

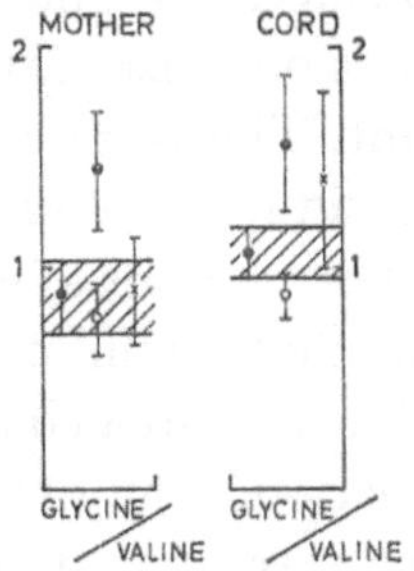

Fig. 10. The quotient between the levels of the amino acids glycine and valine in the mother's venous plasma and the plasma of the cord vein during delivery. The filled circles and the striped area indicate the quotient during normal deliveries (26); the unfilled circles the quotient during delivery after an abnormally short gestation (31); the unfilled circles with a cross the quotient during delivery in the low socio-economic group (36), and the crosses the quotient during delivery after a hypertensive pregnancy where the newborn was SFD (31). Double S.E. is given.

and the SFD syndrome of the newborn. The early born has a low glycine/valine quotient at birth and it seems as if the quotient could be of help in distinguishing low birth weight due to short pregnancy and the SFD syndrome. This is in accordance with what has been found in the Rhesus monkey, where glycine increases and valine decreases in cord plasma during the end of pregnancy (32).

The diagnostic value of the nonessential/essential amino acid ratio has also been re-evaluated because it fails to distinguish between kwashiorkor and marasmus, two clinical forms of malnutrition (22). In experimental calorie restriction the alanine level of plasma promptly decreases, while glycine, which is another non-essential amino acid, increases during the whole experimental period. From Fig. 1 it can be seen, that if the aim is a differential diagnosis between starvation ('marasmus') and hypercaloric low protein intake ('kwashiorkor'), then the alanine/valine quotient could be more helpful.

The glycine/valine and the alanine/valine ratios can be obtained by a simplified, reliable and inexpensive ion-exchange chromatography system such as that described (fig. 2) (27, 28).

The metabolic situation of these SFD newborn infants might be more complex than that of a mere substrate depletion, due to the unknown metabolic adaptations to low nutrient supply. The biochemical alterations responsible for the change in the plasma concentration of free amino acids in response to starvation and protein undernutrition are not known. However, there is one observation of the present investigation that requires comment. The transient 'resistance to decline' of the branch-chained amino acid levels of plasma during the immediate postnatal period of the newborn infants of group A (fig. 9) is of special interest. A catabolism of 'labile protein' can not explain this finding, as the phenylalanine, tyrosine and urea concentrations of plasma were not increased during this period. The observation therefore suggests that there is, at birth, a decreased transport or utilization of branch-chained amino acids.

A transient increase of branch-chained amino acid concentration of plasma is seen in starvation of adults (16, 20). The studies of CAHILL et al suggest that in prolonged starvation there is an attenuation of hepatic gluconeogenesis (45) and an adaptation of the brain to ketone utilization (46). This would enable survival through 'conservation' of body protein stores, while utilizing fat as the primary energy-producing fuel. The mechanisms behind the attenuated gluconeogenesis and the increase of the branch-chained amino acid levels of plasma during starvation are not known.

If there is in these newborn SFD infants a metabolic adaptation comparable to that of starvation, then the increased level of plasma alanine during the first hours of life indicates an inhibited hepatic amino acid uptake or utilization, rather than a decreased peripheral release of amino acids. It seems that an elucidation of the mechanisms whereby the hepatic uptake of amino acids *normally* increases during the immediate postnatal period, as shown by CHRISTENSEN et al in guinea-pigs (47), could provide an insight into these metabolic alterations.

SUMMARY

The present paper summarizes studies aimed at evaluating the possibilities of using the altered homeostasis of plasma free amino acids, characteristic of postnatal undernutrition, as a basis for studies of the effects of foetal undernutrition in man.

The normal venous plasma aminograms of non-pregnant women of fertile age and of pregnant women and cord during delivery are given. During the first hours of life the venous plasma aminogram was found to change to a pattern which is the same as that seen after experimental calorie undernutrition.

In a low socio-economic group of a developing country, maternal plasma and cord plasma showed an increased glycine/valine quotient, which is characteristic both of experimental starvation and experimental protein undernutrition as well as of the clinical syndromes of marasmus and kwashiorkor. In the newborn infants the venous plasma aminogram changed during the first hours of life to a pattern which is the same as that seen after experimental protein undernutrition in infants and in the clinical syndrome of kwashiorkor. The changed pattern was not seen in a short gestation group. The same abnormal pattern was found in 'small for dates' newborns of mothers with hypertension during pregnancy.

The use of the glycine/valine ratio is suggested as an additional 'tool' in the studies of the effects of undernutrition on the metabolic situation of the newborn, the adaptation to extrauterine life and the long-term prognosis concerning physical and mental development.

A simplified and reliable system of ion-exchange chromatography, which is suitable for assessment of the nutritional status is recommended.

REFERENCES

1. WIGGLESWORTH, J. S., (1966) *Brit. Med. Bull.* 22:13.
2. COCHRANE, W. A., (1960) *Am. J. Dis. Child.* 99:476.
3. WAYBURNE, S., (1968) In: *Calorie Deficiencies and Protein Deficiencies*, McCance, R. A. and E. M. Widdowson, eds., J. and A. Churchill Ltd, London, p. 7.
4. DAWKINS, M., (1965) In: Gestational Age, Size and Maturity, *Clin. Develop. Med.* 19:33., Dawkins, M. and W. G. MacGregor, eds., William Heinemann Med. Books Ltd, London.
5. CHOW, B. F. and C. J. LEE, (1964) *J. Nutr.* 82:10.
6. HSUEH, A. M., C. E. AGUSTIN, and B. F. CHOW, (1967) *J. Nutr.* 91:195.
7. WINICK, M. and A. NOBLE, (1966) *J. Nutr.* 89:300.
8. *Nutrition Survey of East Pakistan.* (May 1966) Public Health Service, U.S. Department of Health, Education and Welfare.
9. *World Health Organization Chronicle.* (May 1969) Vol 23, No 5.
10. GRUENWALD, P., (1968) In: *Aspects of Prematurity and Dysmaturity*, Nutricia Symposium, Jonxis, J. H. P., H. K. A. Visser, and J. A. Troelstra, eds., H. E. Stenfert Kroese N.V., Leiden, p. 37.
11. GHOSH, S. and S. DAGA, (1967) *J. Pediat.* 71:173.
12. RAHIMTOOLA, R. J., S. MIR, and S. BALOCH, (1968) *Acta Paediat. Scand.* 57:534.
13. JELLIFFE, D. B., (1966) *World Health Organization monograph series*, No 53, Geneva.

14. WHITEHEAD, R. G., (1965) *Lancet.* II:567.
15. SNYDERMAN, S. E., L. E. HOLT Jr. P. M. NORTON, E. ROITMAN and S. V. PHANSALKAR, (1968) *Ped. Res.* 2:131.
16. ADIBI, S. A., (1968) *J. Appl. Physiol.* 25:52.
17. ARROYAVE, G., (1962) *Am. J. Clin. Nutr.* 11:447.
18. ARROYAVE, G., D. WILSON, C. DE FUNES, and M. BÉHAR, (1962) *Am. J. Clin. Nutr.* 11:517.
19. ENDOZIEN, J. C., E. J. PHILIPS and W. R. F. COLLIS, (1960) *Lancet.* I:615.
20. FELIG, P., O. E. OWEN, J. WAHREN, and G. F. CAHILL, Jr, (1969) *J. Clin. Invest.* 48:584.
21. HOLT, L. E. Jr, S. E. SNYDERMAN, P. M. NORTON, E. ROITMAN and J. FINCH, (1963) *Lancet.* II:1343.
22. SAUNDERS, S. J., A. S. TRUSWELL, G. O. BARBEZAT, W. WITTMAN, and J. D. L. HANSEN, (1967) *Lancet.* II:795.
23. SWENDSEID, M. E., S. G. TUTTLE, W. S. FIGUEROA, D. MULCARE, A. J. CLARK, and F. J. MASSEY, (1966) *J. Nutr.* 88:239.
24. WESTALL, R. G., E. ROITMAN, C. DE LA PENA, H. RASMUSSEN, J. CRAVIOTO, F. GOMEZ, and L. E. HOLT Jr, (1958) *Arch. Dis. Child.* 33:499.
25. SOUPART, P., (1962) In: *Amino Acid Pools,* Holden, J. T. ed., Elsevier Press Inc., New York.
26. LINDBLAD, B. S. and A. BALDESTEN, (1967) *Acta Paediat. Scand.* 56:37.
27. LINDBLAD, B. S. and A. BALDESTEN, (1969) *Acta Paediat. Scand.* 58:252.
28. LINDBLAD, B. S., (1970) *Acta Paediat. Scand.* 59:13.
29. GHADIMI, H. and P. PECORA, (1964) *Pediatrics.* 33:500.
30. PERSSON, B. and J. GENTZ, (1966) *Acta Paediat. Scand.* 55:353.
31. LINDBLAD, B. S. and R. ZETTERSTRÖM, (1968) *Acta Paediat. Scand.* 57:195.
32. KERR, G. R., (1968) *Ped. Res.* 2:493.
33. KRETCHMER, N. (1959) *Pediatrics.* 23:606.
34. BREMER, H. J. and W. NEUMANN ,(1966) *Klin. Wschr.* 44:1076.
35. LEVINE, S. Z., E. MARPLES and H. H. GORDON, (1941) *J. Clin. Invest.* 20:199+209.
36. LINDBLAD, B. S., R. J. RAHIMTOOLA, M. SAID, Q. HAQUE, and N. KHAN, (1969) *Acta Paediat. Scand,* 58:497
37. LINDBLAD, B. S., R. J. RAHIMTOOLA, and N. KHAN, (1970) *Acta Paediat. Scand.* 59:21.
38. ENGSTRÖM, L. and G. STERKY, (1966) *Läkartidningen (Sw.).* 51:4922.
39. MCLAREN, D. S., W. W. KAMEL, and N. AYYOUB, (1965) *Am. J. Clin. Nutr.* 17:152.
40. SWENDSEID, M. E., W. H. GRIFFITH, and S. G. TUTTLE, (1963) *Metabolism.* 12:96.
41. WHITEHEAD, R. G., (1964) *Lancet.* I:250.
42. WHITEHEAD, R. G. and R. F. A. DEAN, (1964) *Am. J. Clin. Nutr.* 14:313+320.
43. DICKINSON, J. C., H. ROSENBLUM and P. B. HAMILTON, (1965) Pediatrics. 36:2.
44. STEIN, W. H. and S. MOORE, (1954) *J. Biol. Chem.* 211:915.
45. OWEN, O. E., P. FELIG, A. P. MORGAN, J. WAHREN, and CAHILL, G. F. Jr, (1969) *J. Clin. Invest.* 48:574.
46. OWEN, O. E., A. P. MORGAN, H. G. KEMP, J. M. SULLIVAN, M. G. HERRERA, and G. F. CAHILL, (1967) *J. Clin. Invest.* 46:1589.
47. CHRISTENSEN, H. N. and J. B. CLIFFORD ,(1963) *J. Biol. Chem.* 238: 1743.

DISCUSSION

Prof. Wolf: Did you find any correlation between the high alanine levels in the small-for-date infants and the blood glucose. Probably there is a connection between gluconeogenesis and this high alanine levels or the low blood glucose in those infants.

Dr. Lindblad: We have studied this in small-for-dates newborns of mothers with hypertension. Up to now we have only had a chance to study three cases with neonatal hypoglycaemia.

One of those small for dates infants had central nervous symptoms. In those three cases the changes were even more pronounced, with very high levels of alanine and proline.*

Prof. Teller: You were referring to the glycine-valine ratio as a parameter to study undernutrition or malnutrition in the newborn. Do you have evidence what this ratio holds true for estimation of undernutrition on later age?

Dr. Lindblad: The figure no. 1 includes studies on infants, children adults and at old age. Also in adults, the glycine level increases and the valine level decreases during undernutrition.

Prof. Teller: This would help the clinician in the rare cases of dystrophy of young children. If one has a valid parameter like glycine-valine ratio, then you can differentiate between malnutrition or dystrophy due to other causes.

* Lindblad, B. S., (1970) *Acta Paediat. Scand.* 59:13.

THE PROTEIN AND ANIMO ACID REQUIREMENTS OF THE PREMATURE INFANT

S. E. SNYDERMAN*

The optimal feeding for the premature infant has yet to be defined and, in particular, the most advantageous intake of protein has been the subject of considerable investigation. Human milk with its low protein content was widely used and considered to be the feeding of choice until the studies of GORDON and LEVINE (1) indicated that premature infants, especially those with birth weights of under 1600 grams, gained weight more rapidly and retained more nitrogen when fed cow's milk mixtures that contained a good deal more protein. These mixtures, however, also contained more minerals and several observers (2–4) suggested that the increased weight gain was the result of fluid retention. With greater appreciation of the strain of an increased solute load on the immature kidney, most recently there has been a tendency to feed a more moderate protein intake, in the range of 3 to 3.5 grams/kilogram/day.

Our studies on the protein requirement of the premature infant were carried out with the two extremes of intake that had been previously utilized in premature feeding – 2 and 9 grams/kilogram/day. Formulas were comparable in every way except for the protein content, and were constituted to provide 130 calories/kilogram/day and 135 cc of fluid per kilogram.

Our experience thus far includes 56 infants fed the high protein formula and 63 given the low protein feeding. The weight gains of all of these infants, with a few exceptions, were quite similar in that they adhered to standard curves which had been established in the premature unit of Bellevue Hospital at a time when the routine feeding provided a high protein intake of, on the average, 5 to 6 grams/

* Department of Pediatrics, New York University Medical Center. Supported by National Institute of Health Grants HD-02064 and HD-02760.

kilogram/day (5). The exceptions were a few babies whose birth weight was less than 1100 grams who gained weight at a slightly reduced rate on the low protein intake and an equal number of babies who received the high protein formula who developed clinical edema and thus gave the false impression of an accelerated rate of weight gain.

Nitrogen balance studies were carried out in 15 low protein and 11 high protein babies (6): striking differences in the amount of nitrogen retained were observed. All of the babies fed the two gram formula retained in the range of 200 milligram/kilogram/day (fig. 1 and 2),

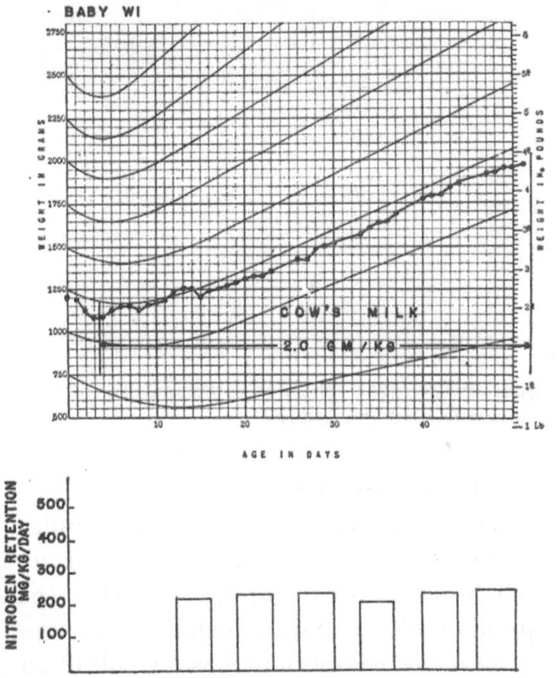

Fig. 1. Weight gain and nitrogen retention of premature infant, birth weight 1200 grams, fed 2 grams protein/kilogram/day.

while the 9 gram/kilogram infants retained at least 2 to 3 times as much (fig. 3 and 4). On the high protein feeding there was much greater variation between individual babies, and there was a greater loss of nitrogen in the stool, but nevertheless, all of the infants on this regime retained considerably more nitrogen than on the lower intake.

These apparently high retentions led us to search for other routes

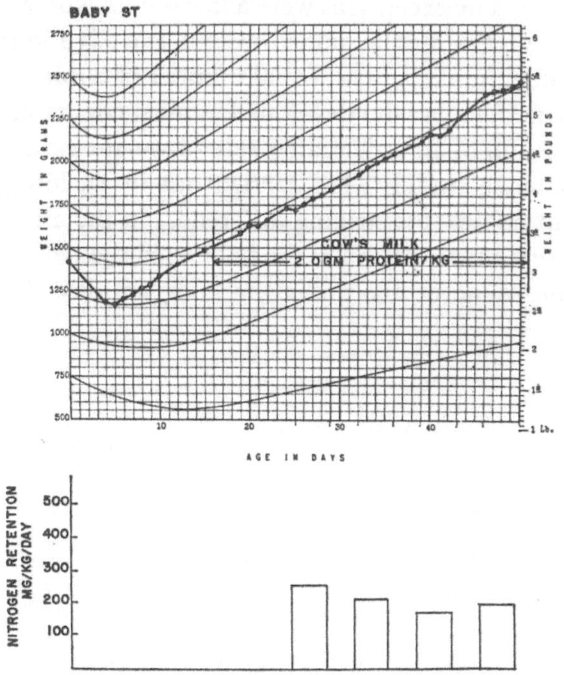

Fig. 2. Weight gain and nitrogen retention of premature infant, birth weight 1420 grams, fed 2 grams protein/kilogram/day.

through which nitrogen might be lost. WALLACE (7) had suggested that such high retentions were the result of a cumulative error: that the amount of nitrogen excreted is underestimated because of failure to measure such losses as occur through the skin (perspiration and epithelial desquamation) and those which occur in wipes in the diaper area; while the intake is overestimated as a result of an undetermined amount lost in drooling and regurgitation. All of these possible sources of error were investigated in 4 high protein infants and were found to account for only 3 to 8% of the total nitrogen retention.

Although even with the most meticulous care, nitrogen balance determinations cannot be regarded as a very precise tool and cannot be utilized to ascertain body composition, these data are very suggestive. The large differences in figures leave little doubt that premature infants on high protein intakes retain more nitrogen than do those on low intakes. The increased retention without a concomitant increase

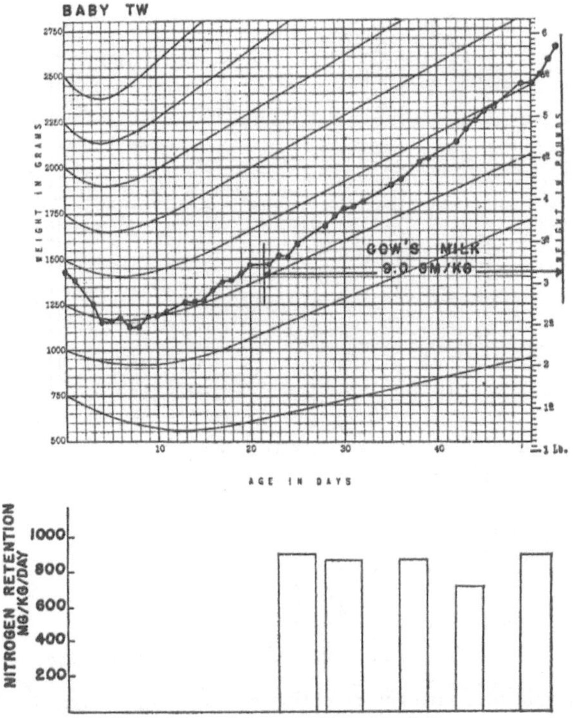

Fig. 3. Weight gain and nitrogen retention of premature infant, birth weight 1430 grams, fed 9 grams protein/kilogram/day. Clinical edema was evident on the 50th day of life.

in body weight allows only one possible conclusion, that there is an alteration in body composition of these infants. The studies of Moulton (8) and of Dickerson and Widdowson (9) all demonstrate a rapid increase in body content of nitrogen during fetal life that is not complete until some time after the seventh postnatal month. It seems quite probable that these infants have an accelerated chemical maturation and attain a more mature body composition at an earlier age. Whether such chemical maturation serves any useful purpose and is accompanied by accelerated development in function has yet to be demonstrated.

These studies give some indication that 2.0 grams of protein/kilogram may be quite close to the minimal requirement for the premature infant. When calculations are made for the biological value,

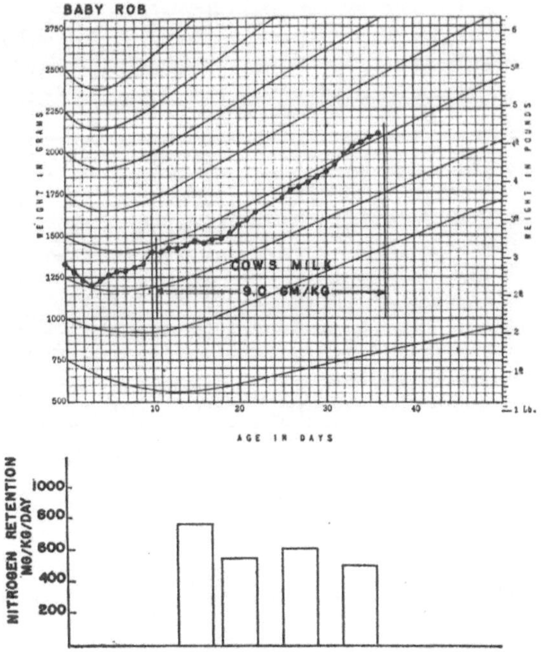

Fig. 4. Weight gain and nitrogen retention of premature infant, birth weight 1330 grams, fed 9 grams protein/kilogram/day.

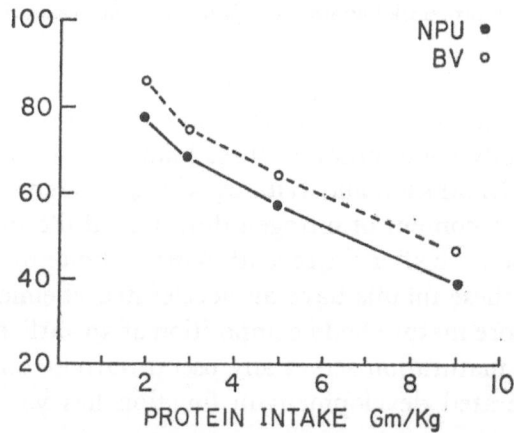

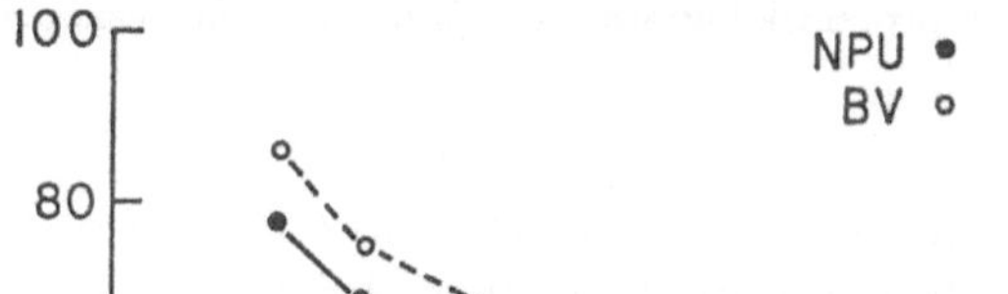

Fig. 5. Relation of the biological value (BV) and net protein utilization (NPU) to the protein intake in the premature infant. The sharp fall in these values between 2 and 3 gram intakes represents the less efficient utilization that occurs after the protein requirement has been met.

which is a measure of the absorbed nitrogen retained in the body, and for the net protein utilized, an index of retained nitrogen related to nitrogen intake, for these as well as for other infants fed 3 to 5 grams protein/kilogram/day, a sharp drop occurs between the 2 and 3 gram intake (fig. 5). Such a drop has been demonstrated to occur in animals after the needs for protein anabolism of the body have been met. (10, 11).

The free amino acid levels of both the plasma and the red blood cells were investigated with two thoughts in mind; that some evidence of deficiency might be found in the infants fed at the lower level, and that some evidence of increased storage might be found in the high protein infants since this intake was invariably accompanied by significant elevations of the blood urea nitrogen and the non protein nitrogen. Plasma amino acids were determined in 24 of these infants and red blood cell levels in 8 high protein and 6 low protein subjects.

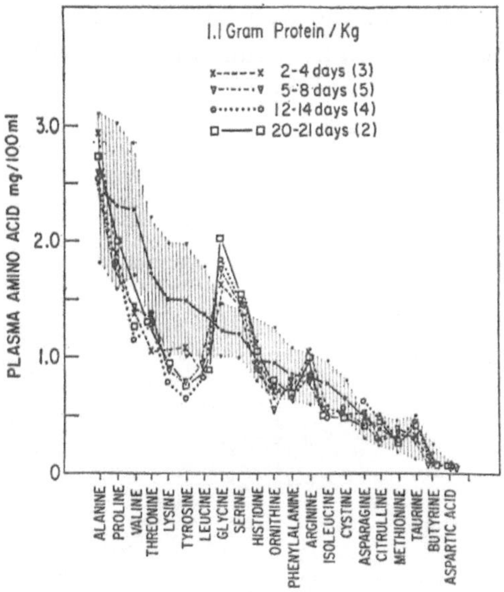

Fig. 6. The plasma aminogram after feeding 1.1 grams protein/kilogram/day for the length of time indicated on the figure. The figures in the parentheses are the number of subjects. The heavy line is the average of 29 infants fed 3 to 3.5 grams protein/kilogram/day, and the shaded area represents one standard deviation above and below this average.

All values were compared to premature infants of the same weight fed 3 to 3.5 grams protein/kilogram.

Before demonstrating the plasma aminogram obtained in the premature infant, I should like to discuss briefly the plasma amino acid levels of full term infants, 2 to 4 months of age, maintained at various levels of restricted protein intake (12). The protein was cow's milk, and all diets were kept constant except for the protein content. The most drastic restriction was 1.1 grams protein/kilogram. Alterations were noted in the plasma aminogram as rapidly as 2 days after the dietary shift and may actually have occurred sooner since bloods were not drawn until that time (fig. 6). The most striking changes were in the depression of the levels of the branched chain amino acids, leucine, isoleucine and valine, of tyrosine and of lysine. In contrast to the depression of these amino acids is the elevation of the glycine level; serine is also elevated; this is a manifestation of the ready interconversion between serine and glycine. Other restricted levels of protein gave similar aminograms (fig. 7). However, when 1.7 grams protein/kilogram was fed, the only change was the elevation of the glycine level, the other amino acids were all within normal limits.

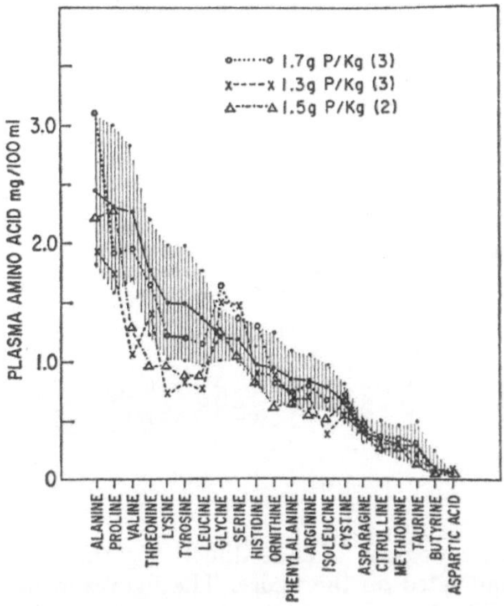

Fig. 7. The plasma aminogram after feeding 1.3, 1.5, and 1.7 grams protein/kilogram/day. The number of subjects are in the parentheses.

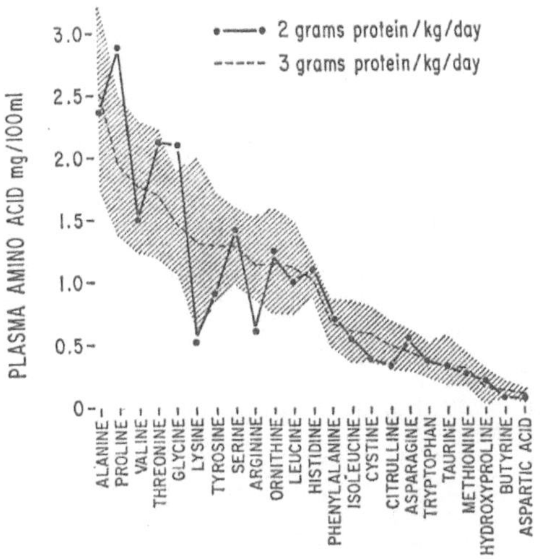

Fig. 8. The plasma aminogram of 12 premature infants fed 2 grams protein/kilogram/day compared to controls fed 3 grams protein/kilogram/day. The shaded area represents one standard deviation above and below the average control.

Since these babies were gaining weight at a normal rate and gave every other indication of good health, the elevation of the glycine level may be the most sensitive indicator of the adequacy of protein intake.

The plasma aminogram of premature infants fed 2 grams of protein/kilogram/day is illustrated in figure 8. The majority of the amino acids are within the normal range. However, there is some depression of the lysine and arginine levels and an elevation of the glycine and proline levels. The elevated proline levels do not seem to be a consequence of the dietary manipulation; we have observed this in a number of premature infants and believe it to be a manifestation of impaired activity of the enzyme system involved in metabolizing this amino acid, and in addition, there was the same degree of elevation in the control bloods of these infants obtained just before the dietary shift. The elevation in glycine level, on the other hand, is the result of the diet, since in every instance it was higher on the diet than in the control blood drawn just before the diet was instituted. The fall in lysine level suggests several possibilities. One is that the lysine requirement of the premature infant is considerably higher than that of the full term infant; we calculated that these infants received 155 milli-

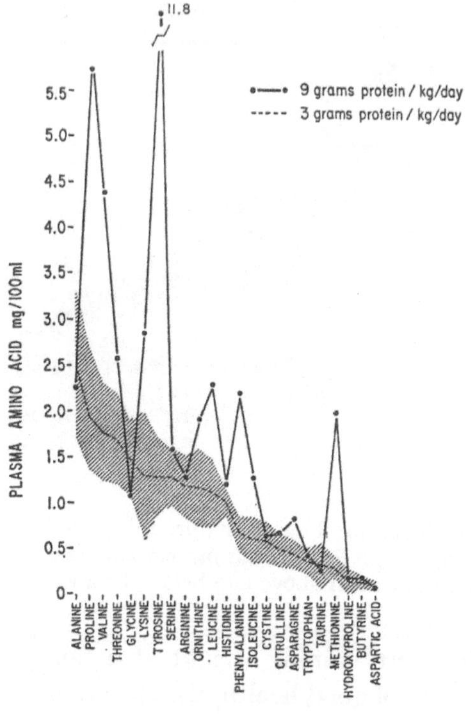

Fig. 9. The plasma aminogram of 12 premature infants fed 9 grams protein/kilogram/day compared to controls given 3 grams protein/kilogram/day. The shaded area represents one standard deviation above and below the average control.

grams/kilogram/day of lysine while our studies on the full term infant demonstrated a requirement of between 88 and 103 milligrams/kilograms/day. (13) Another possibility is that the total lysine content of the diet was not available to the infant because of the formation of a lysine – carbohydrate complex during heat processing; the effect of this may be exaggerated in the premature infant whose digestive processes may be less efficient.

The high protein intake was accompanied by the elevation of the levels of a number of amino acids (Fig. 9). The most marked elevations occurred in the tyrosine and methionine levels and are, no doubt, related to impaired activity of enzymes in their metabolic pathway. In

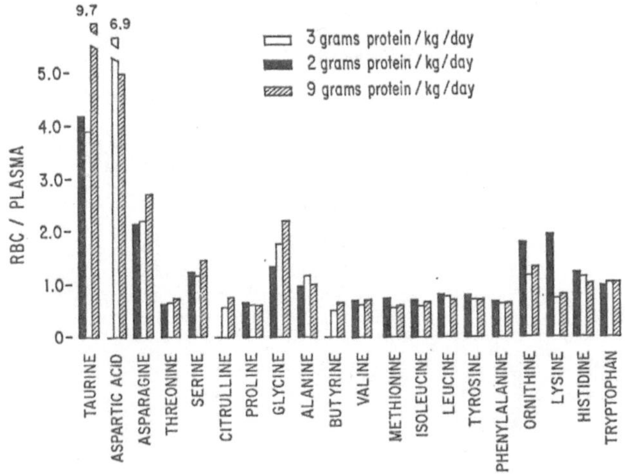

Fig. 10. Amino acid red blood cell-plasma ratios of premature infants given 2, 3 and 9 grams protein/kilogram/day.

contrast to the elevation of the other amino acids is the depression of the glycine to the low normal range.

The free amino acid levels of the red blood cells tended to vary in the same direction as the plasma. Hence the ratio between red blood cell and plasma level was constant despite the changes in protein intake and the striking variation in plasma levels (fig. 10). This indicates that this determination does not have any advantage over the plasma analysis as a criterion of nutritional status. The differences in content between the red cell and plasma, however, pose a number of problems. Simple diffusion processes may explain the one to one ratio between cells and plasma, but the differences on the two sides of the cell membrane suggest the existence of active transport mechanisms into the red cells. The high levels of taurine and aspartic acid suggest possible metabolic differences within the red cell. The combined increase of the amino acid content of both the plasma and the red cells accounted for a very small percentage of the extra nitrogen retained on the high protein diet.

Hydroxyproline peptide excretion, which has been advocated as an index of the growth rate, was determined in 24 hour urines in a group of these infants – 22 low protein and 21 high protein. Excretion of the low protein infants tended to be lower than that of the high protein

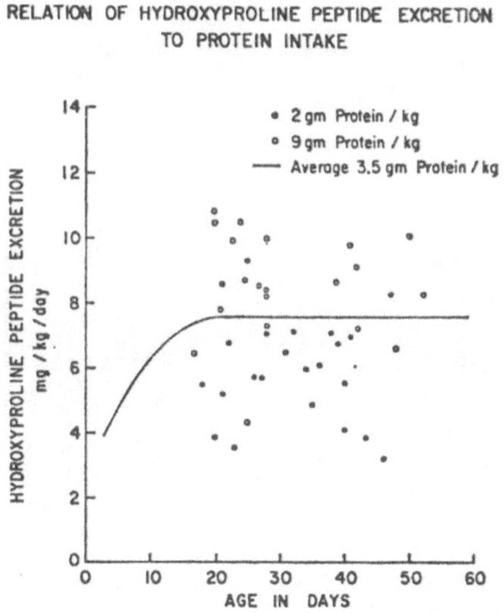

Fig. 11. Hydroxyproline peptide excretion of 22 premature infants fed 2 grams protein/kilogram/day and of 21 premature infants fed 9 grams protein/kilogram/day compared to that of premature infants given a standard feeding providing 3.5 grams protein/kilogram/day.

babies (fig. 11). When compared to the excretion of babies fed the standard milk feeding, the same trends were noted, but the differences were not statistically significant. Free hydroxyproline excretion was similar for both groups. The trends in hydroxypeptide excretion were not due to differences in intake, since there was no detectible hydroxyproline in the milk formula. Also, it was not the consequence of a greater intake of proline. The addition of an equivalent amount of proline to the low protein diet did not influence the hydroxyproline peptide excretion.

We do not know the quantitative amino acid requirements of the premature, but the amounts contained in 2 grams of cow's milk protein may give some indication of the requirements. It seems very probable, with the exception of lysine which we have already discussed, that the amounts are not greater than the amounts listed in table 1. How much these figures are in excess of minimal requirements cannot be answered presently. However, if one can expect the same fall in requirement during the last weeks of prenatal life as there is during the first months of life, then these figures are not greatly in

Table 1. *Amino acids provided by 2 grams of cow's milk protein/kg.*

	Mg/kg/day
Histidine	48
Isoleucine	128
Leucine	216
Lysine	155
Methionine	52
Phenylalanine	104
Threonine	92
Tryptophan	30
Valine	138

excess. Also, one would anticipate that the quantitative amino acid requirements of the premature infant would be greater because of a number of circumstances, including the rapid rate of growth, the impairment in the ability to digest and absorb protein, and the greater loss of amino acids in the urine as a result of impaired renal tubular reabsorption.

Another feature of the amino acid requirements of the premature infant is the possibility that certain amino acids which are not regarded as essential for the more mature individual are required because enzyme systems necessary for their synthesis are not sufficiently developed. We have thus far obtained evidence that tyrosine and cystine are in this category. In the absence of either of these two amino acids, there is impairment in the rate of weight gain, in the amount of nitrogen retained, and there is a depression of the level of the amino acid in the plasma. Twelve premature infants were studied for their requirement of cystine, only two failed to demonstrate the evidences of deficiency that were just mentioned (fig. 12). Of interest too, is the fact that the need may persist for some time; one infant who weighed 1000 grams at birth was restudied when he was 5 months of age and weighed 4.0 kilograms and still manifested a need for cystine. Infants who demonstrated a need for cystine also failed to show an increase in the plasma level of cystine after a load of methionine.

The situation is very similar in the case of tyrosine (fig. 13). We have been able to obtain data that tyrosine is a dietary requirement for the majority of premature infants, that this requirement persists for some months and that a certain number of full term infants also require it.

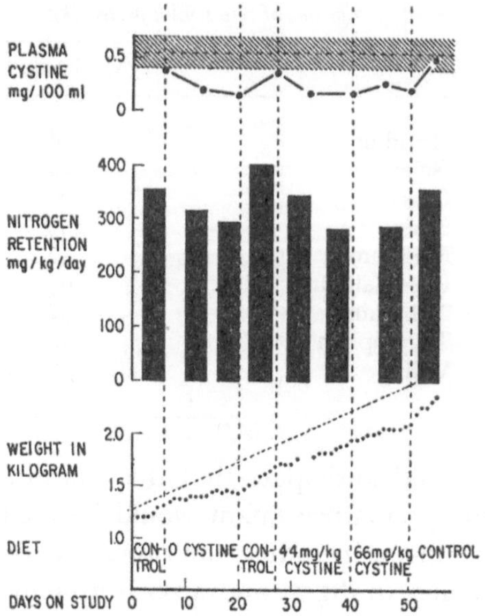

Fig. 12. Protocol of a study demonstrating that cystine is an essential amino acid for the premature infant. The weight gain and nitrogen retention are impaired, and the plasma cystine level falls when cystine is removed from the diet. The criteria of adequacy were not fulfilled by intakes of cystine less than the control which provided 85 milligrams/kilogram/day.

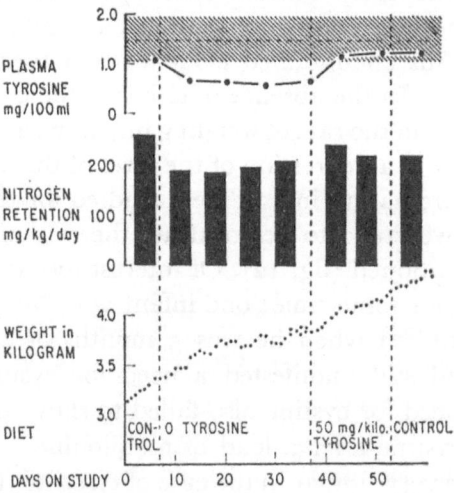

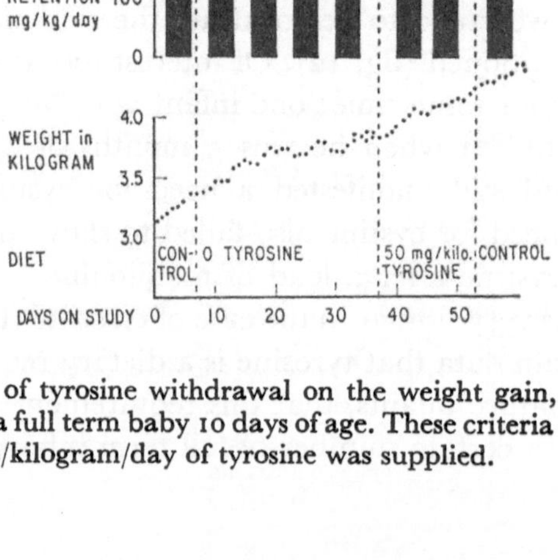

Fig. 13. The effect of tyrosine withdrawal on the weight gain, nitrogen retention and plasma level of a full term baby 10 days of age. These criteria returned to normal when 50 milligrams/kilogram/day of tyrosine was supplied.

SUMMARY

Premature infants gain weight at a similar rate over a wide range of protein intake, however, the amount of nitrogen retained increases with the protein intake. At an intake of 2.0 grams of protein/kilogram, the plasma amino acids are within the normal range except for a slightly depressed level of lysine and arginine and some elevation of the glycine level. This suggests that this level is very close to the minimal requirement. High protein intakes are accompanied by elevation of a number of plasma amino acids, the most striking elevations are of methionine and tyrosine; the glycine level is depressed. Hydroxyproline peptide excretion seems to vary with the protein intake. The essential amino acid requirements of the premature infant are greater in terms of body weight than at other periods of life, and in addition, certain amino acids which are not essential for the mature individual are required by the premature.

REFERENCES

1. Gordon, H. H., S. Z. Levine, and H. McNamara, (1947). *Amer. J. Dis. Child.* 73:442.
2. Crosse, V. M., E. M. Hickmans, B. E. Hawarth, and J. Aubrey, (1954) *Arch. Dis. Child.* 29:178.
3. Kagan, B. M., J. H. Hess, E. Lundeen, K. Shafer, J. B. Parker, and C. Stigall, (1955) *Pediatrics* 15:373.
4. Kagan, B. M., N. Felix, C. W. Molander, R. J. Busser, and D. Kalman, (1963) *Ann. New York Acad. Sc.* 110:830.
5. Dancis, J., J. R. O'Connell and L. E. Holt, Jr., (1948) *J. Pediat.* 33:570.
6. Snyderman, S. E., A. Boyer, M. D. Kogut and L. E. Holt, Jr., (1969) *J. Pediat.* 74:872.
7. Wallace, W. M., (1959) *Fed. Proc.* 18:1125.
8. Moulton, C. R., (1923) *J. Biol. Chem.* 57:79.
9. Dickerson, J. W. and E. M. Widdowson, (1960) *Biochem. J.* 74:247.
10. Platt, B. S. and D. S. Miller, (1958) *Proc. Nutrition Soc.* 17:106.
11. Allison, J. B. (1964) The nutritive value of dietary proteins. In: Munro, H. N. and J. B. Allison; *Mammalian Protein Metabolism.* Academic Press, New York and London.
12. Snyderman, S. E., L. E. Holt, Jr., P. M. Norton, E. Roitman, and S. V. Phansalkar, (1968) *Pediat. Res.* 2:131.
13. Snyderman, S. E., P. M. Norton, D. I. Fowler, and L. E. Holt, Jr., (1959) *Amer. J. Dis. Child.* 97:175.

DISCUSSION

Prof. Fomon: There is at least one additional reason that positive nitrogen balance as measured by balance studies may not really reflect what the body is accumulating. Procedures employed in the balance studies may lead to greater retention of nitrogen *during* these studies than *between* studies.

Dr. SNYDERMAN has stated that the two diets were similar in calories and in components other than protein. Were concentrations of calcium, phosphorus, sodium and potassium similar?

Dr. Snyderman: There is little reason to expect that the amount of nitrogen retained between balance periods would be significantly different than that retained during the balance period since there was only a two day interval between periods, the infants were kept on the same diet, cared for by the same nurses in the same incubators and had the same amount of activity.

The feedings were specially prepared by one of the milk companies. There were only two differences between the feedings, one was the protein content and the other was the additional carbohydrate added to the low protein feeding to keep the two feedings isocaloric.

Prof. Fomon: My second question relates to interpretation: I wonder whether you interpret the abnormal aminogram to be evidence of inadequate nutritional status or merely a reflection of inadequate recent intake of protein. The two things may not be the same.

Dr. Snyderman: The aminogram is a reflection of protein intake and not of generalized nutritional state. It can be related to the level of protein in the diet. The rapid response of the plasma amino acids to a restriction of protein intake is a consequence of the lack of stored protein.

Dr. Widdowson: I am still worried on the high retention of nitrogen from the high protein intake. I have been making some calculations. I have had to make assumptions about the weight of the babies and

I think, but am not sure, that the retention was 200 or 300 mg per kg per day of nitrogen. It seems to me, if this was so, that in 8 weeks one baby would have had half as much nitrogen again in his body as the other although the body weight was the same. This seems impossible.

Dr. Snyderman: I have not tried to make quantitative estimates of the nitrogen content of these babies. The point I wish to make, however, is that the protein content of the body of the high protein baby does contain more protein and that perhaps he is attaining a more mature body composition earlier than the low protein-fed baby.

Dr. Räihä: I was very happy to see Dr. Snyderman's balance studies on the praemature infant requirement for cystine. This was in good agreement with the enzymatic results we got in the human.

Dr. Sereni: Dr. Snyderman, which were the serum urea values in your group of infants fed with 9 grams of proteins/kg/day? We have a series of data in praemature infants with varying protein intake, from 4 till 9 g/kg/day. Over 6 g/kg/day of protein intake there was a significant increase in urea serum concentration.

Second question: Is there any suggestion from your studies that the mean amount of protein requirements is different in small-for-date babies as compared to praemature babies of the same weight.

Dr. Snyderman: The figures for the blood urea nitrogen were quite high in the high protein babies. We have observed elevations in this value when premature infants are fed 4 or more grams of protein/kilogram.

Dr. Lindblad: Do you think, Dr. Snyderman, that you would arrive even closer to the optimum requirement by not just looking at the post-absorptive level, but rather studying the plasma disappearance rates of the individual amino acids after giving an ideal protein, like lacto-albumin?

Dr. Snyderman: The disappearance rates pose many more problems since they are different for different amino acids and also vary with the time interval after a meal.

PROTEIN REQUIREMENT OF NORMAL INFANTS BETWEEN 8 AND 56 DAYS OF AGE

S. J. FOMON*, E. E. ZIEGLER**, L. N. THOMAS, AND L. J. FILER, JR.

In 1967 we published (1) results of a study of normal fullterm infants fed ad libitum a milk-based formula with protein content at or slightly less than the average protein content of human milk. On the basis of these observations, tentative conclusions were drawn concerning requirements for protein and certain essential amino acids during early infancy. Since the time of that publication, we have accumulated additional data on rates of gain in weight and length and serum concentrations of albumin of normal breastfed infants (2). In addition, we have studied other infants fed formulas with relatively low concentrations of protein.

Although we are not yet prepared to speculate further on requirements for essential amino acids, we believe that the newer data permit a more satisfactory statement regarding requirements for protein during the period 8 to 56 days of age.

SUBJECTS AND FEEDINGS

Normal fullterm Caucasian infants with birth weights of 2500 g or more were enrolled in the study during the first nine days after birth. Nearly all were children of students or younger staff members of the University of Iowa and several were siblings of children who had served as subjects of other studies reported from the Infant Metabolic Unit in recent years.

Birth dates ranged from January 1966 to July 1969. Birth weight and certain other data concerning each infant are included in the Appendix.

* Department of Pediatrics University of Iowa. Supported in part by Public Health Service Grant HD 00383 and in part by grants from Ross Laboratories and Mead Johnson and Company.
** Fellow of the Max Kade Foundation, New York.

Table 1. *Composition of formulas.*

	29B	3215A	3200AN
Components			
Protein			
cow milk	×	×	
sodium caseinate			×
Fat (% of total fat)			
corn oil	50	80	80
coconut oil	50	20	20
Carbohydrate			
lactose	×	×	×
Major constituents (g/100 ml)			
protein	*1.15**	*1.30*	*0.99*
fat	3.6	3.7	3.8
carbohydrate	7.8	6.9	7.4
ash	0.25	0.34	0.35
Density (g/ml)	*1.027*	*1.028*	*1.040*
Content of minerals (mg/l)			
calcium	*426*	*552*	*504*
phosphorus	*312*	*459*	*367*
sodium	230	368	272
potassium	507	626	556
chloride	390	461	
magnesium	*56*	*62*	*55*
iron	8.2	1.5	8.0
Content of vitamins per liter			
vitamin A I.U.	1800	1500	1500
thiamine μg	900	400	450
riboflavin μg	1600	1000	500
niacin μg	2900	4000	7000
pyridoxine μg	230	300	330
pantothenate μg	1740	2000	2000
ascorbic acid mg	92	50	50
vitamin D I.U.	400	400	400
vitamin E mg	3.4	5	5

* Italic values indicate our analysis. Other values are manufacturer's analysis.

Data on composition of the feedings are presented in table 1. Two formulas (Formulas 29B and 3215A) were based on fat-free milk solids, a mixture of corn and coconut oils and lactose. These feedings were studied with both male and female infants. Formula 3200AN, studied only with male infants, was generally similar to Formula 3215A except that it contained casein rather than fat-free milk solids; protein concentration of Formula 3200AN was somewhat less than that of Formula 3215A. Caloric density of each of the formulas was 67 kcal/100 ml. Protein concentration of Formula 29B, previously reported (1, 3) as 1.03 g/100 ml (manufacturer's analysis) is reported here as 1.15 g/100 ml (our analysis).

At the time an infant was enrolled in the study, his mother was interviewed by one of us (L.N.T.), details of the program were outlined and written instructions were provided.

Formulas were supplied in 120 or 240 ml ready-to-feed units. A supply of formula sufficient for 48 or 72 hours was weighed and delivered to the family. When a new supply was delivered two or three days later, the bottles from the previous supply (including any unconsumed amounts of formula) were collected and again weighed. At 30 days of age an iron supplement* was introduced into the diet of infants fed Formula 3215A and provided 15 mg of elemental iron daily as ferrous sulfate. As may be noted from Table 1, the other formulas had been fortified with iron by the manufacturer.

During the first 28 days of life, the formula served as the sole source of nutrients. Between 28 and 56 days of age the infants were permitted to receive oatmeal with applesauce and bananas.** Parents of experimental subjects were advised that addition of the strained foods was optional and that the designated formula was a complete food. No attempt was made to encourage feeding of the strained food.

Oatmeal with applesauce and bananas provided 77 kcal and 1.5 g of protein in 100 g of food with a density of 1.08 g/ml. Empty (or partially empty) jars of strained food were collected and weighed. Volume of formula and of strained food was calculated on the basis of weight of each food consumed divided by its determined density.

Data concerning three male and two female infants who received Formula 29B were included in previous reports (1, 3) but are not included in this report because they served as subjects for metabolic balance studies and therefore were managed in a manner somewhat different from that of the infants described here.

* Fer-in-Sol was supplied by the Mead Johnson Company, Evansville, Indiana.
** Gerber Products Company, Fremont, Michigan.

PROCEDURES AND METHODS

The infants were weighed and measured between 6 and 9 days of age and within 2 days of each of the following ages: 14, 28, 42 and 56 days. Weight and length were measured as described by FOMON (4). In describing size and change in size of the infants (Appendix and Table 2), recorded measurements were 'corrected' by parabolic interpolation or extrapolation utilizing three adjacent values to reflect values applicable to ages 8, 14, 28, 42 and 56 days.

Volume of intake per kilogram and intakes of calories and protein per kilogram for the interval 8 to 56 days were calculated in the following manner: The average daily intake (e.g., volume in ml/day) for each interval (i.e., 8–14, 14–28, 28–42 and 42–56 days of age) was divided by the average weight for that interval (assumed to be one-half the sum of initial and final weights) to yield intake per kilogram (e.g., ml/kg/day) for that interval. The weighted average of the values for all four intervals represents the value for the interval 8 to 56 days.

Blood for determination of albumin concentration in serum was obtained by venipuncture of the external or internal jugular vein. With few exceptions, 6 ml of blood were obtained between 1:00 and 1:30 pm; there was no restriction relating to the time of feeding.

Concentrations of albumin in sera were calculated from total protein concentrations and percentage of albumin as determined electrophoretically. Concentrations of total protein in serum were determined by the biuret method. The method was standardized with control sera which were, in turn, standardized by determinations of nitrogen using the Dumas method utilizing a nitrogen analyzer.* Separation of serum proteins into the various fractions was carried out by electrophoresis on cellulose acetate.**

Determinations of total protein content of sera from fasting normal adult subjects yield similar values whether determined by the biuret method or by the Dumas method. However, lipemia influences results of the biuret method and in recent studies we have found that with

* Coleman Instruments, Inc., Maywood, Ill.

** Model R-101, Microzone Electrophoresis Cell. Cellulose acetate membranes were scanned with Model RB, Analytrol, using Model R-102 Microzone Scanning Attachment with speed control set at 30. These instruments are from Beckman Instrument Company, Fullerton, Calif.

sera of infants obtained (as in this study) at variable intervals after feeding, lipemia occurs in some samples and may result in falsely high values. The error can be corrected by including a serum blank but this was not done in the present study. Nevertheless, all results reported here were obtained with the same method and we believe that comparison of results from the various feeding groups is not affected.

RESULTS

Fifty-nine infants were enrolled in the study and all but four completed 56 days of observation. The analysis to be presented pertains only to the 55 infants for whom complete data are available. However, information about all infants is presented in the Appendix, including reasons that four infants did not complete the study and comments on performance of these infants to the time of their withdrawal from the study.

Although strained oatmeal with applesauce and bananas was introduced into the diet as an optional food at 28 days of age, in most instances this food contributed only a small percentage of caloric intake. During the interval 28 to 56 days of age, six infants (one male and three female infants fed Formula 29B, one male infant fed Formula 3215A and one fed Formula 3200AN) received more than 10% of caloric intake (10.6 to 16.9%) and of protein intake (10.4 to 17.4%) from the strained food. Nine infants (one female infant fed Formula 29B, two male and three female infants fed Formula 3215A and three male infants fed Formula 3200AN) received between 5 and 10% of caloric and protein intakes from the strained food. All other infants received less than 5% from this source or no strained food at all. Average intakes of calories from the strained food were similar in the various feeding groups, ranging from 4.1% of calories by males fed Formula 3215A to 6.4% of calories by females fed Formula 29B. Thus, differences in performance of the various groups of infants can be interpreted primarily on the basis of differences in the formulas.

Data from a previous study of breastfed infants (2) have been included as a reference for evaluation of data on gains in weight and length and serum concentrations of albumin of infants receiving the various formulas.

Table 2. *Summary of results.*

	Males				Females		
	Breast-fed	29B	3215A	3200AN	Breast-fed	29B	3215A
Number of subjects	58	10	11	11	46	8	15
Volume of intake (ml/day)		701 (82)*	791 (137)	710 (104)		625 (66)	661 (82)
Volume of intake (ml/kg/day)		170 (21)	178 (31)	168 (16)		147 (18)	158 (19)
Caloric intake (kcal/day)		470 (55)	539 (93)	497 (72)		421 (42)	451 (56)
Caloric intake (kcal/kg/day)		114 (14)	121 (21)	117 (11)		99 (11)	108 (13)
Intake of protein (g/day)		8.7 (1.0)	10.6 (1.8)	7.5 (1.1)		7.8 (0.8)	8.9 (1.1)
Intake of protein (g/kg/day)		2.11 (0.26)	2.39 (0.41)	1.76 (0.16)		1.82 (0.21)	2.11 (0.25)
Gain in weight (g/day)	37.4 (8.4)	35.8 (6.7)	41.1 (6.1)	38.8 (8.1)	31.0 (7.1)	29.1 (6.3)	32.6 (7.3)
Gain in weight (g gain/100 kcal)		7.44 (1.10)	7.55 (1.07)	7.60 (0.85)		6.71 (0.97)	7.04 (1.05)
Gain in length (mm/day)	1.25 (0.17)	1.24 (0.13)	1.33 (0.09)	1.16 (0.12)	1.18 (0.17)	1.13 (0.14)	1.17 (0.17)
Gain in length (mm/100 kcal)		0.260 (0.028)	0.247 (0.042)	0.231 (0.038)		0.262 (0.028)	0.255 (0.035)
Albumin** (g/100 ml)	4.14 (0.34) N=36	3.90 (0.29) N=8	4.08 (0.41) N=8	3.58 (0.47) N=5	4.03 (0.35) N=27	4.13 (0.24) N=6	4.23 (0.30) N=14

* Values in parentheses are standard deviations.
** Concentration of albumin in serum at age 52–58 days; N indicates the number of determinations.

Table 3. *Statistical comparisons* of selected data from the various feeding groups.*

	Males			Females	
	29B	3215A	3200AN	29B	3215A
Gain in Weight					
Breastfed	NS	<0.01	NS	NS	NS
29B	–	<0.01	NS	–	<0.05
3215A	–	–	NS	–	–
Gain in Length					
Breastfed	NS	<0.01	<0.01	NS	NS
29B	–	<0.01	<0.05	–	NS
3215A	–	–	<0.01	–	–
*Albumin***					
Breastfed	NS	NS	<0.05	NS	<0.01
29B	–	NS	NS	–	NS
3215A	–	–	<0.05	–	–

* P values derived from Student's 't' test. N.S. indicates that the P value was greater than 0.05.
** Serum concentration of albumin at 54 to 58 days of age.

INFANTS FED MILK-BASED FORMULAS

Forty-four infants (21 males and 23 females) were fed formulas based on fat-free milk solids, corn oil, coconut oil and lactose. As may be seen from Table 1, protein concentration was slightly greater in Formula 3215A than in Formula 29B.

Summary data on mean daily volumes of intake, caloric intakes and intakes of protein between 8 and 56 days of age are presented in Table 2. Volumes of intake (ml/day or ml/kg/day), caloric intakes (kcal/day or kcal/kg/day) and, especially, intakes of protein (g/day of g/kg/day) were greater by infants fed Formula 3215A than by those fed Formula 29B.

Data on gains in weight and length of the infants are presented in Figure 1 and summarized in Table 2. Mean gain in weight by infants of the same sex was significantly greater by those fed Formula 3215A than by those fed Formula 29B (table 3). Mean gain by male infants fed Formula 3215A was significantly greater than that by male breastfed infants. Mean gain in weight per 100 kcal consumed was 7.44 g for males fed Formula 29B and 7.55 g for those fed Formula 3215A. Corresponding values for females were 6.71 and 7.04 g.

Mean gains in length were 1.24 mm/day for males fed Formula 29B and 1.33 mm/day for males fed Formula 3215A. Mean gain in length of breastfed males was 1.25 mm/day. The difference between mean gain in length by male breastfed infants and that by infants fed Formula 3215A was statistically significant (table 3). The difference between mean gain in length by male infants fed Formula 29B and by those fed Formula 3215A was also statistically significant. As may be seen from figure 1 and table 2, rates of gain in length were somewhat less by female infants fed Formula 29B than by breastfed females or by those fed Formula 3215A. However, these differences were not statistically significant (table 3).

The ranges of values for serum concentrations of albumin at 56 days of age were similar for male breastfed infants and for those fed Formulas 29B and 3215A (fig. 2). Mean values were also similar (table 2)

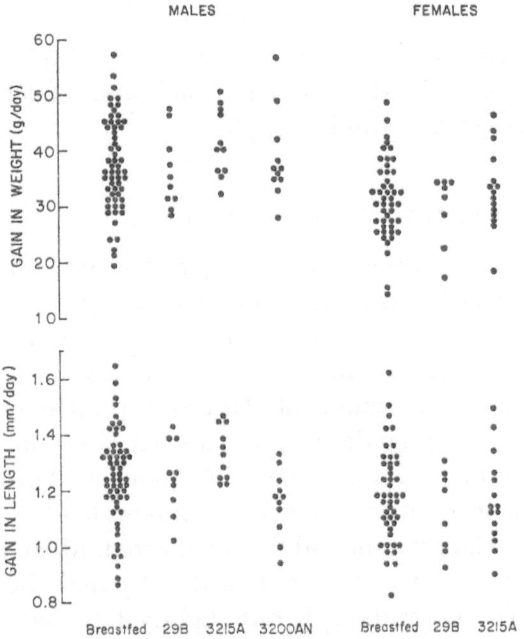

Fig. 1. Gains in weight and length in relation to feeding. Each point indicates the gain in weight (upper panel) or gain in length (lower panel) of one infant during the interval 8 to 56 days of age. The infants were breastfed or received experimental Formulas 29B, 3215A or 3200AN.

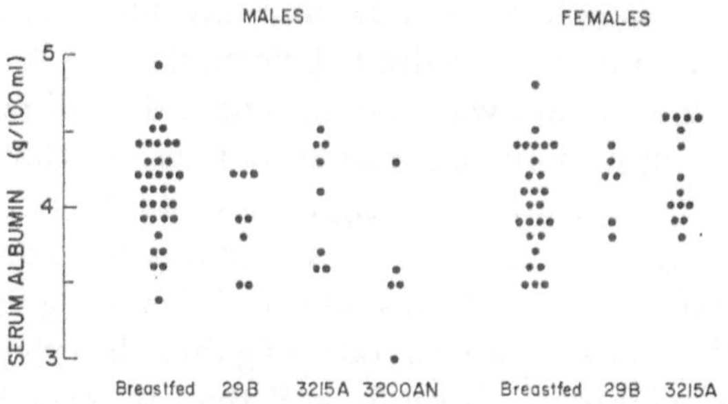

Fig. 2. Serum concentrations of albumin in relation to feeding. Each point indicates the serum concentration of albumin of one infant between 54 and 58 days of age. The experimental formulas are the same as in figure 1.

and the differences between the means were not statistically significant (table 3). Mean serum concentration of albumin of female infants fed Formula 3215A was significantly greater than that of female breastfed infants (table 3).

Mean serum concentrations of albumin of female infants fed Formula 29B were not significantly different from those of female breastfed infants or of those fed Formula 3215A.

INFANTS FED CASEIN-BASED FORMULA

Eleven male infants received Formula 3200AN. Protein concentration of this formula was less than that of Formula 29B or Formula 3215A (table 1). As may be seen from Table 2, mean volume of intake and mean intake of calories by infants fed Formula 3200AN were similar to those by infants fed Formula 29B. However, protein intakes averaged only 7.5 g/day (1.76 g/kg/day) by infants fed Formula 3200AN compared with 8.7 g/day (2.11 g/kg/day) by infants fed Formula 29B.

In spite of the lower protein intakes by infants fed Formula 3200AN, rate of gain in weight was not adversely affected. Mean gain in weight (38.8 g/day) was slightly greater than that by male breastfed infants and by those fed Formula 29B but slightly less than that by male infants fed Formula 3215A. The differences were not statistically significant (table 3). Mean gain in weight per 100 kcal consumed by infants fed Formula 3200AN was 7.60 g, a value similar to that for male infants fed Formula 29B or for those fed Formula 3215A.

Mean gain in length by infants fed Formula 3200AN was 1.16 mm/day, a value significantly less than that by male breastfed infants or by male infants fed Formula 29B or Formula 3215A (table 3).

As may be seen from figure 2, concentrations of albumin at 56 days of age were generally somewhat less in sera of infants fed Formula 3200AN than in those of breastfed infants or of infants fed Formula 29B or Formula 3215A. Mean serum concentrations of albumin are presented in Table 2. The mean value for male breastfed infants was significantly different from that of male infants fed Formula 3200AN. Similarly, the difference between the mean values for male infants fed Formula 3215A and for those fed Formula 3200AN were statistically significant (table 3).

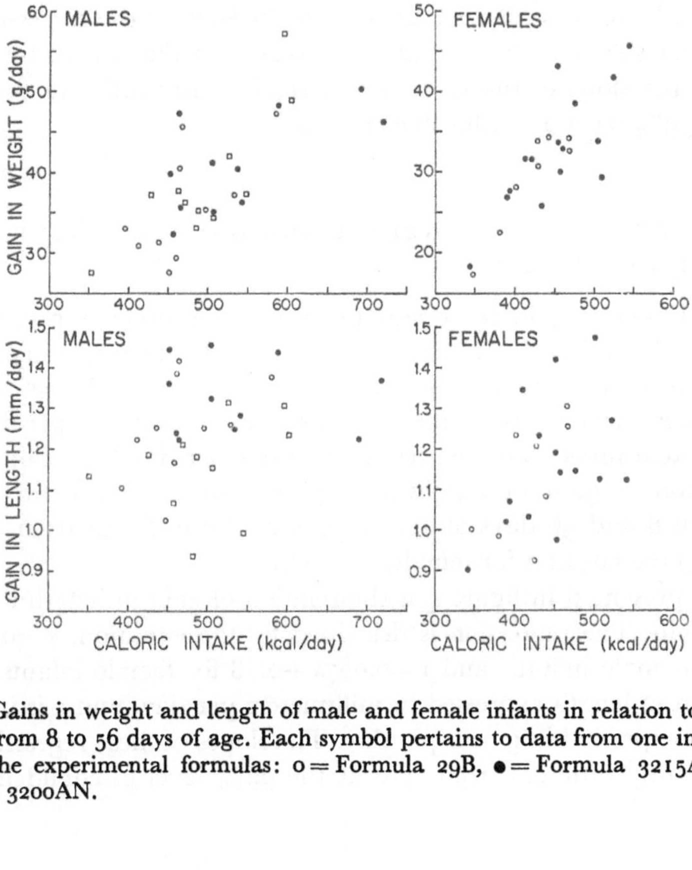

Fig. 3. Gains in weight and length of male and female infants in relation to caloric intakes from 8 to 56 days of age. Each symbol pertains to data from one infant fed one of the experimental formulas: o = Formula 29B, • = Formula 3215A, □ = Formula 3200AN.

RELATION OF GAIN IN WEIGHT AND GAIN IN LENGTH TO CALORIC INTAKE

As may be seen from figure 3, gain in weight between 8 and 56 days of age generally increased in relation to caloric intake. The regression of gain in weight on caloric intake is described for males by the equation, $y = 0.065x + 5.8$, where y is gain in weight expressed as grams per day for the interval 8 to 56 days of age and x is caloric intake, expressed as kilocalories per day during the same interval. The corresponding equation for female infants is $y = 0.109x - 16.5$. The slopes of these regressions differ significantly from zero at the 99% level of confidence ($r = 0.61$ and $r = 0.82$, respectively).

The regression of gain in length on caloric intake is described for males by the equation, $y = 0.0004x + 1.02$ and for females by the equation, $y = 0.0014 + 0.52$, where y is gain in length expressed as millimeters per day and x is caloric intake expressed as kilocalories per day. In the case of the male infants the slope of the regression does not differ significantly from zero ($r = 0.28$). In the case of the female infants the slope of the regression is significantly different from zero at the 99% level of confidence ($r = 0.47$).

RELATION OF GAIN IN WEIGHT AND GAIN IN LENGTH TO INTAKE OF PROTEIN

The relation of gain in weight to intake of protein is presented in figure 4. The relationship between gain in weight and intake of protein is described by the equation, $y = 2.1x + 20.1$ for males and $y = 5.1x - 11.9$ for females, where y is gain in weight expressed as grams per day, and x is protein intake, also expressed as grams per day. The slope of the regression of gain in weight (g/day) on intake of protein (g/day) between 8 and 56 days of age is significantly different from zero for males ($r = 0.50$) and for females ($r = 0.81$).

Also presented in figure 4 is the relation of gain in length to intake of protein. The regression is described by the equation, $\gamma = 0.032x + 0.97$, for male infants, and $y = 0.067x + 0.58$ for female infants, where y is gain in length expressed in millimeters per day, and x is intake of protein expressed in grams per day. The slopes of these regressions are significantly different from zero at the 99% level of confidence ($r =$

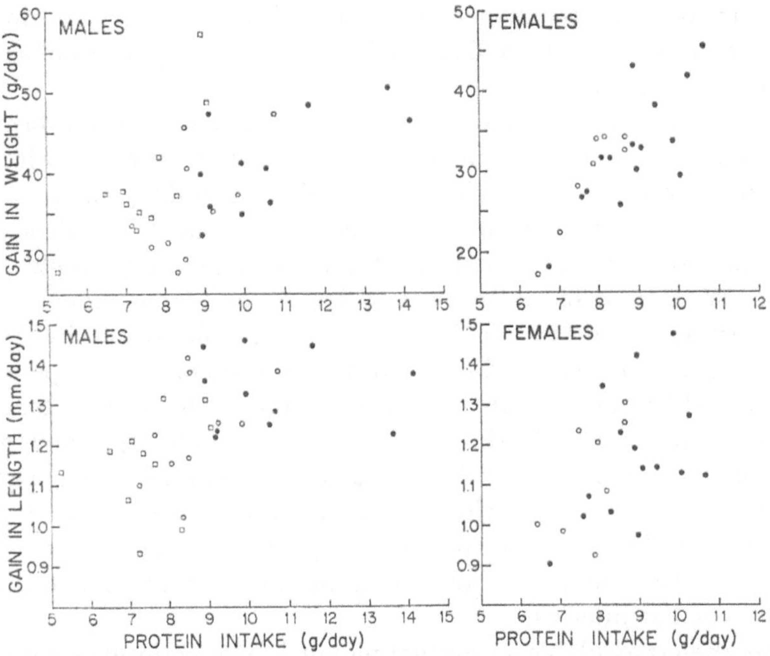

Fig. 4. Gains in weight and length of male and female infants in relation to protein intakes from 8 to 56 days of age. Each symbol pertains to data concerning one infant as indicated in Figure 3.

0.46 and r = 0.47, respectively). The statistically significant nature of the regression of gain in length of male infants on intake of protein is particularly noteworthy in view of the lack of a statistically significant regression of gain in length on caloric intake in these infants.

DISCUSSION

When infants are observed over a sufficient period of time while receiving a specified diet and demonstrate normal performance with respect to nutritional parameters, it is reasonable to assume that the diet is adequate in providing total calories and specific essential nutrients. For this statement to be meaningful with respect to the observations reported here, it is necessary to consider whether (a) the duration of our observations represent 'a sufficient period of time', (b) whether available parameters for evaluating nutritional performance are adequate, and (c) whether satisfactory reference values are available for these parameters.

Because it was anticipated that each of the experimental formulas would provide adequate intakes of all essential nutrients with the possible exception of protein, the duration of study (i.e., from 8 to 56 days of age) was chosen in the belief that it would be sufficient for detection of minimal evidences of protein deficiency, should these occur. We cannot, of course, exclude the possibility that a longer interval of study would have disclosed abnormalities not discernible in the present study. However, the period 8 to 56 days of age is a period of particularly rapid growth and there is reason to assume that the requirement for protein (in terms of grams of protein per day, gram of protein per kilogram per day or, during ad libitum feeding, of grams of protein per 100 kilocalories) is somewhat greater during this interval than during subsequent periods of less rapid growth. Thus, there would appear to be some reason for examining protein requirement during this particular interval.

Parameters available for evaluating nutritional performance include rates of gain in weight and length and serum concentrations of albumin. Data from our previous study (2) of normal breastfed infants may be used as a reference for evaluating results of the present study with respect to these three parameters. Other parameters include gain in weight and gain in length per unit of calorie intake or per unit of protein intake. Because food intake data are not available for the breastfed infants, these parameters are suitable only for comparisons between groups of formula fed infants.

In comparing mean gains in weight and length and mean serum concentrations of albumin of the various groups of formula fed infants with those of breastfed infants of the same sex, the only statistically significant differences observed were lower mean values for gain in length and serum concentration of albumin of male infants fed Formula 3200AN and higher mean gain in length and weight of male infants fed Formula 3215A.

The relation of gain in weight or gain in length to calorie intake is of value in assessing protein nutritional status only when absorption of nutrients is good. Whereas urinary losses are relatively unimportant in energy balance, fecal losses may account for a substantial percentage of calorie intake, especially in relation to loss of fat (5). With respect to the formulas fed in this study, data from metabolic balance studies with other infants receiving these same formulas (5, 6) indicate that fat absorption was good. Therefore, the lack of correlation between caloric intake and gain in length by male infants cannot be attributed to excessive losses of fecal fat.

On the basis of available data, it seems reasonable to conclude that Formula 3200AN was nutritionally inferior to Formulas 29B and 3215A. Two observations suggest that the inferiority was based on deficient quantity or quality or protein: (a) the low mean serum concentration of albumin, and (b) the observation that gain in length was more closely related to protein intake (fig. 4) than to calorie intake (fig. 3). Mean intake of protein and mean gain in length were less but mean calorie intake was slightly greater by infants fed Formula 3200AN than by those fed Formula 29B. Although these observations do not necessarily indicate that protein was the limiting essential nutrient in Formula 3200AN ,we believe that this explanation of the data is the most likely.

Even if one accepts the conclusion that protein was the limiting nutrient in Formula 3200AN, there appears to be little basis for speculation about whether the deficiency applies to total protein, to one or more essential amino acids or to both.

Because the observations reported here strongly suggest that Formulas 29B and 3215A provided adequate intakes of total calories and of all essential nutrients, it may be concluded that the requirement for cow milk protein was no greater than that provided by these feedings.

By expressing intakes of protein in terms of grams per kilogram of body weight, data from the present study may be compared with the 1.78 g/kg/day estimate of protein requirement (calculated by the 'factorial method') by the Joint FAO/WHO Expert Group (7) for infants from birth to 3 months of age. Mean protein intake by infants fed Formula 29B was 2.15 g/kg/day for males and 1.82 g/kg/day for females. In view of the presumably greater average daily requirement for protein per kilogram between 8 and 56 days of age than between birth and 90 days of age, the protein intakes by infants fed Formula 29B (which we interpret as no less than the requirement) appear to agree reasonably well with that calculated by the Joint FAO/WHO

Expert Committee. However, we are unwilling to assume, as does the Expert Committee, that requirement for protein per kilogram is the same for male and for female infants.

Mean intake of protein by male infants fed the casein-based Formula 3200AN was 1.81 g/kg/day. This intake of protein, almost identical to the FAO/WHO calculated value, was found to be inadequate. As already mentioned, we do not know whether the unsatisfactory performance of this group of infants was related to the quantity of protein, to its quality or to both.

The most satisfactory method of expressing protein requirement of infants will undoubtedly remain a matter of dispute. For infants fed ad libitum, we prefer to state protein requirement in terms of grams of protein per unit of calorie intake. This approach offers the simplicity of designating a single value rather than a range of values and yet allowing a greater absolute intake of protein for more rapidly growing infants who consume greater intakes of calories.

We therefore conclude that the requirement for protein from cow milk is no greater than 1.15 g per 67 kcal (1.72 g per 100 kcal). Because this ratio of protein intake to calorie intake appears adequate during the period of most rapid growth, there is every reason to believe that it will also be adequate during subsequent periods of infancy when growth is less rapid.

SUMMARY

Fifty-five normal fullterm infants, 32 males and 23 females, were studied from 8 to 56 days of age while receiving one of three experimental formulas of relatively low protein content. Food intakes were recorded for each day of study. Gains in weight and length and serum concentrations of albumin were determined and results were compared with those from a previous study of breastfed infants.

Mean gains in length and weight and serum concentrations of albumin of infants fed a milk-based formula providing 1.15 g of protein per 67 kcal (Formula 29B) were not significantly different from those of breastfed infants of the same sex. Gains in length and weight of infants fed a milk-based formula providing 1.30 g of protein per 67 kcal (Formula 3215A) were significantly greater than those of breastfed infants in the case of males but not in the case of females. Serum concentrations of albumin were not significantly different between infants fed Formula 3215A and breastfed infants of the same sex. It is concluded that the requirement for protein of normal fullterm infants is no greater than that provided by Formula 29B, i.e., 1.15 g of protein per 67 kcal (1.72 g of protein per 100 kcal).

Mean gain in length (but not in weight) and mean serum concentration of albumin of infants fed a casein-based formula providing 0.99 g of protein per 67 kcal were significantly less than those of breastfed infants. On this basis it is concluded that the formula was nutritionally inadequate, presumably in relation to protein quantity, protein quality or both.

REFERENCES

1. Fomon, S. J., and L. J. Filer, Jr., (1967) In: *Amino Acid Metabolism and Genetic Variation*, Nyhan, W. L., ed., McGraw-Hill, New York, p. 391.
2. Fomon, S. J., L. J. Filer, Jr., L. N. Thomas and R. R. Rogers, (1970) *Acta Paediat. Scand.*, Suppl. 202.
3. Fomon, S. J., L. J. Filer, Jr., L. N. Thomas, R. R. Rogers and A. M. Proksch, (1969) *J. Nutr.* 98:241.
4. Fomon, S. J., (1967) *Infant Nutrition*, W. B. Saunders, Philadelphia, Pa.
5. Fomon, S. J., E. E. Ziegler, L. N. Thomas, R. L. Jensen and L. J. Filer, Jr., (1970) *Amer. J. Clin. Nutr.* 23: (1299).
6. Fomon, S. J., E. E. Ziegler, L. N. Thomas, R. L. Jensen and L. J. Filer, Jr. Manuscript in preparation.
7. Joint FAO/WHO Expert Group on Protein Requirements (1965) *Protein Requirements*, WHO Technical Report Series, No. 301.

APPENDIX

Formula	Subject Number	Birth Weight (g)	Size: 8 days length (cm)	Size: 8 days weight (g)	Size: 56 days length (cm)	Size: 56 days weight (g)	Intake 8–56 days calories (kcal/day)	Intake 8–56 days protein (g/d)	Albumin* (g/100 ml)
				Males					
29B	126	3160	50.2	3226	56.2	4725	438	8.1	4.2
	127	3100	50.8	3280	56.8	4964	499	9.2	4.2
	130	3130	49.1	3285	55.7	5550	581	10.7	3.5
	132	3530	51.4	3545	–	–	–	–	–
	133	3350	50.8	3420	–	–	–	–	–
	134	3500	53.2	3640	–	–	–	–	–
	136	3720	52.4	4000	58.4	5779	533	9.9	3.9
	137	3380	52.3	3545	57.9	4950	460	8.5	–
	140	4150	53.8	3960	59.7	5444	413	7.6	–
	145	2550	47.5	2577	54.1	4521	465	8.6	3.9
	149	3800	52.7	3850	57.6	5178	450	8.3	4.2
	150	2550	48.8	2655	54.1	4245	395	7.3	3.8
	153	2860	49.2	2835	56.0	5022	466	8.5	3.5
3215A	950	3910	51.7	3797	57.6	6066	463	9.1	3.6
	951	3120	48.2	3307	54.1	5020	466	9.2	–
	952	3760	55.2	3955	62.2	5932	505	10.0	4.3
	953	3760	54.1	3665	60.6	5215	454	8.9	3.6
	954	3420	51.8	3578	58.2	5255	506	10.0	4.5
	955	3350	51.8	3385	57.8	5330	536	10.6	4.4
	956	3460	52.3	3600	58.5	5336	541	10.7	4.4
	958	3910	53.1	3840	59.0	6253	692	13.6	4.1
	960	3230	52.1	3380	58.7	5599	720	14.2	–
	962	3010	49.5	2878	56.5	4789	453	8.9	3.7
	963	2860	49.5	2940	56.4	5255	589	11.6	–
3200AN	1301	2940	50.2	3000	55.3	4816	462	6.9	3.5
	1303	3810	51.4	3800	57.2	5533	470	7.0	3.5

	[illegible]	[illegible]	[illegible]	[illegible]	[illegible]	[illegible]	[illegible]	[illegible]	
	1305	3230	52.0	3227	57.6	4912	488	7.3	3.6
	1306	3560	51.0	3474	57.2	6221	598	9.0	–
	1307	3160	48.9	3162	53.7	4946	549	8.3	–
	1308	3250	51.0	3175	56.7	4964	429	6.5	–
	1310	3370	49.4	3490	53.9	5074	484	7.2	–
	1311	2930	49.2	2728	54.6	4057	353	5.3	3.0
	1313	3500	52.9	3700	58.8	6048	604	9.1	4.3
	1314	3600	51.4	3607	56.9	5265	507	7.7	–
				Females					
29B	135	3180	49.3	3130	55.2	4473	400	7.4	–
	139	3180	51.8	3295	58.1	4862	469	8.7	3.8
	143	3600	51.9	3600	57.1	5242	443	8.2	4.2
	144	3680	51.7	3796	57.7	5435	468	8.6	3.9
	147	3290	50.7	3340	55.1	4818	427	7.9	–
	148	3900	52.3	3785	58.1	5413	428	8.0	4.3
	151	3540	49.4	3530	54.1	4604	381	7.0	4.2
	152	4080	51.8	4080	56.6	4903	347	6.4	4.4
3215A	975	4540	53.9	4400	58.2	5269	343	6.7	4.2
	976	3540	51.8	3670	58.4	5188	411	8.1	4.0
	977	4020	54.2	4275	59.6	5686	510	10.0	4.6
	978	3430	51.7	3710	57.2	5289	460	9.1	3.9
	979	3100	50.7	3289	56.6	4528	432	8.5	4.5
	980	3240	50.2	3275	55.7	5110	479	9.4	4.0
	981	3295	50.8	3350	56.5	4951	452	8.8	–
	982	2730	48.0	2814	53.1	4134	386	7.6	4.1
	983	3370	51.4	3325	56.1	4772	455	9.0	4.0
	984	3220	49.5	3297	55.6	5310	524	10.3	4.6
	985	3420	52.1	3385	57.1	4899	421	8.3	4.4
	986	2740	49.2	2820	–	–	–	–	–
	987	3360	50.9	3481	56.3	5672	545	10.7	3.8
	988	2780	47.8	2905	54.6	4976	454	8.9	3.9
	989	3240	49.8	3345	56.9	4960	502	9.9	4.6
	990	2910	48.9	2913	53.8	4197	385	7.6	4.6

* Concentration of albumin in serum at age 56 days

APPENDIX

The Appendix presents weight at birth and length and weight at age 8 days for each of the 59 infants. For the 55 infants who completed 56 days of observation, length and weight at age 56 days are also included. In instances in which serum concentration of albumin was determined at age 56 days, this value is also presented.

An attempt was made to determine the reasons that four infants failed to complete 56 days of observation and to evaluate performance of each of these infants to the time of withdrawal from the study. Three male infants fed Formula 29B failed to complete 56 days of observation. One of these infants (subject 132) was lost to follow-up for reasons that could not be determined after the visit at age 14 days. Gain in weight between 8 and 14 days of age was 15.8 g/day. Subjects 133 and 134 moved from town after the visit at age 28 days. Gains in weight between 8 and 28 days of age were 30.6 and 30.2 g/day, respectively, values slightly below the 25th percentile value (31.4 g/day) for male breastfed infants (2). Subject 986, a female infant fed Formula 3215A ,was withdrawn from the study by her parents after the visit at age 42 days because they did not wish to have blood obtained from her. Gains in weight and length between 8 and 42 days of age were 32.5 g/day and 1.09 mm/day, respectively.

DISCUSSION

Prof. McCance: I have two points.

The first is that protein requirements as you know depend upon the total caloric intake. So that the relation between your protein and your calorie intake per day is very important.

The other point is that your figure that approximates to 2 g protein per kg per day is an interesting one because Waterlow, and other people, think that that figure is quite sufficient to a child from extreme protein deficiency and provide for growth at a high rate.

Prof. Fomon: Dr. WATERLOW and I have discussed this point. We agreed that an intake of 10 grams of protein per day, most of it of high quality, should be adequate. Then the younger babies would receive more protein per kg and the older infants would get less.

Prof. Teller: What was the birth weight of your infants. Was there a great variation from just above praemature weight to full term infants? I ask this question because milk companies claim that it is good practice to feed praemature babies a high protein milk. Do you feel that from your data this is justified.

Prof. Fomon: Our data do not really help to answer that question. Birth weights of the infants are given in the Appendix of our paper. If I were to design an experiment to study the protein requirements of praemature infants in the fashion we have employed for study of fullterm infants, I would begin with greater protein intakes per kilogram and then gradually work down to lesser intakes.

Prof. Bickel: We are not only interested in your statement 'not greater than', but also in your other statement, which after all you put in; this is a little too low probably.

And for this statement, which may be very important for instance for treatment of infants with inborn errors, how much protein does a child really need and what is too little. I must say once more that

I think the criteria of length or albumin in plasma alone seem to me rather scanty. I just wondered if you had considered this question. Yesterday Dr. SNYDERMAN discussed aminoacid pattern in blood. That is another very sensitive criterium for too little protein which really went a little beyond your relatively crude statement of protein requirement.

Prof. Fomon: Our criteria are in a sense quite gross. On the other hand, Dr. SNYDERMAN pointed out that the aminoacid pattern of the blood changed within two days of changing the diet and therefore must primarily reflect recent dietary intake rather than nutritional status per se. I do not think that I would have great confidence in plasma aminoacid levels as a measure of protein nutritional status. We are interested in other measures that might be used in study of normal babies and should be anxious to receive your suggestions.

PROTEIN STATUS OF 'SMALL FOR DATE' ANIMALS

E. M. WIDDOWSON*

A baby or animal may be small at term for a variety of reasons, which are not all nutritional. Table 1 illustrates this. The weight of girl babies averages less than that of boy babies, and the work of LUBCHENCO, HANSMAN, DRESSLER and BOYD (1) showed that the mean weight of the male foetus was already greater than that of the female by the 24th week of gestation and that the average boy was heavier than the average girl from then onwards till term. This is true of other species too, the guinea pig for example, and it has been suggested that it may be due to greater antigenic dissimilarity when the foetus is a male (2). Whether this is the explanation or not, there seems no reason to suppose that females are more likely than males to be undernourished *in utero*.

Table 1. *Some causes of a small weight for gestational age.*

I. *Mother well-nourished*	
1. *Hormonal*	Females smaller than males
2. *Nutritional*	Slow foetal growth due to small blood flow to placenta and foetus. This may be caused by:
	a. Small size of mother
	b. A large number of foetuses competing for limited supply of nutrients
	c. Hypertension and toxaemia
	d. Intermittent constriction of blood vessels e.g. due to smoking
	e. Unfortunate siting in the uterus
II. *Mother malnourished*	
	a. Reduced blood flow
	b. Alteration in composition of blood?

* Dunn Nutritional Laboratory, Infant Nutrition Research Division, University of Cambridge and Medical Council.

All the evidence goes to show that the most usual reason why a foetus grows less rapidly than is usual and consequently becomes small for its gestational age, is because it has been provided with a small maternal blood flow. The placenta is usually correspondingly undersized. Foetal growth is often retarded if the number of foetuses in the uterus, or in one uterine horn, is large (3), because the blood flow in the uterine artery has to be shared among them. It may also be retarded if the foetus is in an unfortunate position in the uterus, where the blood supply is particularly poor (4, 5, 6, 7, 8). Growth is limited by a deficiency of all the nutrients, and the effects are similar to those of undernutrition after birth.

In species that generally have only one foetus a small mother tends to produce small young. When a large Shire horse was crossed with a tiny Shetland pony (9), the newborn foal was appropriate to the size of the mother in whichever direction the cross was made. The small foal received less blood *in utero*, but it is a nice point whether one considers it dysmature or not. It had not achieved its full growth potential for it immediately began to grow very rapidly after birth. It was undoubtedly small, but there is no evidence that it was less mature or less normal than the large foal.

An animal that has had too little food during pregnancy, or a diet containing little or no protein, may also produce small young. We do not yet know whether this also is entirely due to a reduced blood flow, or whether some alteration in the composition of the mother's blood plays some part. We are investigating this at the present time. Be that as it may, the extent of the effect depends not only upon the nature and degree of deprivation, but also upon the species. In rats the weight of the young at birth can be reduced by severe dietary restriction of the mother (10, 11, 12) but the effect is small, because the young are born relatively immature after a short gestation period. In guinea pigs, which have a much longer period of gestation, and which are much more mature when they are born, the weight at birth can be halved if the pregnant animal is suitably undernourished. Whether undernutrition of the mother is likely to have much effect on the growth of the foetus also depends on the relative size of the mother and young at term (table 2). A newborn guinea pig weighs about one eighth as much as its mother, so a litter of four amounts to half her total weight. A newborn pig, on the other hand, is only one two-hundredth

Table 2. *Size of young compared with size of mother.*

Species	Rat g	Guinea pig g	Pig kg	Sheep kg	Man kg
Weight of mother	300	800	200	80	60
Usual number of young	10	4	10	1 or 2	1
Total weight of young at birth	50	400	10	8 or 12	3.5
Mean weight of 1 young at birth	5	100	1	8 or 6	3.5
Total weight of young as % mother's weight	25	50	5	10 or 15	6
Mean weight of 1 young as % mother's weight	2.5	12.5	0.5	10 or 7.5	6

of its mother's weight, so a litter of 10 is only one twentieth of her weight, which is approximately the same fraction of its mother's weight as one full term human baby. In neither pigs nor human beings does maternal undernutrition greatly reduce the size of the young at birth.

STUDIES ON 'SMALL FOR DATE' PIGS

I have used runt pigs weighing only one third to one half as much as the rest of the litter at term as examples of dysmature animals born of well-nourished mothers. I have used two controls for these animals which are runts because they were implanted at a bad site in the uterus. a. Animals of the same age, that is large littermates of the full-term runts, and b. animals of the same size, that is well grown foetuses of about 90 days gestation. Full term in the pig is 120 days.

Our pigs that were 'small for date' had less than the normal amount of protein in their bodies, first because they were small, and second because the percentage of protein in the body was lower than that in their littermates (table 3). Both of these are signs of immaturity. The runt pigs, however, contained more protein than foetuses of the same size because the percentage of protein in their bodies was higher. They were therefore more mature than the foetuses in this respect. The difference between the amount of protein in the foetus and that in the full-term runt was entirely a matter of concentration, while the difference between the amount in the runts and in their littermates was mostly a matter of size.

Table 3. *Protein in body of pigs.*

	Foetus	Runt	Large littermate of runt
Gestational age days	90	120	120
Body weight g	576	578	1586
Total protein in body g	42	66	180
Protein in body (g/100 g)	7.3	9.7	11.3

All the organs of the runts were small and consequently contained less protein than those of their larger littermates. Table 4 shows that the muscle was affected more than the kidneys and the kidneys more than the brain. Most of the organs in the runts contained more protein than those of the foetuses of the same body weight, but the muscles did not. The quadriceps muscles of the dysmature pigs were smaller, and contained less protein than those of the foetal control.

Table 4. *Total protein in organs of pigs g.*

	Foetus	Runt	Large littermate of runt
2 Quadriceps muscles	0.42	0.32	1.20
Liver	1.55	1.52	5.45
Heart	0.27	0.49	1.02
2 Kidneys	0.28	0.35	0.85
Brain	0.87	1.39	2.05

Winick and Noble (13) have made the generalisation that early growth of all tissues is brought about by rapid cell division without any increase in the size of each cell. At a particular age for each organ the cells begin to increase in size while continuing to increase in number. When cell division has slowed down and eventually ceased growth is due entirely to an increase in the size of each cell. Finally this too stops and growth of the organ is over. Thus the number and size of the cells in an organ can be taken as an index of its maturity.

Like Winick and Noble I am using the amount of DNA in the organs as a measure of the number of cells, and the ratio of protein/DNA as a measure of their size. This is valid if we make three assumptions. 1. that the cells are mononucleated, 2. the nuclei are diploid and 3. that the amount of DNA in a diploid nucleus is constant – the value usually taken is 6.2 pg DNA per nucleus. Muscle fibres are multinucleated, and the amount of DNA does not measure the number of fibres, but it does measure the number of nuclei, and the protein/DNA ratio is an index of the average amount of cytoplasm with which each nucleus is associated.

Table 5. *Total DNA in organs of pigs mg.*

	Foetus	Runt	Large littermate of runt
2 Quadriceps muscles	22.0	15.9	31.0
Heart	16.1	30.0	46.3
2 Kidneys	28.5	37.7	65.8
Brain	25.5	35.2	48.3

Table 5 shows the total amount of DNA in the quadriceps muscles, heart, kidneys and brain of the pigs. If we compare the values for the well grown foetus of 90 days gestation and the large full-term animal we see that normal development during the last quarter of gestation is associated with a large increase in the amount of DNA and hence the number of cells in the heart, kidneys and brain, and a smaller increase in the number of nuclei in skeletal muscle. The small full-term runts had less DNA in all their organs than their age controls. Cell division had been hindered but not stopped entirely by the inadequate nutrition before birth, for the weights of DNA in the heart, kidneys and brain of the runt lay between those of the foetus which was of the same size, and the larger full-term animal of the same age.

Table 6. *Ratio protein mg/DNA mg in organs of pigs.*

	Foetus	Runt	Large littermate of runt
2 Quadriceps muscles	18.7	19.7	38.0
Heart	16.7	16.1	21.8
Kidneys	9.9	8.4	12.7
Brain	34.0	39.4	42.3

Not so, however, in the muscle. There nuclear division had not yet reached the stage of development found in the normal foetuses of 90 days gestation.

Table 6 shows the ratio of protein to DNA in the same tissues. The cells in all of them grew in size between 90 days gestation and full-term when growth of the foetus was normal, but in the runts growth in size was so delayed that the cells of the heart and kidneys were no larger at term than they were in a normal 90 day foetus. The same was true of the amount of cytoplasm per nucleus in skeletal muscle. In the runts' brains the cells were a little larger, but smaller than those in their normal littermates.

STUDIES ON 'SMALL FOR DATE' GUINEA PIGS

I am using guinea pigs to compare the effects of an unfortunate position in the uterus with those of severe undernutrition of the mother. Large newborn animals born of well-nourished mothers have been used as controls. Table 7 shows the weights of the organs of the three groups of animals at birth. It is known that in guinea pigs litters of more than 4 tend to be born prematurely, and the animals providing the data shown in table 5 all came from litters of 4 or less, and the mean number in the litter was the same in each group. Both ways of retarding growth produced small organs and, as in the pigs, the muscles were affected more than the brain. The 'small for date' animals born of well-nourished mothers had smaller muscles and hearts than those born of undernourished mothers, and these organs contained a little

Table 7. *Weights of organs of guinea pigs.*

	Mother undernourished	Mother well-nourished	
	Newborn small-for-dates	Newborn small-for-dates	Newborn normal size
Body weight g	62	62	114
Weight quadriceps muscles g	0.41	0.33	0.85
Weight heart g	0.33	0.26	0.48
Weight kidneys g	0.69	0.69	1.19
Weight brain g	2.30	2.35	2.62

Table 8. *Total protein in organs of guinea pigs.*

	Mother undernourished	Mother well-nourished	
	Newborn small-for-dates	Newborn small-for-dates	Newborn normal size
Body weight g	62	62	114
Protein in quadriceps muscles mg	63	58	133
Protein in heart mg	50	40	73
Protein in kidneys mg	93	93	161
Protein in brain mg	210	216	241

less protein (table 8). This may have been related to their gestational age when they first felt the effects of undernutrition. All the organs of both groups of 'small for date' animals contained less protein than those of the newborn animals of normal size.

Table 9 shows the amount of DNA in the organs. The muscles, heart and kidneys of the 'small for date' animals contained less DNA than the corresponding organs of the newborn of normal size, indicating that

Table 9. *Total* DNA *in organs of guinea pigs.*

	Mother undernourished	Mother well-nourished	
	Newborn small-for-dates	Newborn small-for-dates	Newborn normal size
Body weight g	62	62	114
DNA in quadriceps muscle mg	1.08	0.97	1.27
DNA in heart mg	0.97	0.89	1.24
DNA in kidneys mg	4.78	4.60	7.30
DNA in brain mg	4.67	4.80	4.80

nuclear division had been hindered by undernutrition before birth, whichever way the undernutrition had been brought about. The brains of the animals in all three groups on the other hand had similar amounts of DNA. It is known that the brain of the guinea pig has its full quota of DNA at the time of birth (14), and cell division in the brain of this species was evidently not hindered by the degree of undernutrition imposed by us before birth.

The size of the cells of the heart, kidneys and brain of the guinea pigs, as measured by the protein/DNA ratio, was not affected by the slow growth before birth as much as it was in the runt pigs (table 10 cf table 6). One reason for this may have been that the growth retardation was less – the 'small for date' guinea pigs weighed half as much as the larger newborn animals with which they were compared, whereas the runt pigs weighed only one third as much as their larger littermates. Furthermore, the cells in the organs of the guinea pig at birth are larger, and nearer their mature size than the cells in the organs of the newborn pigs.

The protein/DNA ratio was low in the skeletal muscle of both groups of 'small for date' guinea pigs, as it was in the muscle of the runt pigs (table 6). The development of muscle fibres, and the incorporation of nuclei into them after they have been formed from the myotubes, is a different process from the division of mononucleated cells. It was

Table 10. *Ratio protein mg/DNA mg in organs of guinea pigs.*

	Mother undernourished	Mother well-nourished	
	Newborn small-for-dates	Newborn small-for-dates	Newborn normal size
Body weight g	62	62	114
Quadriceps muscles	58	60	104
Heart	52	45	59
Kidneys	20	20	22
Brain	44	45	50

believed for a long time that once the myoblasts had fused to form myotubes there was no further mitosis, so that the number of nuclei in the myotube determined the number of nuclei in the fibre right on into adult life. During the past 10 years those concerned with the structure of muscle have been puzzled as to how the comparatively few nuclei that exist in foetal muscle are sufficient for the bulk of muscle in the adult, and it is now known that there is an increase in sarcolemmal nuclei throughout muscle growth in man (15). It now seems that this is brought about, not by mitosis of the original nuclei and DNA synthesis within the muscle fibre, but by the incorporation into the fibre of so-called 'satellite' cells (16). These are mononucleated and they divide like other mononucleated cells. The nett result is an increase in DNA in the individual muscle. There is also an increase in the protein/DNA ratio, and both these changes in the muscle are more severely affected by undernutrition before birth than they are in other organs with mononucleated cells.

One further point. The muscle of the normal newborn guinea pig, with a protein/DNA ratio of 104, is more mature in this respect than the muscle of the newborn rat or pig, but less mature than that of the human baby (table 11). Undernutrition before birth has hindered this aspect of maturation, but the muscle of the 'small for date' guinea pig is still more mature than that of the normal pig, and the muscle of the 'small for date' pig more mature than that of the normal rat.

Table 11. *Amount of protein (mg) associated with each mg of* DNA *in skeletal muscle.*

Species	Newborn	Adult
Rat	15	400
Pig		
Small-for-dates	20	380
Normal	38	
Guinea pig		
Small-for-dates	60	390
Normal	104	
Man	175	300

REFERENCES

1. Lubchenco, L. O., C. Hansman, M. Dressler, and E. Boyd, (1963) *Pediatrics* 32:793.
2. Ounsted, C. and M. Ounsted, (1970) *Lancet* 2:857.
3. Eckstein, P., T. McKeown, and R. G. Record, (1955) *J. Endocr.* 12:108.
4. Ibsen, H. L., (1928) *J. exp. Zool.* 51:51.
5. Rosahn, P. D. and H. S. N. Greene, (1936) *J. exp. Med.* 63:901.
6. Waldorf, D. P., W. C. Foote, H. L. Self, A. B. Chapman and L.E. Casida, (1957) *J. Anim. Sci.* 16:976.
7. McLaren, A. and D. Michie, (1960) *Nature*, Lond. 187:363.
8. Perry, J. S. and J. G. Rowell, (1969) *J. Reprod. Fert.* 19:527.
9. Walton, A. and J. Hammond, (1938) *Proc. Roy. Soc. B.* 125:311.
10. Chow, B. F. and C. Lee, (1964) *J. Nutr.* 82:10.
11. Zeman, F. J., (1967) *J. Nutr.* 93:167.
12. Hohenauer, L. and W. Oh, (1969) *J. Nutr.* 99:23.
13. Winick, M. and A. Noble, (1965) *Devel. Biol.* 12:451.
14. Dobbing, J. and J. Sands, (1970) *Brain Res.* 17:115.
15. Cheek, D. B., (1968) *Human Growth*, Lea and Febiger, Philadelphia, Pa.
16. Holtzer, H. (1970) In: *The Physiology and Biochemistry of Muscle as a Food*, 2, Briskey, E. J., R. G. Cassens, and B. B. Marsh eds., University of Wisconsin Press, Madison, p. 585.

DISCUSSION

Dr. Lindblad: You said that undernutrition of the pregnant woman has a 'small' effect on the foetus. Is the time factor in this situation of some influence? If you look at the world today, it is certainly a long-standing pre-pregnant undernutrition that is relevant. Are there any experiments in animals to study the influence on the foetus of long-standing pre-pregnant undernutrition?

Dr. Widdowson: I can tell you something about this in guinea pigs. When we start to undernourish the mother, or make her protein-deficient, as soon as she is mated she often produces no live young at all. Since our experiments depend on getting live young we now deprive the mother from halfway through gestation. This is sufficient to reduce the weight of each individual young by half.

Prof. Fomon: It was fascinating to see objective evidence of maturity of individuals based on skeletal-muscle. What would you consider the best organ or tissue to use for looking at greater versus lesser maturity in different species?

Dr. Widdowson: The muscle is the organ that is most affected, as it is in undernutrition after birth. The brain is the organ that is always least affected.

Prof. Fomon: Among species of animals delivered normally at term would you consider the protein/DNA ratio of skeletal-muscle, of brain or of kindey to be most useful in indicating maturity?

Dr. Widdowson: I think any of these. Also the physiological development of the animal is a very good index.

Dr. Schröter: You have shown that most of the organs are affected in the small for date animals. The postnatal increase of free fatty acids is much more marked in small-for-date infants than in well grown infants. If most organs are affected we have to assume that also the white and brown adipose tissue is deminished. How can we explain then the high increase of free fatty acids in human infants?

Dr. Widdowson: The human infant is exceptional in having so much fat in its body at birth. The pig has only 1% of fat when it is born, so it can hardly have a diminished content. The guinea pig does have fat, both white and brown fat. I am investigating the effect of prenatal undernutrition on the deposition of both kinds of fat at the present time.

Dr. Hull: I hope the one main point in my presentation will explain why free fatty acids go up more rapidly in dysmature infants. The question I wanted to ask is related to the previous question. How many of the findings that you described are reversible? How many are permanent? Is it possible to influence the loss by giving extranutrition?

Dr. Widdowson: As far as my evidence goes at present the organs of the adult that has been born small have less DNA and less protein than the orgens of animals that were large at birth.

INFANTILE MALNUTRITION: ITS PRODUCTION AND EFFECTS

R. A. MCCANCE*

Malnutrition may have numerous causes and affect all ages. Some of these causes alter amino acid metabolism and protein synthesis in highly specific ways. A deficiency of iodine is one and a deficiency of iron is another, but these must be relatively well known to you. Others may not be so familiar, but this is not the meeting at which to discuss them: only to point out that they exist.

I propose to devote the time at my disposal to the forms of malnutrition which are so widespread in the developing countries. Basically there are two quite separate metabolic syndromes. One is due to a deficiency of food as a whole, no matter how good the food may be, and this is best thought of as a deficiency of calories: the other is due to a deficiency of protein in a diet in which unlimited calories are available. These two syndromes affect amino acid metabolism in quite different ways, and it is these differences we shall be considering. Clinically the syndromes often appear to merge if the children, who are not getting enough protein, can not get or will not take plenty of carbohydrate. The cure for both syndromes is plenty of good food.

Malnutrition may affect children soon after birth but in most underdeveloped countries it is commonly a disease of toddlers from one to four years of age, and the age incidence varies for local reasons from one country to another. The cause is always a failure on the part of the child to pass smoothly from the milk of its mother to the household diet. If the mother has no milk the child is likely to reach in a starving marasmic state in a very short time. A similar fate commonly befalls twins towards the end of their first year even if their mother had plenty of milk at first, for children of this age can make little or nothing of the household food. In some parts of the world, and this

* Sidney Sussex College, Cambridge.

I think applies particularly to Jamaica and Johannesburg, the mother may try to eke out her meagre supply of milk with a very sweet cereal – or arrowroot – pap, and if so the children may be brought up at this relatively early age suffering from a deficiency of protein rather than one of calories, i.e. of total food.

At older ages the children have more chance of being weaned reasonably successfully on to the household diet, particularly if the mother continues to feed the child at the breast, and in Uganda it is at these ages that children are very apt to suffer from a deficiency of protein in areas where the staple food, e.g. cassava or bananas, contains very little protein.

Gastroenteritis may accentuate the child's difficulties. If it is severe it may injure the mucosa of the intestine and prevent it functioning as it should. The lactase is the enzyme most likely to be destroyed and this may make it impossible to treat the child with milk (1), (2). The children in some ethnic groups lose their lactase for genetic reasons soon after weaning, and if they then become malnourished the same problem of how to feed them will arise (3). Even if the enteritis is mild, the mother may feed the child on a very sweet pap as the only thing it will take and continue to do so long after the diarrhoea has cleared up. This is the reason why protein deficiencies are common in places such as Morocco where the staple is wheat, which is an excellent cereal containing 10 times as much protein as the banana and a far higher protein/calorie ratio. It has often occurred to me that CZERNY and KELLER's 'Mehlnährschaden' may well have fallen into this category and that 'Zuckernährschaden' might have been a happier name. Calorie deficiencies and protein deficiencies in young children were studied by KERPEL FRONIUS (4) and his colleagues many years ago, and his findings and judgements have been extended rather than modified by subsequent work. The following account of the effects of these two deficiencies on amino acid and protein metabolism is taken largely from his writings and three recent reviews of the subject (5,6,7). Only the most recent references and those not mentioned in these reviews have as a rule been quoted individually.

CALORIE DEFICIENCIES

The essential features of nutritional marasmus are 1. a diminished rate of growth with normal or high levels of growth hormone in the plasma. The degree of the diminution varies with the severity of the deficiency. The protein mass of the body is always small for a child of the same age and the weights of some organs relatively more affected than others. The fat and the skeletal muscles are most reduced. The result is a tiny wasted child without any subcutaneous fat and always hungry in the absence of complications. 2. A low metabolic rate and a slow protein turnover. This leads to a low rate of cell renewal in the gut and to a diminished excretion of hydroxyproline peptides in the urine. This has been made the basis of a test to find out whether a child, seen for the first time is growing at a satisfactory rate (8). The test usually gives an abnormal result if a child is not getting enough food, but is is not a specific test for this and, as it is based upon the hydroxyproline/creatinine ratio in a casual specimen of urine multiplied by the weight of the child, the result hinges upon a ratio and three variables. This makes for a wide normal range which lowers its diagnostic value in individual cases and precludes its use as an early sign of trouble. It should have a place in survey work but some authors have been dissatisfied with it. Another abnormality in calorie deficient children, which is also found in protein deficient children, is their poor response to tuberculin, even to 10 times the normal dose, which has been taken to indicate diminished cellular immunity (9).

In spite of this falling off in the rate of growth and the changes in protein turnover there are few alterations in the protein structure of the body, or in the amino acid equilibria inside and outside the cells. The volume of the extracellular fluids is increased relative to the weight of the body (10,11,12) but the percentages of the plasma proteins are not consistently changed. Anaemia is not a problem, the enzymes in the pancreatic juice (4) and succus entericus are present in normal amounts. It is in these respects that deficiencies of calories differ so strikingly from those of protein. There is no evidence of the retention of waste products, but hypoglycaemia is often a problem (13). The heart is small and histological changes of a non specific nature have been found in it but, in the absence of intercurrent infections and the necessity for fluid replacement, failure must be rare.

PROTEIN DEFICIENCIES

If the daily food of a child contains too little protein to meet its amino acid requirements for maintenance and growth before its energy requirements have been satisfied by the dietary carbohydrates and fat, a state of protein deficiency develops. The body becomes depleted of those amino acids which it cannot synthesise for itself, for there is always some wastage of these as they move into and out of the metabolic pool. This leads to characteristic alterations in the structure of the body consisting of a. a failure to grow at the normal rate in spite of high growth hormone levels in the plasma, and therefore to a fall in the intricate hydroxyproline index (14) in the urine, and other signs of delayed growth similar to those found in calorie deficiencies. b. A lower metabolic rate than normal (because the child is not growing) but usually a higher one than in the marasmic child who is not only not growing, but also deprived of the normal sources of energy. c. A fall in the albumin (4), β globulin and particularly in the siderophilin in the circulating plasma. This is probably due, or at any rate associated with, a fall in the turnover rate of these proteins in the absence of sufficient available amino acids. The rate of cell renewal in the mucosa, however, and the turnover of other proteins may be normal. The γ-globulins, for example, may be quite normal and their rate of production high in the presence of an infection. Differences may emerge in the way the different immunoglobulins are implicated or affected by protein deficiencies or calorie deficiencies, but recent work has not clarified the issue (15,16,17,18). d. The proportion of the lean body mass occupied by extracellular fluids is increased in all protein deficient animals – as it is in the calorie deficient ones, but in children it is usual for the increase to be extensive and oedema to be an important diagnostic sign. e. Peeling lesions of the skin, which are often moist in the flexures. f. Anaemia-sometimes associated with a megaloblastosis (19,20) g. A fall in the production of melanin leading to reddish hair. h. Differential changes in the amino acids in the circulating plasma and metabolic pool which lead to a fall in the normal ratio of essential to non essential ones (21,22,23). i. Subnormal amounts of copper but not of zinc (24) in hair and very low concentrations of copper and to a lesser extent of zinc in the dry fat free liver. These low concentrations are probably due to subnormal quantities of the specific binding proteins. j. Unusual metabolic pathways (25), a risk of hypoglycaemia and a disordered carbohydrate metabolism, and the appearance of abnormal metabolites in the urine.

The result of all these lesions is an anorexic, apathetic, miserable child, too short for its age, often quite fat, with a fatty liver, extensive skin lesions and reddish friable hair.

We have just been thinking about the protein status of animals – and babies – that are small for dates. The babies have many of the signs of an older child that is calorie deficient, but with a relatively normal protein 'Haushalt'. Thus, compared with their age controls, they a. have failed to grow and have a low excretion of hydroxyproline peptides (26). b. Contain more extracellular water per 100 g of lean body mass (27), but are not oedematous. c. Contain little or no fat. d. Have relatively normal serum proteins so far as they have been studied – while e. they do not have complete anorexia, skin lesions, anaemia, or discoloured friable hair. The children of women in poor socio-economic circumstances in Africa and elsewhere may have amino acid ratios after birth that suggest a deficiency of protein (28), (29), (30), (31) but aminograms and amino acid ratios require careful interpretation, and the time at which the specimens are taken is clearly critical. If the children are functionally protein deficient, moreover, their mothers must have been protein deficient also. While such mothers in my experience have often been on low protein diets, this does not necessarily imply that they have been protein deficient and they are usally capable of lactating for a year or more which does not suggest to me a deficiency of any kind.

REFERENCES

1. WHARTON, B., G. HOWELLS, and I. PHILIPS, (1968) *Brit. Med. J.* 4:608.
2. KERPEL FRONIUS, E., L. JÁNI, and M. FEKETI, (1966) *Ann. Paediat.* 206:245.
3. KEUSCH, G. T., F. J. TRONCALE, B. THAVARAMARA, P. PRINYANONT, P. R. ANDERSON, and N. BHAMARAPRAVATHI, (1969) *Am. J. Clin. Nutr.* 22:638.
4. KERPEL FRONIUS, E., (1957) *Mod. Probl. Paed.* 2:146.
5. Various authors, (1968) In: *Calorie deficiencies and protein deficiencies.* eds. Mc Cance, R. A. and E. M. Widdowson, Churchill, London.
6. WATERLOW, J. C., (1969) In: *Mammalian protein metabolism.* Vol. 3 eds. Munro, H. N. and J. B. Allison, Academic Press, London and New York p. 325.
7. MCCANCE, R. A. (1970) In: *Recent advances in paediatrics.* Gairdner, D. and D. Hull, eds. Churchill, London. p.

8. Whitehead, R. G., (1965) *Lancet*, 2:567.
9. Smith, N. J., (1970) Personal communication.
10. Kerpel Fronius, E. and S. Kovach, (1948) *Pediatrics* 2:21.
11. Kerpel Fronius, E. and F. Varga, (1953) *Acta Paediat.* 42:256.
12. Kerpel Fronius, E., (1960) *J. Pediat* 56:826.
13. Kerpel Fronius, E. and E. Kaiser, (1967) *Acta Paediat. Scand. suppl.* 172.
14. McLaren, D. S., H. Loshkajian, and A. A. Kanawati, (1970) *Brit. J. Nutr.* 24:641.
15. Aref, G. H., M. K. B. El Din, A. I. Hassan, and I. I. Araby, (1970) *J. Trop. Med. Hyg.*, 73:186.
16. El-Gholmy, A., O. Helmy, S. Hashish, R. H. Aly and V. El-Gamal, (1970). *J. Trop. Med. Hyg.* 73:192.
17. El-Gholmy, A., O. Helmy, S. Hashish, H. A. Ragan, and Y. El-Gamal, (1970) *J. Trop. Med. Hyg.* 73:196.
18. Simbeye, A. G. A., (1970) *J. Trop. Med. Hyg.* 73:200.
19. Adams, E. B., (1969) *Am. J. Clin. Nutr.* 22:1634.
20. Lynch, S. R., D. Becker, H. Seftel, T. H. Bothwell, K. Stevens, and J. Metz, (1970) *Am. J. Clin. Nutr.* 23:792.
21. Grimble, R. F. and R. G. Whitehead, (1970) *Brit. J. Nutr.* 24:557.
22. Arroyave, G., (1970) *Am. J. Clin. Nutr.* 23:703.
23. Weller, L. A., S. Margen and D. H. Calloway, (1969) *Am. J. Clin. Nutr.* 22:1577.
24. Bradfield, B. R., T. Yee and J. M. Baertl, (1969) *Am. J. Clin. Nutr.* 22:1349.
25. Read, W. W. C., D. S. McLaren, M. Tchalian, and S. Nassar, (1969) *J. Clin. Invest.* 48:1143.
26. Younoszai, M. K. and J. C. Haworth, (1968) *Pediat. Res.* 2:17.
27. Cassady, G., (1970) *Ped. Clin. North Amer.* 17:79.
28. Lindblad, B. S., (1970) *Acta Paediat. Scand.* 59:13.
29. Lindblad, B. S., J. Razia, Rahimtoola and Nafees Khan, (1970) *Acta Paediat. Scand.* 59:21.
30. Mestyán, J., M. Fekete, Gy. Soltész, L. Lajos, L. Gáti, J. Preisz and J. Doszpod, (1969) *Biol. Neonat.* 14:153.
31. Mestyán, J., M. Fekete, I. Járai, E. Sulyok, S. Imhof, Gy. Soltész, (1969) *Biol. Neonat.* 14:164.

DISCUSSION

Dr. Papadatos: What is the commonest cause of death in the two groups of babies you have described: in the starved babies and in the protein deficient babies.

Prof. McCance: The cause of death during treatment in marasmic children is usually intercurrent infection. They shouldn't die. They are hungry. The important thing is to give them enough to eat. Most people fail to do this and this prolongs their time in hospital or their exposure to intercurrent infections. The protein deficient children are very vulnerable and you have to treat them with great care. The commonest cause of death is heart failure. It is due partly to the fact that they are oedematous which is itself partly due to a fall in plasma albumin and partly to an element of low cardiac output. The danger of heart failure is especially high when they are anaemic. When you treat these children with a high protein diet they synthesize albumin very fast, expand their plasma volume, and this is accentuated if the food contains salt. There may be no change in plasma albumin but the haemoglobin may fall two grams per cent in the first three days. This is enough to induce heart failure. They get sudden enlargement of the liver and die.

Prof. Bickel: I'm very interested in the aspect of brain function and mental retardation. Recently there has been a lot of speculation, that in slum areas where the children are protein deficient there will be later on insufficient brain development and brain damage. You have here some extreme situations as I understood of protein deficiency versus caloric deficiency. I just wondered if you have found differences of mental development between those two groups. Have you paid attention to the development of mental function in children, who were born to very protein deficient mothers.

Prof. McCance: I personally have not, but there is a big litterature about this. I have tried to summarize this in my paper. The great difficulty here is that it is almost impossible to establish a satisfactory control.

Dr. Veeger: May I ask you a question about the lactase defiency. Lactase deficiency is a racial factor in Uganda people after weaning. Secundary lactase deficiency does occur in protein deficiency. It is becoming increasingly common to send milk and milkpowder to those countries. The question is if they should send normal cow milk or milk without lactose. What is your opinion about this very practical question?

Prof. McCance: You can demonstrate a lactase deficiency in these children by giving a lactose load. We gave adults and children lactose and found it easy to show that they were often partially or wholly lactase-deficient. Milk, however, is on the whole well tolerated, because the milk given does not contain so much lactose as the test dose and its absorption is slower. All the children with protein deficiency were given milk. We had only one period when many children had gastro-enteritis and some of these children we had to treat on diets containing no lactose. I think that this is the answer. You can treat with milk and in 9 cases of the 10 the children will have enough lactose to deal with the lactose given them. The cost of taking out lactose is very great, and too expensive to make it necessary.

The other point I would like to make is this. The child gets diarrhoea, the mother puts it on a very sweet food mixture. When the child gets better the mother maintains it on this diet. Some months later the child comes in with kwashiorkor. Protein deficiency is not only common in Uganda but also in Johannesburg where they eat maize and in Morocco where they eat wheat. Sugar is the reason for this protein deficiency, it is not primarily the fault of the basal diet.

Prof. Visser: May I come back Sir to the small for date babies. I think you are quite right in saying that those babies are suffering from a calorie-deficiency syndrome. This may have practical implications. Would you recommend calories or proteins for such a group of pregnant women. What about treatment of small for date babies after birth? How much calories would you recommend, how much protein?

Prof. McCance: A good diet will cure both protein-deficiency and calorie-deficiency. This has confused the clinician, for as he is often faced with mixed syndromes and knows that good food will cure both he has ceased to diagnose whether the child is calorie-deficient or protein-deficient. This has greatly delayed our understanding of the metabolic picture or biochemical findings. People have investigated the aminoacid ratio in malnutrition without bothering to make the differential diagnosis and then, after finding normal and abnormal figures they have concluded that the test was no good. The figures should be normal in the marasmic child, and abnormal in the protein-deficient child. I don't think I could choose a diet for the small for date infants other than good food and a protein intake appropriate for a child of that size.

SESSION II

GENERAL DISCUSSION

Dr. Young: I would be very interested to know why foetuses have such a high plasma glycine level. I think it is known more or less why there is a high alanine level. High plasma alanine levels occur when a lot of transamination is taking place and low alanine levels are present when gluconeogenesis takes place.

Dr. Lindblad: The characteristic change in protein undernutrition is a plasma glycine, alanine and proline increase. Collagen is a polypeptide of primarily these three aminoacids. The changed homeostasis of free aminoacids might reflect an increased breakdown and decreased synthesis of collagen.

I studied hypopituitary dwarfs. The thought was what we were actually registering was not malnutrition but decreased growth. Those dwarfs however had only an increase of proline and not of alanine and glycine.

Prof. Fomon: It is increasingly common to provide complete parenteral nutrition through a centrally placed venous catheter to babies who are seriously ill. Aminoacids in the infusion are provided by hydrolysates of either fibrin or casein. The aminoacid pattern is therefore quite unlike that of human plasma. Do you think that this may offer some potential problems?

Dr. Lindblad: I think we know very little about the optimal aminoacid requirements. Today, the best we can do is probably to compose a mixture with an aminoacid composition as close to human lactalbumin as possible. This means the use of synthetic mixtures rather than hydrolysates.

Prof. Wolf: Could I make a comment on the question of parenteral feeding with aminoacids. We did some studies with so-called blood-pattern aminoacid mixtures, which resembled the plasma aminoacid composition. Those solutions were given to praemature and small for date infants. We didn't see major excretion of aminoacids in urine. With another mixture of aminoacids, a requirement-adapted composition, we saw a high excretion of aminoacids in the urine.

Dr. Widdowson: To Dr. YOUNG. You mentioned, and I know you have pointed this out before, that there is a much bigger difference between maternal and foetal plasma aminoacid levels in the guinea pig then in other species. In the guinea pig very peculiar in this respect? And why? Has it something to do with the rate of growth of the foetus or with the type of placenta?

Dr. Young: I think the foetal-maternal plasma aminoacid ratio in the guinea pig is particularly high due to the very low maternal levels. I have already mentioned that the low maternal levels which one usually finds in pregnant women, the erve or the guinea pig must be partly due to the high circulating oestrogen and progesteron. The foetal to maternal weight ratio is particularly large in guinea pigs at term. A part of the low aminoacid levels in the maternal guinea pig may be due to a relatively high foetal uptake.

Dr. Henssen: Prof. McCANCE has spoken about babies that were small for date on account of malnutrition. In our country we have babies that are small for date babies due to placental insuffieciency. The uterine blood flow has been too low. Do these children born after pregnancy with placental insufficiency grow up normally?

Prof. McCance: If the delay has been relatively small, children whose growth has been delayed by calorie or protein deficiency will get back on their normal growth. But if the delay has been severe, and you must remember that the delay is often very severe and not necessarily entirely nutritional; for malaria, parasites, hookworms and so on, may come into it and the children may have fallen very behind by the age of 3 or 4. Then they may grow at a normal rate, as fast as children in this country, but they exhibit no 'catch up' growth and remain small at every age compared with children in Holland.

When the children in Holland reach the age of 18 however, they stop growing, for by this age they can reach their full genetic stature. But the children who have not reached that stature as in the underdeveloped countries can go on growing until they are 20, 22, 24 years of age and maybe by that age may reach it. There was a very fine piece of statistical work done in Holland on this subject by Dr. Oppers. Very interesting figures have been published recently about this from the Congo by Dr. Vis.

Dr. Lindblad: You were saying that a high protein intake could lead to heart failure. Do you advice a low protein intake in kwashiorkor? Is that correct, Prof. McCance?

Prof. McCance: No, not quite. I must have put my case badly. These children who come in with protein deficiency have got oedema and they are vulnerable to feeding. But it is the salt that is the main cause of the trouble, it is not the amount of protein. If you take all salt out of these children diet you can feed them much more safely.

Dr. Troelstra: Our group has observed a child with hyperglycinaemia from the first weeks of life. In stead of protein we were giving a mixture of aminoacids in total amount of 1.5 to 2.0 g per kg per day, without glycine and serine. After a few months we decreased the amount of aminoacids because glycine level in blood was still high. The total amount of aminoacid was lowered to 0.75 g per kg per day. There were two remarkable points: the glycine level was still higher and the plasma protein was going down. The child developed oedema and his general condition deteriorated. So we had to give again the higher amount of aminoacids. With this intake of aminoacids her growth in respect to gain in length and weight was satisfactory during an observation period of one year or more. This may be of some interest in regard to minimal requirements of aminoacids in artificial feeding.

Prof. Fomon: It is important to remember that the requirement for nitrogen provided as a mixture of amino acids is almost surely not the same as the requirement for nitrogen provided as whole protein.

Dr. Hull: I understand this was a patient with non-ketotic hyperglycinaemia. We have a child with ketotic hyperglycinaemia with propionicacidaemia in which we had the same problem, namely rearing a child on as low protein diet as we could. We were also assessing serum glycine levels. In fact there seems to be very little correlation between the amount of glycine the child was fed and the amount in the blood. I would like to ask the experts whether a high level of glycine is toxic or not? Does it matter if the glycine level in the blood is high? This child was given protein 0.75 g per kg per day for a long period. Its growth in length appeared to be satisfactory, its weight however was not.

It proved a very difficult child to assess the effect of his low nutrition on his intellectual development, because we don't know how much of his delay was a consequence of the basic defect and how much was a consequence of the diet we have been giving.

We have in fact treated this child with biotin, in the hope that this will stimulate the enzyme that has been lazy. This has produced a biochemical improvement, it has not produced a clinical improvement.

Prof. Jonxis: Does anybody know about the toxicity of high glycine levels in the blood?

Dr. Hommes: I don't think the glycine as such is toxic. The fact that you observe a high glycine level in blood certainly means something. The normal metabolism is somehow disturbed, which may be toxic. This is however different from a glycine toxicity per se.

SESSION III

CARBOHYDRATE-FAT METABOLISM

THE DEVELOPMENT OF INSULIN SECRETION IN MAN

R. D. G. MILNER*

The function of the β cell of the islets of LANGERHANS in the human foetus and newborn has, for obvious reasons, been more difficult to study than the morphology of endocrine pancreatic development. In many mammalian species islets develop in two 'generations' (1): a primary generation that grows out from the solid cords of cells which will form the primitive pancreatic tubules and a second generation that appears after the acini have formed and arises either from the acinar cells (2) or, in common with acinar cells, from the cells of the pancreatic ductules (3). Only LIU and POTTER (4) have described two definite generations of islets in human tissue, the first beginning at the eighth week of gestation from the primitive ducts and the second, during the third month of intra-uterine life, from the terminal ducts. The histological and histochemical development of the interacinar or secondary islets has been described in detail (5, 6, 7, 4, 8, 9, 10). Granulated β cells are first seen at nine weeks (7). Electron microscopy at this stage of development has shown the islets to contain β cells and two kinds of α cells, α_1 cells containing faint globular granules of unknown function and α_2 cells with electron dense granules containing glucagon (11, 12). The spatial and numerical relationship of β and α cells changes through the second and third trimesters. In foetal life α cells are always more numerous than β cells but the proportion of β cells increases with development so that at birth the ratio of α:β cells is approximately unity (13, 14). In contrast the α:β cell ratio in adult man is between 1:3 and 1:9 (15, 16). The changing ratio could be explained by a differential rate of development of α and β cells or by more rapid involution of the α cell population. Changes suggestive of degeneration of the α cells during the last three months of intrauterine

* Department of Child Health, University of Manchester, St. Mary's Hospital, Manchester 13, England. This work was supported by grants from the Medical Research Council and the British Diabetic Association.

life have been noted (4) as has degeneration of whole islets (17) but the significance of these observations remains unexplained. Early in pregnancy the α and β cells exist in adjacent clusters in a bipolar islet. Later the β cells are enveloped by α cells in a mantle islet and after 30 weeks the two cell types become intermingled as they are in the mature adult islet (8).

Correlation of islet histology with pancreatic insulin content offers another method of assessing β cell development. GRILLO and SHIMA (18) found insulin in the pancreas of a human foetus of 80 mm crown-rump length but not in a 35 mm foetus, which led them to conclude that insulin synthesis occurred before β cell granulation. The pancreatic insulin content rises later in pregnancy to much above adult levels, being 6.3 ± 1.1 U/g between 20 and 32 weeks and 12.7 ± 3.2 U/g between 34 and 40 weeks whereas in the adult it is 2.1 ± 0.3 U/g (43).

Insulin secretion *in utero* has been studied by the injection of various substances into foetuses at operation for termination of pregnancy. Neither glucose nor arginine stimulates insulin release under these conditions between weeks 13 and 19 of foetal life (83, 19). Insulin has been detected in amniotic fluid beyond 16 weeks gestation in concentrations similar to those found in normal adult blood (20). It has not proved possible to state definitely whether the hormone is foetal or maternal in origin, or whether the concentration changes meaningfully in response to glucose loading.

The sampling of blood from the foetal scalp for glucose and insulin measurements during labour, before and after giving the mother intravenous glucose, (21, 22, 23) has confirmed the results of earlier work (24) in which the effect of hyperglycaemia on plasma insulin levels in mother and baby at the time of birth was studied. Intravenous glucose given to the mother during the second stage of labour caused maternal and foetal hyperglycaemia, a rise in maternal plasma insulin levels but only a small and slow rise in foetal plasma insulin levels (table 1). The variable metabolic and hypoxic stress of labour on the foetus makes it difficult to assess whether observations made at this time reflect accurately the physiological competence of the developing β cell.

Work has been reported indicating that the human placenta has a limited permeability for insulin in both directions (80) or from foetus to mother only (25) but the balance of evidence suggests that the placenta is impermeable or of such limited permeability that the in-

Table 1. *Maternal and umbilical cord concentrations of blood sugar and plasma insulin.*

Group	No. of cases	Blood sugar (mg/100 ml)		Plasma insulin (micro units/ml)	
		Mean ± S.E.	Range	Mean ± S.E.	Range
Control patients:	31				
Mother		97 ± 3	74–128	29 ± 4	<6–79
Baby		82 ± 3	52–122	9 ± 1	<6–19
Glucose infusions:	17				
Mother		120* ± 7	76–181	36 ± 6	10–110
Baby		100* ± 6	53–147	18* ± 5	<6–89
Glucose injection-birth interval:					
4–20 (mean 12) minutes	12				
Mother		196* ± 11	143–284	44* ± 4	27–68
Baby		160* ± 10	90–216	13* ± 1	<6–19
21–60 (mean 40) minutes	9				
Mother		163* ± 11	107–204	50* ± 6	19–75
Baby		155* ± 10	99–193	11 ± 2	<6–28
61–100 (mean 84) minutes	9				
Mother		119* ± 9	80–174	58 ± 14	23–170
Baby		109* ± 9	80–164	28* ± 5	9–64

* Denotes $P < 0.05$ in comparison with control patients.
Taken from reference (24)

sulin transported is of no functional importance (26, 22, 19, 27, 28).

Glucose is a relatively poor stimulus of insulin secretion in the premature or full-term normal newborn (29, 30, 31, 32, 33) but this does not mean that the β cell is unresponsive to all stimuli, Milner and Wright (34) showed that glucagon caused insulin release in the full term newborn. In the premature infant both glucagon and a mixture of nine essential amino acids are potent stimuli of insulin release (31). Measurements of urinary insulin exretion suggest that there is a sixfold rise in insulin production over the first five days of life in the normal newborn (35).

Hypersecretion of insulin in infants of diabetic mothers and haemolytic disease of the newborn is considered in detail below. Rarer causes include insulinoma of the pancreas (36) and it has been suggested that hyperinsulinism may be associated with a congenital absence of α cells (37, 38, 39).

MATERNAL DIABETES MELLITUS

The precocious development of the foetal β cell in maternal diabetes mellitus is well understood (see reviews: 79, 82). The foetus of a diabetic woman well controlled with insulin is intermittently hyperglycaemic and has maternal insulin antibodies in the circulation (40, 41). Hypertrophy and hyperplasia of the foetal islets occurs (42), accompanied by an increase in pancreatic insulin content (43). The islet hyperplasia may be accompanied by eosinophilic infiltration and fibrosis, changes which have been called sub-acute interstitial pancreatitis (44). The lesion may be the result of prolonged exposure of the foetal β cell to insulin antibodies, for if mice are given repeated intraperitoneal injections of insulin antibody there is rapid and persistent β cell degranulation followed by infiltration of the islets with eosinophils, neutrophils and monocytes (45).

Hypersecretion of insulin occurs *in utero* causing increased lipogenesis (46) and persists for a variable time following birth. Hyperinsulinaemia in the baby is difficult to quantitate because of interference by circulating antibody in the immunoassay system used for the measurement of insulin (47). The offspring of women with diabetes who are not treated with insulin have postnatal hypoglycaemia intermediate in severity between that of normal babies and that of insulin-treated diabetics, indicating a modest hypersecretion of insulin (48) which has been confirmed by plasma insulin measurements during glucose tolerance tests (33, 49). The insulin response to sustained hyperglycaemia indicates however that there may be no difference in insulin secretion between infants of normal and diabetic mothers when the glucose stimulation is chronic (50). In one study of the long-term effect on β cell function of this abnormal intrauterine experience (49) the offspring of diabetic women were investigated at birth and again when two years old. Six of the nine two-year old infants tested had abnormally high blood glucose responses to intravenous glucose. In four this was associated with hyperinsulinaemia and in two with hypoinsulinaemia.

The infant of a diabetic woman treated with oral sulphonylureas may be at a particular disadvantage. Not only is the foetus exposed to hyperglycaemia but also to the sulphonylurea drugs which cross the placenta (51) and stimulate further the secretion of insulin by the foetal β cell. Such an infant is born hyperinsulinaemic and with therapeutic levels of an insulinotropic drug which is degraded slowly because of the immaturity of the foetal liver (52). These babies may suffer profound intractable hypoglycaemia for which treatment by exchange transfusion is necessary to remove the drug and restore the blood glucose level to normal (53, 54). Glucose tolerance tests in these babies

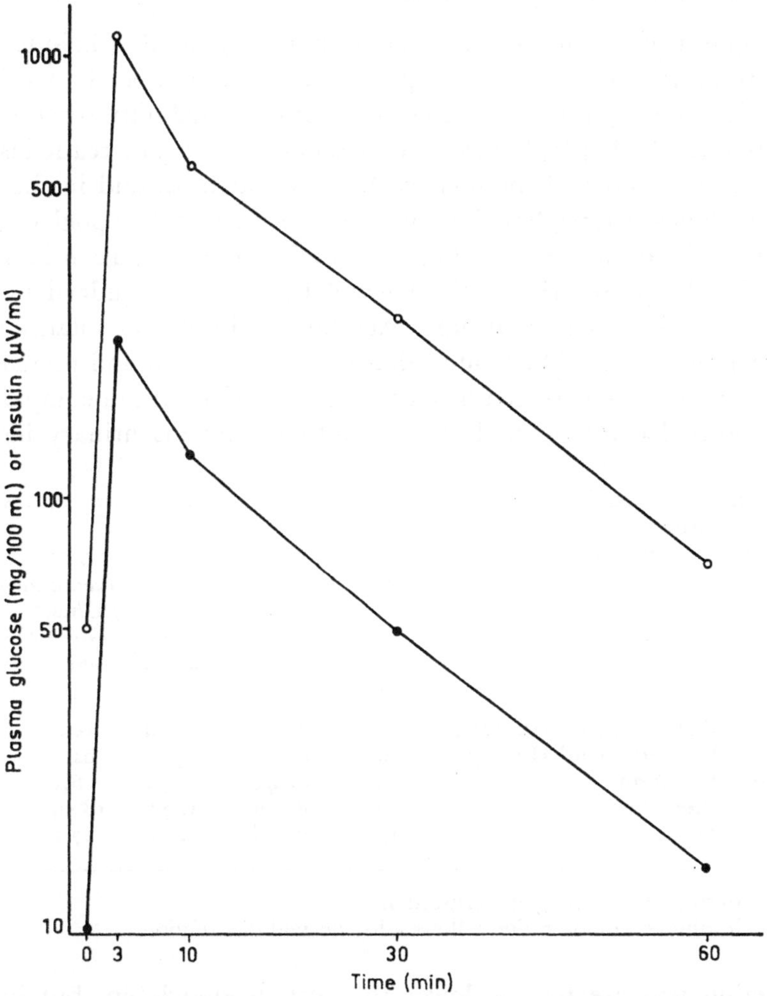

Fig. 1. Intravenous glucose tolerance (0.5 g glucose/kg body weight) at age of 30 hour in the infant of a diabetic mother who had been treated with tolbutamide during pregnancy. Note logarithmic scale on vertical axis. Open circles: plasma insulin; solid circles: plasma glucose. Taken from reference (53).

have resulted in the highest plasma insulin levels yet recorded in the newborn (fig. 1) (53) and although not all such infants become hypoglycaemic (55) it seems prudent to avoid maternal therapy which can cause foetal disease (56).

ERYTHROBLASTOSIS FOETALIS

Although it has been known for more than 30 years that infants with erythroblastosis foetalis have hyperplasia of the islets of Langerhans (57, 58, 59) its significance has not been appreciated until recently. In addition to islet hyperplasia such babies have a high pancreatic insulin content (60) and high plasma insulin levels at birth and in the succeeding hours (61, 62, 63). This may be associated with hypoglycaemia (64, 65). Schiff and Lowy (66) have studied the association between gestational age, severity of the haemolytic process as judged by the cord haemoglobin and urinary excretion of insulin of infants with haemolytic disease. They found that in both full-term and premature infants there was increased urinary excretion of insulin in comparison with normal controls (table 2). In full-term infants urinary insulin

Table 2. *Urinary insulin excretion in normal infants and infants with haemolytic disease (HDN).*

Babies		Number	Gestation wk	Insulin/creatinine ratio μU/mg*		
				mean	+SEM	−SEM
HDN:	Full term, cord Hb > 13 g	6	36–39	6.9	10.0	4.7
:	Full term, cord Hb < 13 g	6	36–39	47.0	64.4	34.4
Control:	Full term	45	36–42	5.4	6.1	4.9
HDN:	Premature	10	30–36	129.7	186.9	90.1
Control:	Premature	13	29–36	21.9	27.2	17.9

Taken from reference (66) by permission.
* The insulin/creatinine ration follows a log normal distribution.

excretion was greater the lower the cord haemoglobin, but in the premature infants there was no correlation between insulin excretion and the severity of the haemolytic process. None of the infants was large for its gestational age, suggesting that chronic hyperinsulinaemia

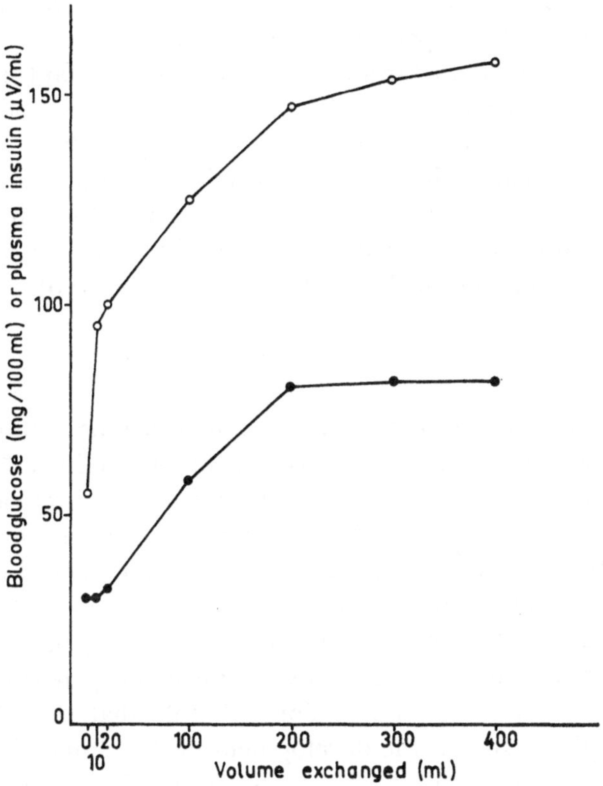

Fig. 2. Mean blood glucose (open circles) and plasma insulin levels (closed circles) during exchange transfusion with ACD blood in 22 infants with haemolytic disease of the newborn. Taken from reference (67).

had not occurred *in utero*. Six of the ten premature infants became hypoglycaemic in the first day of life but only one of the 12 full term infants was so affected.

Hypoglycaemia is even more likely to occur after exchange transfusion when blood preserved with citrate and glucose is used. In the latter part of such an exchange performed by conventional methods both the blood glucose and plasma insulin of the baby rise to a high plateau (fig. 2) (67). At the moment the transfusion stops the infant is in a metabolic situation, akin to that of the baby of the diabetic mother when the umbilical cord is cut, but without the energy reserves of such a baby. There is a rapid fall in blood glucose and hypoglycaemia may occur (D. Schiff – personal communication).

The reason for increased insulin secretion in such infants is not clear The placenta is known to be a site of active insulin degradation (68, 69) and it has been suggested that placental hyperplasia in erythroblastosis foetalis causes increased destruction of insulin and thereby compensatory hypersecretion (66). An alternative hypothesis is that haemolysis causes raised circulating levels of glutathione which split the disulphide bonds of the A and B chains of insulin (70).

ANENCEPHALY

Insulin secretion in the human anencephalic has not aroused much interest among investigators and yet is important in a full understanding of the development of insulin secretion. Foetal rabbits, decapitated *in utero* on day 24 or 26, have higher plasma insulin levels and a lower pancreatic insulin content on day 29 than control littermates (71). If the decapitated foetuses are given 1 mg ovine growth hormone the pancreatic insulin content rises to normal levels, but 1 mg ovine growth hormone and 2.5 mg cortisol reduce the pancreatic insulin content more than decapitation alone. A clue that the adenohypophysis may play a role in the development of the human foetal endocrine pancreas is provided by Van Assche, De Gasparo and Gepts (72) who studied the morphology of the endocrine pancreas and hypothalamo-hypophyseal system in anencephalics and correlated this with the umbilical cord plasma insulin level. A functional hypophysis is not necessary for normal development of the endocrine pancreas to occur. In anencephalics born to women with a reduced glucose tolerance there was a difference between those without a hypothalamo-hypophyseal system and those with a functional hypophysis (table 3). Those with a functional hypophysis resembled intact infants born to women with an abnormal glucose tolerance in having a high percentage of endocrine tissue in the pancreas, a high percentage of β cells in the islets of Langerhans and a raised umbilical cord plasma insulin level. Anencephalics with no hypothalamo-hypophyseal system born to women with an abnormal glucose tolerance did not show these changes. The data do not allow speculation on which facet of hypophyseal function is responsible for the difference but the observations

Table 3. *The endocrine pancreas in anencephalics correlated with the presence or absence of the hypothalamo-hypophyseal system (H.H.) and maternal glucose tolerance.*

Clinical description	Cases	β cell development		
		% endocrine tissue in pancreas	% β cells in islet	insulin in cord blood μU/ml
Anencephalics without a H.H. system –				
a. Normal maternal GTT	9	4.7±1.7	40 ± 6.1	12±1.0
b. Abnormal maternal GTT	8	5.0±1.6	38 ± 9.7	9±2.3
c. No maternal GTT	9	4.9±1.7	37 ± 9.1	10±3.3
Anencephalics with a H.H. system –				
a. Normal maternal GTT	3	3.2±0.4	41 ± 2.3	11±1.5
b. Abnormal maternal GTT	4	14.2±7.7	60 ± 7.1	34±2.6
Normal infants –				
a. Normal maternal GTT	40	5.1±1.6	40 ± 7.5	—
b. Abnormal maternal GTT	18	11.1±4.9	58.5±11.4	—

Reproduced with permission from reference (78).

on decapitated rabbit foetuses (71) suggest that growth hormone may be among the causative factors.

INSULIN RELEASE FROM HUMAN FOETAL PANCREAS IN VITRO

An obvious gap in the above description of the development of insulin secretion in man is the absence of information on the secretory behaviour of the human foetal β cell *in vitro*. The availability of fresh tissue from dead foetuses aborted by hysterotomy has made it possible to investigate this facet of β cell development. The body weights of the foetuses studied varied between 50 and 625 g and the period of gestation between 14 and 24 weeks. The design of the experiments was based on that used for the study of the development of insulin secretion in the rabbit (73) and the mechanism of action of various stimuli and inhibitors of insulin release (74, 75). In a typical experiment a pancreas would be divided into four to ten pieces of approximately 5 mg each. Each piece was incubated separately in a physiological buffer solution and was transferred to a new flask at 30 min. intervals. To

Table 4. *Stimulation of insulin release from human foetal pancreas in vitro by glucose, arginine, leucine or tolbutamide.*

Stimulus	Body wt. g	No. of observ-ations	Mean ± SE insulin release ng/mg pancreas 30 min.		Level of signifi-cance*
			Basal	Stimulated	
Glucose					
(3 mg/ml)	50	5	0.51±0.11	0.42±0.15	N.S.
	84	6	0.28±0.08	0.29±0.09	N.S.
	94	4	0.56±0.15	0.83±0.10	P<0.05
	146	8	0.22±0.09	0.33±0.13	N.S.
	243	7	2.47±1.62	2.32±1.55	N.S.
	254	8	0.45±0.18	0.77±0.32	P<0.005
	358	5	1.41±0.42	0.76±0.19	
	379	5	0.82±0.37	0.85±0.31	N.S.
	625	10	0.55±0.65	1.59±1.24	P<0.001
Leucine					
(5m M)	84	6	0.28±0.08	0.67±0.31	P<0.02
	145	8	0.41±0.18	0.77±0.32	P<0.02
	146	8	0.22±0.09	0.51±0.07	P<0.001
	358	5	1.94±0.71	1.50±0.40	N.S.
	379	5	1.11±0.64	1.13±0.47	N.S.
	625	4	0.61±0.22	0.96±0.56	N.S.
Arginine					
(5m M)	94	4	0.56±0.15	0.54±0.10	N.S.
	243	3	3.34	8.30	—
	358	5	0.79±0.36	2.29±1.04	P<0.01
	379	5	0.74±0.34	1.25±0.31	P<0.01
Tolbutamide					
(400μg/ml)	243	4	1.89±0.81	2.38±1.89	N.S.
	254	4	0.44±0.13	0.45±0.06	N.S.

* Statistical analysis by Student's *t* test for difference in means between two groups or significance of difference of (stimulated – basal) for paired data.

some flasks stimuli of insulin secretion were added. Insulin released into the incubation medium was measured by immunoassay. It was thus possible to measure insulin release from a group of pieces of pancreas first under basal conditions and then in the presence of a stimulus. Alternatively, insulin release could be studied from two groups of pieces from the same pancreas simultaneously, one group being incubated in control medium while the other was in medium containing a stimulus of insulin secretion.

Of the stimuli, glucose was studied most frequently. It caused a variable and modest release of insulin, being effective in three out of nine experiments (table 4). Leucine contrasted with arginine in that stimulation of insulin release by leucine occurred in the smaller foetuses while arginine was effective only in the larger ones. Tolbutamide did not cause insulin secretion in either of two experiments.

Stimuli which act by raising intracellular levels of 3′, 5′ – cyclic adenosine monophosphate (cyclic AMP) are effective in the rat and

Table 5. *Stimulation of insulin release from human foetal pancreas in vitro by glucagon, theophylline or dibutyryl cyclic* AMP.

Stimulus	Body wt. g	No. of observ- ations	Mean ± SE insulin release ng/mg pancreas. 30 min.		Level of signifi- cance*
			Basal	Stimulated	
In 3.0 mg/ml glucose:					
Glucagon (5μg/ml)	99	8	1.58±0.48	2.58±0.63	P<0.01
	145	8	0.43±0.16	0.87±0.23	P<0.005
	243	4	1.69±0.83	3.72±2.23	P<0.05
Theophylline (1 mM)	254	4	0.61±0.21	2.98±0.82	P<0.005
	625	5	1.03±0.26	3.10±1.90	P<0.05
Dibutyryl-cyclic AMP (1 mM)	254	4	0.92±0.37	3.08±0.89	P<0.025
	625	5	2.15±1.61	4.49±3.19	P<0.025
In 0 or 0.6 mg/ml glucose:					
Glucagon (5μg/ml)	243	4	1.82±0.81	2.59±1.04	P<0.005
	358	5	0.99±0.30	1.29±0.39	N.S.
	379	5	1.07±0.37	1.61±0.43	P<0.01
Theophylline (1 mM)	379	5	1.19±0.48	1.98±0.66	P<0.02
	625	5	0.38±0.06	3.04±0.49	P<0.001
Dibutyryl-cyclic AMP (1 mM)	625	5	0.71±0.93	2.39±0.65	P<0.01

* Statistical analysis by Student's *t* test for difference in means between groups or significance of difference of (stimulated – basal) for paired data.

rabbit only in the presence of extracellular glucose (76, 77), in contrast to the stimuli already described. Glucagon was a uniformly effective stimulus from 15 weeks onwards as were the two other stimuli, theophylline and dibutyryl cyclic AMP, which are thought to act by the same mechanism (table 5). Each stimulated insulin release in the presence or absence of glucose. Transmembrane ionic fluxes in the β cell have been shown to play a fundamental part in the release of insulin (74, 81) and it was of interest, therefore, to find that potassium, ouabain and barium were effective from 14 weeks gestation onwards and were the most potent of the three groups of stimuli tested (table 6).

Table 6. *Stimulation of insulin release from human foetal pancreas in vitro by potassium, ouabain and barium.*

Stimulus	Body wt. g	No. of observ-ations	Mean + SE insulin release ng/mg pancreas. 30 min.		Level of signifi-cance*
			Basal	Stimulated	
Potassium					
(60mM)	84	4	0.39+0.25	1.30+0.86	P<0.05
	426	8	0.49+0.35	2.08+0.57	P<0.001
Ouabain					
(10^{-5} M)	358	5	2.79+0.74	7.61+2.18	P<0.001
	426	8	0.41+0.26	1.05+0.41	P<0.005
Barium					
(2.54mM)	116	8	0.54+0.26	5.68+1.64	P<0.001
	358	5	2.81+0.38	14.53+1.80	P<0.001

* Statistical analysis by Student's *t* test for difference in means between two groups or significance of difference of (stimulated − basal) for paired data.

It is apparent that the β cell is functionally competent at an early stage in foetal life: 14 weeks, but that at this time the spectrum of stimuli which will cause the secretion of insulin differs from that characteristic of adult man. It is unlikely that ionic events are a primary cause of insulin release *in utero* but it is possible that foetal insulin release may be governed at this stage of development by metabolites such as amino acids and hormones such as glucagon, while glucose is a relatively poor or completely ineffective stimulus of secretion.

SUMMARY

The morphological and functional development of the β cell of the islets of Langerhans in the normal human foetus and newborn is described. The abnormal development of β cell function in infants of diabetic mothers, infants with haemolytic disease and anencephalics is contrasted with the normal to illustrate various factors that influence insulin secretion *in utero*. Studies of insulin release from human pancreas *in vitro* indicate that, between 14 and 24 weeks gestation, glucose is an indifferent stimulus of insulin secretion and tolbutamide is ineffective. The β cell is functional at this stage of development however. Three groups of stimuli are effective: the amino acids: leucine and arginine; the ionic stimuli: potassium, ouabain and barium; and stimuli which act by raising intracellular cyclic AMP concentrations: glucagon, theophylline and dibutyryl cyclic AMP.

The experiments described here were carried out in collaboration with Mr. M. A. Ashworth. It is a pleasure to thank Professor J. A. Davis for his encouragement and support.

ADDENDUM

(18 March 1971): Further experiments and a more rigourous analysis of the results have revealed that glucose (3.0 mg/ml) never definitely stimulated insulin release from pieces of human pancreas *in vitro*. All other results described above have been confirmed.

REFERENCES

1. Laguesse, E., (1896) *J. Anat. et Physiol.* 32:209.
2. Laguesse, E., (1906) *Revue generale d'histologie* 2:1.
3. Diamare, V., (1905) *Int. Mschr. Anat. Physiol.* 22:129.
4. Liu, H. M. and E. L. Potter, (1962) *Archs. Path.* 74:439.
5. Conklin, J. L., (1962) *Amer. J. Anat.* 111:181.
6. Ferner, H. and W. Stoeckenius Jr., (1950) *Z. Zellforsch. mikrosk. Anat.* 35:147.

7. JIRÁSEK, J. E., (1965) *Acta Histochem.* 22:62.
8. ROBB, P., (1961) *Quart. J. Exp. Physiol.* 46:335.
9. VAN ASSCHE, F. A., (1968) *Biol. Neonat.* 12:331.
10. VAN ASSCHE, F. A., (1969) *Biol. Neonat.* 14:19.
11. BJÖRKMAN, N., C. HELLERSTROM, B. HELLMAN and B. PETERSSON, (1966) *Z. Zellforsch. mikrosk. Anat.* 72:425.
12. HELLMAN, B., (1966) *Biol. neonat.*, 9:263.
13. FERNER, H., (1951) *Virchows Arch.* 319:390.
14. SCHULTZE-JENA, B. S., (1953) *Virchows Arch.* 323:653.
15. HESS, W., (1946) *Schweiz. Z. Path.*, 9:46.
16. MCLEAN, N. and R. F. OGILVIE, (1955) *Diabetes* 4:367.
17. EMERY, J. L. and H. P. R. BURY, (1964) *Biol. neonat.* 6:16.
18. GRILLO, T. A. I. and K. SHIMA, (1966) *J. Endocrin.* 36:151.
19. SCHWARTZ, R., (1968) *Proc. R. Soc. Med.* 61:1231.
20. CASPER, D. J. and F. BENJAMIN, (1970) *Obstet. Gynec.* 35:389.
21. COLTART, D. M., R. W. BEARD, R. C. TURNER and N. W. OAKLEY, (1969) *Brit. med. J.* 4:17.
22. PATERSON, P., P. PAGE, P. TAFT, L. PHILLIPS and C. WOOD, (1968) *J. Obst. Gynec. Br. Cmmwlth.* 75:917.
23. TOBIN, J. D., J. F. ROUX and J. S. SOELDNER, (1969) *Pediatrics* 44:668.
24. MILNER, R. D. G. and C. N. HALES, (1965) *Brit. Med. J.* 1:284.
25. KELLER, J. M. and J. S. KROHNER, (1968) *Obstet. Gynec.* 32:77.
26. BUSE, G. B., W. J. ROBERTS and J. BUSE, (1962) *J. Clin. Invest.* 41:29.
27. SPELLACY, W. N., F. C. GOETZ, B. Z. GREENBERG and J. ELLS, (1964) *Am. J. Obst. Gyn.* 90:753.
28. WOLF, H., V. SABATA, H. FRERICHS and P. STUBBE (1969), *Horm. Metab. Res.* 1:274.
29. BAIRD, J. D. and J. W. FARQUHAR, (1962) *Lancet*, 1:71.
30. GENTZ, J. C. H., R. WARRNER, B. E. H. PERSSON and M. CORNBLATH, (1969) *Acta Pediat. Scand.* 58:481.
31. GRASSO, S., N. SAPORITO, A. MESSINA and G. REITANO, (1968) *Diabetes*, 17:306.
32. ISLES, T. E., M. DICKSON and J. W. FARQUHAR, (1968) *Pediat. Res.* 2:198.
33. PILDES, R. S., R. J. HART, R. WARRNER and M. CORNBLATH, (1969) *Pediatrics*, 44:76.
34. MILNER, R. D. G. and A. D. WRIGHT, (1967) *Clin. Sci.* 32:249.
35. LOWY, C. and D. SCHIFF, (1968) *Lancet* 1:225.
36. SALINAS Jr., E. D., H. H. MANGURTEN, S. S. ROBERTS, W. H. SIMON and M. CORNBLATH, (1968) *Pediatrics*, 41:646.
37. GOTLIN, R. W. and H. K. SILVER, (1970) *Lancet*, 1:1346.
38. GROLLMAN, A., W. E. MCCALEB and F. N. WHITE, (1964) *Metabolism* 13:686.
39. MCQUARRIE, I., E. I. BELL and B. ZIMMERMAN, (1950) *Fedn. Proc.* 9:337.
40. JØRGENSEN, K. R., T. DECKERT, L. M. PEDERSEN and J. PEDERSEN (1966) *Acta Endocr. Kbh.* 52:154.
41. SPELLACY, W. N. and F. C. GOETZ, (1963) *Lancet* 2:222.
42. CARDELL, B. S., (1953) *J. Obstet. Gynec. Br. Emp.* 60:834.
43. STEINKE, J. and S. DRISCOLL, (1965) *Diabetes* 14:573.
44. D'AGOSTINO, A. N. and R. C. BAHN, (1963) *Diabetes*, 12:327.
45. LOGOTHETOPOULOS, J. and E. G. BELL, (1966) *Diabetes* 15:205.
46. FEE, B. A. and W. B. WEIL, (1963) *Ann. N. Y. Acad. Sci.* 110:869.
47. ISLES, T. E. and J. W. FARQUHAR, (1967) *Pediat. Res.* 1:110.

48. McCann, M. L., P. A. J. Adam, B. F. Likly and R. Schwartz, (1966) *New Engl. J. Med.* 275:8.
49. Velasco, M. S. A. and E. P. Paulsen, (1969) *Pediatrics* 43:546.
50. King, K. C., P. A. J. Adam, G. A. Clemente and R. Schwartz, (1969) *Pediatrics*, 44:381.
51. Miller, D. I., H. Wishinsky and G. Thompson, (1962) *Diabetes* (supplement), 11:93.
52. Nitowsky, H. M., L. Matz and J. A. Bezofsky, (1966) *J. Pediat.* 69:1139.
53. Kemball, M. L., C. McIver, R. D. G. Milner, C. H. Nourse, D. Schiff and J. Tiernan, (1970) *Archs Dis. Childh.* 45:696.
54. Zucker, P. and G. Simon, (1968) *Pediatrics* 42:824.
55. Sutherland, H. W., P. D. Bewsher, J. D. Cormack and J. M. Stowers, (1970) *Diabetologia* 6:50.
56. Adam, P. A. J. and R. Schwartz, (1968) *Pediatrics*, 42:819.
57. Liebegott, G., (1938) *Beitr. path. Anat.* 101:606.
58. Potter, E. L., H. P. G. Sickel and W. A. Stryker, (1941) *Arch. Path.* 31:467.
59. Van Assche, F. A., M. de Gasparo and M. Renaer, (1970) *Biol. Neonat.* 15:176.
60. Driscoll, S. G. and J. Steinke, (1967) *Pediatrics*, 39:448.
61. From, G. L. A., S. G. Driscoll and J. Steinke, (1969) *Pediatrics* 44:549.
62. Raivio, K. O. and K. Österlund, (1969) *Pediatrics* 43:217.
63. Thorell, J. I., (1970) *Acta. Endocr. Kbh.* 63:134.
64. Barrett, C. T. and T. K. Oliver, Jr., (1968) *New Engl. J. Med.* 278:1260.
65. Hazeltine, F. G., (1967) *Pediatrics*, 39:696.
66. Schiff, D. and C. Lowy, (1970) *Pediat. Res.* 4:280.
67. Milner, R. D. G. and A. D. Wright, (1966) *Clin. Sci.* 31:309.
68. Freinkel, N. and C. J. Goodner, (1960) *J. Clin. Inv.* 39:116.
69. Freinkel, N. and C. J. Goodner, (1962) *Arch. Int. Med.* 109:163.
70. Steinke, J., F. A. Gries and S. G. Driscoll, (1967) *Blood* 30:359.
71. Kervran, A., A. Jost and G. Rosselin, (1970) *Diabetologia*, 6:51.
72. Van Assche, F. A., M. de Gasparo and W. Gepts, (1969) *Biol. Neonat.* 14:374.
73. Milner, R. D. G., (1969) *J. Endocrinol.* 44:267.
74. Hales, C. N. and R. D. G. Milner, (1968) *J. Physiol.* 194:725.
75. Milner, R. D. G. and C. N. Hales, (1969) *Biochem. J.* 113:473.
76. Malaisse, W. J., F. Malaisse-Lagae and D. Mayhew, (1967) *J. Clin. Invest.* 46:1724.
77. Milner, R. D. G., (1970) *J. Endocrinol.* 47:347.
78. Van Assche, F. A., W. Gepts and M. de Gasparo, (1969) *Horm. Metab. Res.* 1:251.
79. Baird, J. D., (1969) *J. Endocr.* 44:139.
80. Gitlin, D., J. Kumate and C. Morales, (1965) *Pediatrics*, 35:65.
81. Hales, C. N. and R. D. G. Milner, (1968) *J. Physiol.* 199:177.
82. Hoet, J. P., (1967) *Bull. Acad. Royal Med. Belg.*, 7:85.
83. King, K., K. Yamaguchi, J. Butt, K. Teramo, K. Raivio, J. Roux and R. Schwartz, (1970) *abstract Am. Soc. Pediat. Res.*

DISCUSSION

Dr. Rappaport: I was very much impressed by your presentation, mainly on the growth hormone problem. I would like to know if you have some information on the action of growth hormone on insulin secretion in utero. The interest in this comes from the clinical observation that some hypopituitary dwarfs, but not all, do not secrete insulin when you inject glucose i.v. or tolbutamide or arginine.

But this does not occur after hypophysectomy. I wonder but it is probably only a speculation, if the lack of insulin secretion in those hypopituitary dwarfs can be traced back to lack of growth hormone in utero.

Dr. Milner: I think the speculations you made are very interesting.

Prof. Villee: I think you have demonstrated that by 14 weeks of development the foetal pancreas has the ability to synthesize insulin and holds it there and will release it if you give an appropriate stimulus. My question is which of these stimuli may actually be present in the foetal pancreas to produce a release of insulin.

Dr. Milner: We are now completely in the field of speculation. An interesting difference between the foetal islet and the adult islet is in the ratio of alpha to beta cells. In the adult there are 3 to 9 beta cells for every alpha cell. At birth the ratio is approximately 1 to 1. Earlier in gestation there may be more alpha cells than beta cells. Where do the alpha cells go? Do the beta cells come more slowly? It is a very provocative thought, that in fact glucagon may be do something in utero we are not yet aware of.

Prof. Teller: People are studying the dynamics of insulin secretion by perfusing of the pancreas. The question is what about information on perfusion of foetal pancreas or neonatal pancreas. As you know there is an early peak of insulin release. Is this apparent in the newborn pancreas as well or is there a different dynamics, which would be very important to explain some of the contradictory glucose-insulin relationship in the newborn.

Dr. Milner: The question is very pertinent. If you give a constant glucose stimulus, say 300 mg per cent glucose solution, into a perfused pancreas, you get a spike and wave of insulin secretion after respectively 2 and 30 minutes. There are two phases in the insulin release. This pattern of release cannot be reproduced in the type of experiments we have performed.

Dr. Young: I could try to explain your results by an analogy with some work we have done on the release of aminoacids by the perfused placenta, which is also biphasic. There is always some time during which the organ is without a blood supply while you are putting in the cannulae. Do you think the insulin is just released into the tissue during its preparation and is washed out during the first 1 or 2 minutes of perfusion? The second curve could be your real response.

Dr. Milner: That is very interesting. I never had an association with those sort of experiments. I have heard many other interpretations to explain those curves. We have to make an experiment to exclude it. I don't know if this hypothesis has ever been considered.

PANCREATIC GLUCAGON, AND GLUCAGON-LIKE MATERIAL IN TISSUES AND PLASMAS FROM HUMAN FOETUSES 6–26 WEEKS OLD

R. ASSAN, AND J. BOILLOT*

INTRODUCTION

Determination of the first appearance of glucagon in the human fetal pancreas is of some interest from an organo-genetic point of view.

The evolution of the concentration of this hormone in pancreatic tissue and plasma, raises the problem of glucagon secretion and its possible physiological role during fetal life.

In the present work, pancreatic, gastric, and enteric extracts from 65 freshly collected human foetuses were prepared; glucagon (from pancreas), and a glucagon-like immuno-reactive (GLI) material (from gut and stomach) were characterized and assayed by 2 radio-immunological systems.

In plasma, glucagon and GLI of 3 foetuses aged 15, 23 and 26 weeks were assayed.

MATERIAL AND METHODS**

81 human foetuses were collected from surgical and gynecological wards, mostly on occasion of self induced abortion. Only 65 foetuses proved usable for hormonal study, after analysis of the conditions of collection, and medical investigation of the maternal anamnesis (mainly for diabetes, nephropathy, rhesus iso-immunisation). The age of pregnancy was carefully determined by comparison of maternal anamnesis, and weights of fetus, pancreas, and stomach. The ages in the

* Hôtel-Dieu – Place du Parvis Notre-Dame – 75 – PARIS – FRANCE.

** We gratefully thank for technical assistance MRS A. DELAGE, J. DUCLOUX and for help in collecting samples, DR. NATHALIE JOSSO, PR. CATHERINE TCHOBROUTSKY, and the medical staffs and nurses of the Clinique Chirurgicale de l'Hôtel-Dieu and Service de Gynécologie et Obstétrique de l'Hôtel-Dieu de Paris.

group studied here, range between 6 and 26 weeks after the last maternal menses.

The foetuses were kept at low temperature (+4 °C) from emission until dissection and weighing (from 1 to 12 hours). Dissected organs were kept at —20 °C until extraction; then crushed in 3 ml of acid alcohol (pure ethanol 250 ml, water 78 ml, HCl (10^N): 5 ml), in the presence of washed sand, kept overnight and centrifuged; the precipitate was washed twice with 1 ml of acid alcohol. All operations were performed at low temperature; special attention was paid to glassware contamination. The recovery of glucagon was estimated by addition of labelled glucagon and was found to be between 75 and 80%.

Acid alcohol extracts were rediluted 1/10 to 1.10.000 in veronal buffer plus albumin 5‰ and protease-inhibitors (trasylol, epsilon amino-caproïc acid). The absence of interference with the immunoassay system was checked for acid alcohol without tissue extract diluted in the same way; extracts were also prepared with foetal striated muscle and placental fragments and they showed no interference with the assay.

Two different immunoassay systems for glucagon were used, both including purified glucagon for tracer and standards. For the first system, a rabbit anti-beef-pork anti glucagon antiserum (PVP8) was used: it has been demonstrated previously that in this system human pancreatic extracts, serially diluted, follow the pork glucagon standard curve (1); this system is sensitive to addition of 30 pg of glucagon; gastric and enteric extracts interfere with this assay system, with an immunological behaviour (in serial dilution) different from purified glucagon and from human pancreatic extracts. The second immunoassay system used is specific for pancreatoglucagon: this includes the K-47 antiserum, generously gifted by LISE HEDING (2): *in this system extra pancreatic digestive extracts gave no interference at all.*

All the extracts were checked in 4 dilutions at least.

RESULTS

The population studied appeared homogeneous in evolution of body-weight and respective weights of pancreas, stomach, gut (figures 1, 2, 3, 4); the evolutions of body weights and pancreas weights are very comparable to those found by other workers (3, 4).

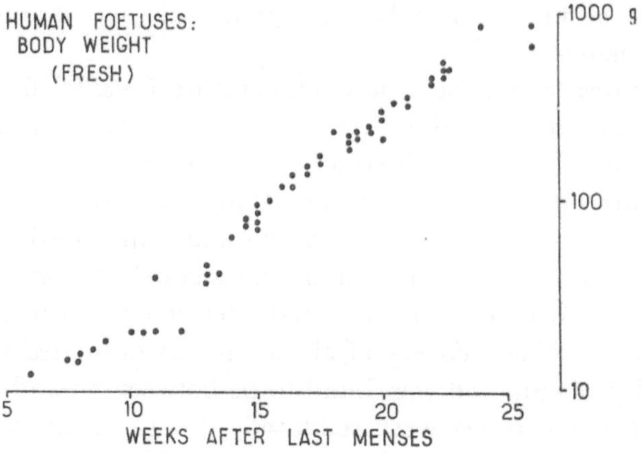

Fig. 1. Human foetuses: body weight (fresh).

1. *Pancreatic glucagon*

Immunoassayable glucagon, absent when pregnancy is six weeks old, is detectable at the end of the 8th week; the absolute amount found then is one nanogramme for one pancreas (30 times higher than the limit of sensitivity of the assay); the pancreatic content measured at 8½ weeks attains 5 nanogrammes; then it increases according to a

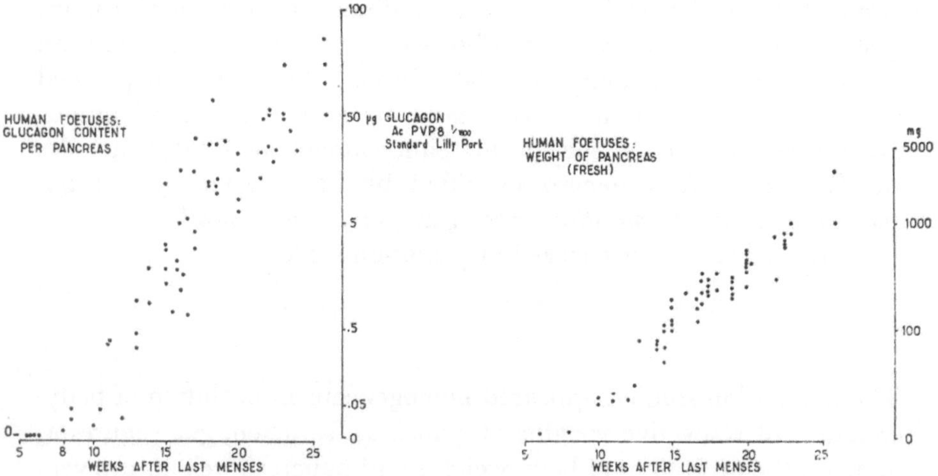

Fig. 2. Weight of pancreas (fresh) and glucagon content per pancreas.

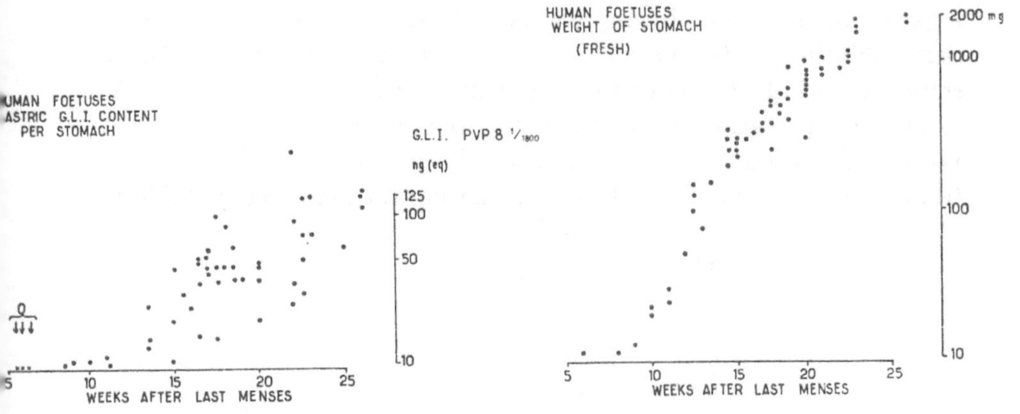

ig. 3. Weight of stomach and G.L.I. content.

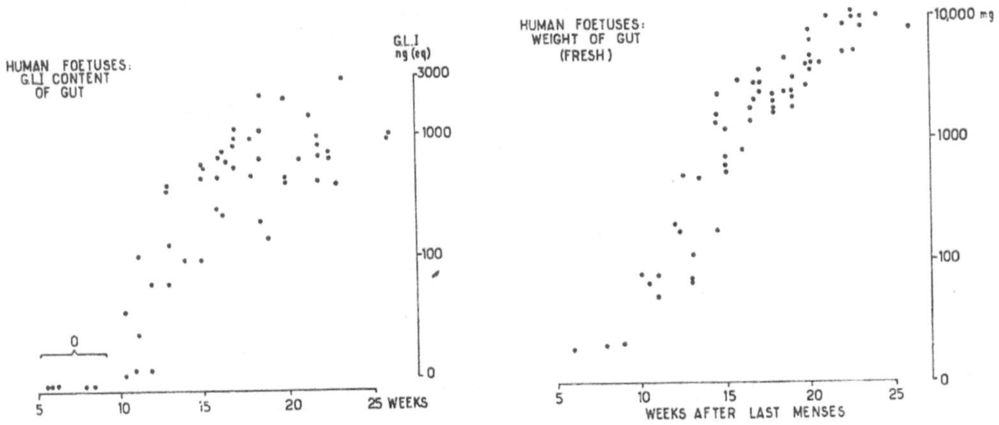

Fig. 4. Weight of gut and G.L.I. content.

Table 1. *Glucagon concentration increases strongly from 8th to 26th week; in adult pancreas, glucagon concentration was found 1–3 ng/mg (with same extraction procedure).*

Weeks after last menses	Weight of pancreas (mg)	Glucagon content (μg)	Glucagon concentration in fresh tissue (μg/mg)
10	21	27	1.28
12	40	60	1.50
15	90	220	2.45
17	150	500	3.33
20	350	1800	5.15
22	600	4000	6.65
25	1400	10000	7.15

logarithmic function during the period studied (up to 26 weeks). Serial dilution study shows that this material always behaves like the standard and like human adult pancreatic extract (figure 5).

The concentration of glucagon per weight-unit of fresh tissue was not found constant: it increases regularly during the periods studied, from 1,28 ng/mg (10th week) to 7,15 ng/mg (at 25th week) (table I).

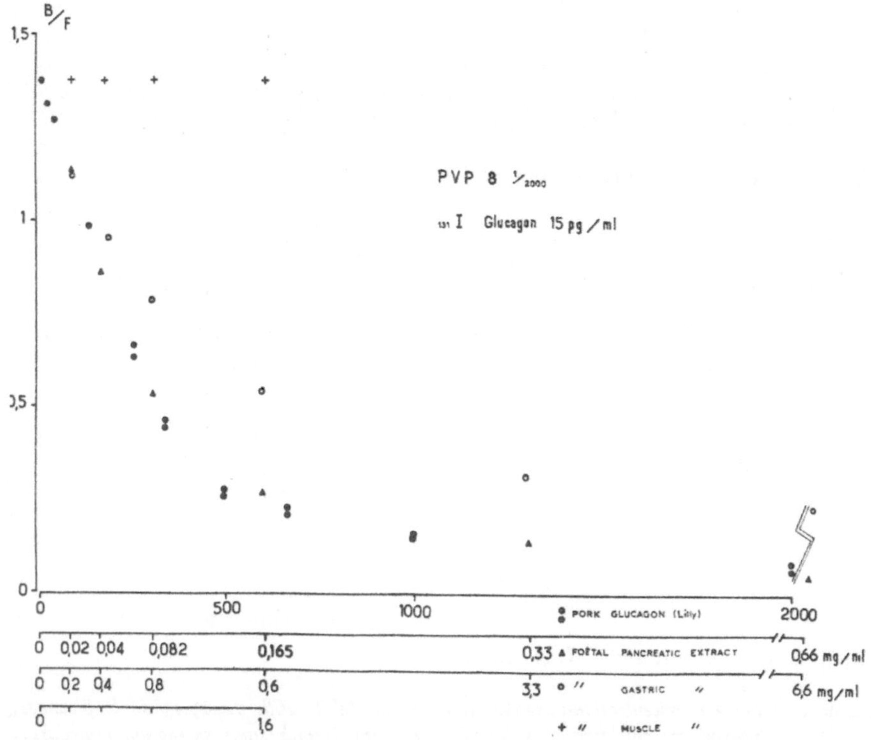

Fig. 5. Radio immunological behaviour of extracts (pancreas-stomach-muscle) from a 13 weeks old human foetus, compared to purified pancreatic pork glucagon, when matched with the PVP-8 antiserum.

2. *G.L.I. in stomach and gut*

An interference with the PVP-8 immunoassay system appears for gastric and enteric tissues from the 10th week of gestation (figures 3 and 4); the interfering material does not follow the glucagon standard curve when serially diluted (figure 5); the results can be expressed here only in terms of glucagon equivalents and for comparable dilutions as long as a standard of G.L.I. is not available. No interference was obtained with these digestive materials in the K47 immunoassay system. With this important restriction, it seems possible to assert progressive increase of the amounts evaluated in gut and stomach; this interference with the assay system is always much lower than the corresponding glucagon value found for the same age in the pancreas (about 1/100 in terms of concentration).

Table 2. *Basal levels for blood glucose, and hormones in 2 foetuses, living and kept at room temperature.*

	Foetus 15 weeks	Foetus 26 weeks			
	Immediatly after emission	After emission	+60′	+120′	+180′
Glycemia mg %	46	–	55	45	45
G.L.I. (PVP8) pg/ml equiv.	610	900	750	750	725
Glucagon (K-47) pg/ml	80	240	180	180	180
Insulin μu/ml	21	22	25	23	26
Growth hormone ng/ml	–	>30	>30	–	–

Table 3. *Glucose, glucagon, G.L.I., in a 25 weeks old foetus, kept at room temperature, before and after arginine intra peritoneal administration. (0,3 mg/Kg),*

	—15′	0	15′	30′	45′	60′	90′
Glycemia mg %	65	46	48	65	85	83	62
G.L.I. (PVP8) pg/ml equiv.	585	765	630	765	720	840	840
Glucagon (K-47) pg/ml	indetectable	90	120	120	90	90	100

3. *Glucagon and G.L.I. activity in plasma*

Three living foetuses, aged 15, 23, 26 weeks were studied: blood was collected by cardiac puncture and matched against the 2 immunoassay systems; from one of these 3 foetuses (26 weeks) blood was collected every hour for 4 hours at room temperature; from another (23 weeks) blood was collected every 15 minutes after intraperitoneal administration of arginine hydrochloride (0,3 mg/kg). Table 2 shows that measurable levels of glucagon and G.L.I. activity could be assayed in these plasmas.

Levels for glucagon and G.L.I. are within the range found in adults. No significant increase for glucagon but a slight increase for G.L.I. occurred after arginine administration.

DISCUSSION

The results of radio immunological detection of glucagon in the human fetal pancreas are in agreement with the results of histologic techniques, for the period of appearance, as well as for the evolution: 2 successive generations of islets are usually described by histologists, the first appearing at the 8th week and the second approximately at the 5th month (5, 3, 4); the first generation is submitted to a progressive involution after the 3rd month. It seems that that alpha cells are detectable with specific histologic stainings, as soon as the islet is clearly recognizable, that is, around the 8th week (4). Several works using histologic and electronmicroscopic techniques confirm this early appearance of alpha cells (at least upon morphological criteriums) in man (3) as well as in rats (6, 7, 8); however, until now the presence of glucagon-like immunoreactive material in fetal pancreas has been described only in later ages in rats (6, 9) and not at all in the human foetus.

The progressive increase of the glucagon concentration per unit of weight of fresh tissue which is found here seems to correlate with some histological well-known data and with radio-immunological data obtained in the rat: from a histological point of view, alpha cells clearly out-number the beta cells in the islet from 10 weeks to 5 months, then they are submitted to a progressive reduction in number (3, 4). This is strikingly correlated by radio immunoassay in rat fetal pancreas (9): in this species the concentration of glucagon per gram of pancreatic tissue attains a maximum around the 2nd third of gestation, then decreases, and is finally lower in adult pancreas than the maximal values found in fetal life. The group of human foetuses studied here does not include samples older than 26 weeks: however it seems obvious that the concentrations reached at this period are much higher than those found in the adult pancreas (1–3 μg/mg). The physiological significance of this high pancreatic glucagon content around the 2nd third of gestation is not known.

The presence of a G.L.I. content in stomach and gut, distinct from glucagon, can be detected as early as glucagon in the pancreas (or a little later). No absolute quantitative values can be attributed to the results found with the PVP-8 system for this material. Similar features are well known for adult gastric and enteric extracts (1). The nature and physiological significance of this material are still obscure.

The presence of glucagon and G.L.I. in circulating plasma as early as the 15th week, although supported up till now by few samples, has been demonstrated. This circulating glucagon cannot be maternal glucagon: no transplacenrol transfer occurs when exogenous glucagon is infused either into the foetus or into the mother, in the sheep species (10). Everything about the regulation, and eventual action, of this fetal glucagon secretion is still to be investigated. During the 2 isolated experiments performed here no significant glucagon increment was detected during 4 hours of fasting and after arginine intraperitoneal infusion.

CONCLUSION AND SUMMARY

Data are presented about the concentration of glucagon and G.L.I. in tissues of 65 human foetuses 6–26 weeks old, and plasmatic glucagon and G.L.I. of 3 living human foetuses (15, 25, 26 weeks old). The results of a short fast (4 hours) and of arginine infusion, are presented.

REFERENCES

1. Assan, R., Glucagon and glucagon cross-reacting substances in gastric (G.E.) and pancreatic (P.E.) extracts from 12 animals species. 3rd Intern. Congress of Endocrinol. – Mexico 1968, *Abstract Excerpta Med. Found*, Amsterdam 1968.
2. Heding, L. G., (1969) The production of glucagon antibodies in rabbits. *Hormone Metab. Res.* 1:87–88.
3. Liu, h. m.-Potter E. L., (1962) Development of the human pancreas. *Arch. Pathol.* 74:439–452.
4. Robb, R., (1961) The development of the islets of Langerhans in man. *Arch. Dis. Child.* 36:229–230.
5. Emery, J. L., H. P. R. Bury, (1964) Involutionary changes in the islets of Langerhans. *Biol. Neonatorum* 1964, 6:15–26.
6. Orci, L., E. Lambert, Ch. Rouiller, A. E. Renold, E. Samols, (1969) Evidence for the presence of A-cells in the endocrine fetal pancreas of the rat. *Hormone Metab. Res.* 1:108–110.
7. Perrier, H., A. Porte, R. Jacquot, (1969) Présence de cellules A dans le pancréas foetal de rat. *C. R. Acad. Sc. Paris* 269:841–843.
8. Zagury, D., (1961) Contribution à l'étude morphologique des secrétions pancréatiques chez le rat. *Ann. Sci. Nat. Zool.* 12ème série, 111:186–296.
9. Rutter, W. J., (1969) Independantly regulated synthetic transitions in fetal tissues in: '*Fetal Atonomy*', Ciba Found. coll. Churchill, J. A., London, Ed. Wolternholme, G. E. W., M. O'Connor, p. 59–78.
10. Alexander, P., R. Assan, D. Nixon, and coll. under press.
11. Barnes, A. C. (1968) *Intra-uterine development*, vol. 1, Lea Febiger Ed., Philadelphia, p. 530.
12. Blum, D., J. Dodion, H. Loeb, P. Wilkin, P. O. Hubinon, (1969). Studies on hypoglycemia in small-for-dates newborns. *Arch. Dis. Child.* 44: 304–310.
13. Brock, L. C., W. R. Clark, R. H. Williams, W. Rutter, (1969) Embryonic development of the endocrine pancreas: I Analysis of hormonal levels. *Diabetes*, 18, 321.
14. Conklin, J. S., *The development of the pancreas of the human foetus.* Ann Arbor, Michigan University Microfilm Inc., Cat no 61, 2739.
15. Cornblath, M., R. Schwartz, (1966) *Disorders of carbohydrate metabolism in infancy.* Saunders., Philadelphia, p. 297.
16. Dawes, G. S., H. J. Shelley, (1968) Carbohydrate metabolism in foetus and newborn. In '*Carbohydrate metabolism and its disorders*', vol. 2, Dickens, F. P. J. Randle, Ed. Wheelan, Academic Press, London, New-York, p. 87–121.
17. Ferner, H., W. Stoeckenius, (1951) Die cytogenese des Inselsystems beim Menschen. *Z. Zellforsch Mikr. Anat.* 35:147–175.
18. Girard, J., D. Bal, (1970) Effets du glucagon-zinc sur la glycémie et la teneur en glycogène du foie foetal du rat en fin de gestation. *C. R. Acad. Sci. Paris*, 271: 777–779.
19. Grillo, T. A. I., K. Shima, (1966) Insulin content and enzyme histochemistry of the human fetal pancreatic islet. *J. Endocrinol.* 36:151–158.
20. Maclean, N., R. F. Ogilvie, (1955) Quantitative estimate of pancreatic islet tissue in diabetic subjects. *Diabetes*, 4/5:367.
21. Messina, A., G. Reitano, S. Grasso, N. Saporito, (1968) Effetti del glucagone solla secrezione insulinica del neonato immaturo. *Voll. Soc. Ital. Biol. Sper.*, XLIV:2015–2018.

22. MILNER, R. D. G., (1969) The secretion of insulin from fetal and post natal rabbit pancreas in vitro in response to various substances. *J. Endocrinol.* 44:267–272.
23. MUNGER, B. L., (1958) A light and electron microscopic study of cellular differentiation in the pancreatic islet of the mouse. *Amer. J. Anat.* 103:275–311.
24. PEARCE, R. M., (1903) The development of the island of Langerhans in the human embryon. *Amer. J. Anat.* 2:445–455.
25. SCHULTZE-JENA, B. S., (1953) Das quantitative und qualitative Inselbild menschlicher feten und neugeborenen. *Virchows Arch. Path. Anat. Physiol.* 323:653–663.
26. VAN ASSCHE, F. A., (1968) A morphological study of the Langerhans islets of the fetal pancreas in late pregnancy. *Biol. Neonatorum,* 12:331–342.
27. WEICHSELBAUM, A., J. KYRLE, (1909) Uber das verhalten der Langerhansschen insulin der menschlichen pankreas im fötalen und post fötalen leben. *Arch. Mikrosk. Anat. Int. Med.* 74:223–258.

DISCUSSION

Dr. Rappaport: I would like to know if there is a correlation between this increment in content of glucagon of the pancreas and the histological observation of the foetal pancreas.

Dr. Assan: I cannot answer you. We have very few histological data. The measurement of alpha cells was not done for the whole pancreas but for a part of it. As far as I know the repartition of alpha cells could be variable from one point to another in the pancreas. No conclusions can be drawn from these figures.

Dr. Hommes: Many of the actions of glucagon are mediated via cyclic AMP. If you study the development of glucagon secretion you should also know the activity and perhaps the development of adenyl cyclase. Do you know anything about it?

Dr. Assan: This is not my special field. I completely agree that to demonstrate an intervention of glucagon during foetal life we need not only the presence in tissue, the presence in blood but also the target cell able to receive information.

As far as I know phosphorylase activity was demonstrated in the liver after 10 weeks. Glucose-6-phosphatase activity comes out after 18 to 20 weeks. All that I can say that is that with very unphysiological doses of glucogon (0.1 mg) injected in a foetus of 25 weeks an increase of glucose level could be obtained (from 40 to 60 mg per cent after 20 minutes, measured with glucose-oxydase method). But I have no idea of the sensibility of the target cells.

Dr. Hull: I have always been interested in the suggestion that an infusion of glucagon is given for hypoglycaemia. In experimental animals glucagon doubles the metabolic rate. Glucagon is a lipolytic hormone which stimulates lipolysis in brown adipose tissue and heat production. By so doing it will increase glucose uptake by brown adipose tissue. Although it will cause a rise in the circulating level of glucose, it also causes a considerable increase in glucose utilisation. Therefore I think one might loose in the long term by injecting glucagon into babies.

FUNCTIONAL DEVELOPMENT IN BROWN ADIPOSE TISSUE

D. HULL AND M. J. HARDMAN*

Brown adipose tissue is prominent in newborn and young mammals including man and our experimental animal – the rabbit. It has two important functions. Firstly, it is a store and supply of fatty acids, and secondly, it is a site of extra heat production during cold exposure. Structurally the tissue is formed of a single cell type surrounded by a rich capillary network. The relationship between the size of any organ and its functional capacity is bound to be complex, however, in view of the relatively simple structure of brown adipose tissue it seems probable that there is a close and direct relationship between the tissue's weight and its capacity to produce heat or release fatty acids. It is therefore of interest that the size of brown adipose tissue relative to body weight in rabbits reaches a maximum about the time of birth. In absolute terms it continues to increase in size to maturity (fig. 1). This observation alone suggests that brown adipose tissue has a special function in the newborn period. We have been interested in the factors determining its function and development.

THERMOGENESIS OF BROWN ADIPOSE TISSUE

As a consequence of cold exposure, sympathetic activity releases noradrenaline close to the cells. Noradrenaline activates tissue lipase which in turn increases the rate of hydrolysis of triglyceride to fatty acids and glycerol. It is possible that the intracellular release of fatty acids itself increases the rate of heat production (1). However, noradrenaline will stimulate thermogenesis in brown adipose tissue which is deplete of fat. In this situation brown adipose tissue produces heat by drawing glucose and fatty acids from the circulation (2). Thus nor-

* Institute of Child Health, 30 Guilford Street, London, U.K.

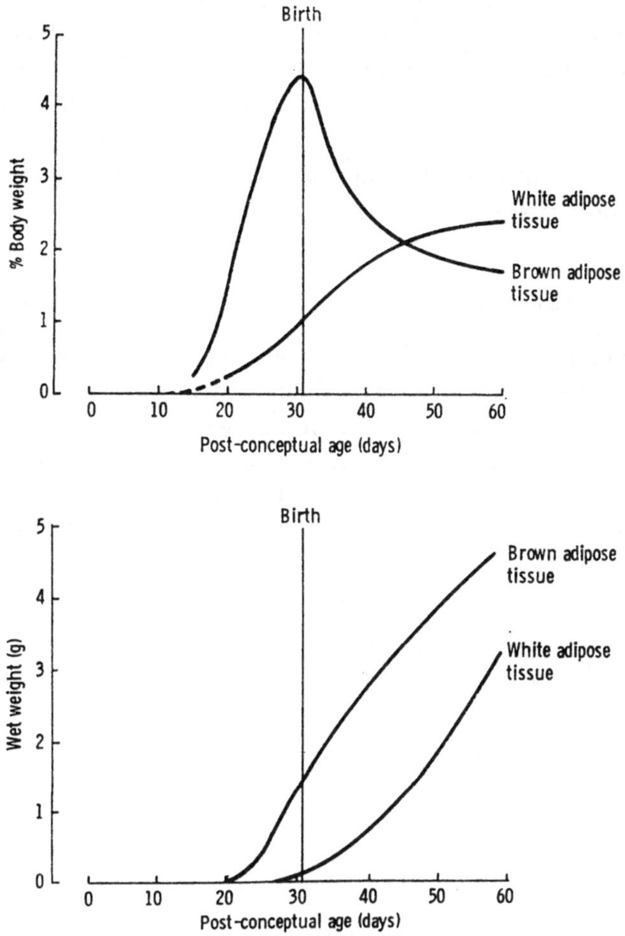

Fig. 1. The absolute and relative weights of brown and white adipose tissue of rabbits before and after birth are shown plotted against post-conceptual age.

adrenaline has at least two separate actions on brown adipose tissue: it increases fatty acid mobilisation and it stimulates intracellular oxidation and heat production. The fraction of fatty acids released by lipolysis which are oxidized in the tissue varies with the animals' previous environmental conditions (*cf. infra.*).

The biological effects of noradrenaline infusion are similar to those of cold exposure in newborn rabbits with respect to changes in circulating levels of free fatty acids and glycerol as well as the increase in thermogenesis. For this reason and for technical convenience noradrenaline infusions have been used to mimic cold induced thermogenesis in many of our experiments. In newborn rabbits brown adipose tissue is the major site of thermogenesis during both cold exposure and noradrenaline infusion (3), thus the increase in the whole rabbit's rate of oxygen consumption is a fair measure of heat production in its brown adipose tissue.

ONSET OF THERMOGENESIS AFTER BIRTH – THE SWITCH ON

In utero developing mammals enjoy constant warm ambient conditions and yet within minutes of birth their brown adipose tissue produces heat in response to the mammals first experience of cold exposure (4) (fig. 2). In the rabbit, the maximum rate of heat production gradually increases over the first few hours. This rise may reflect increasing enzymic activity in brown adipose tissue but it could also be due to an

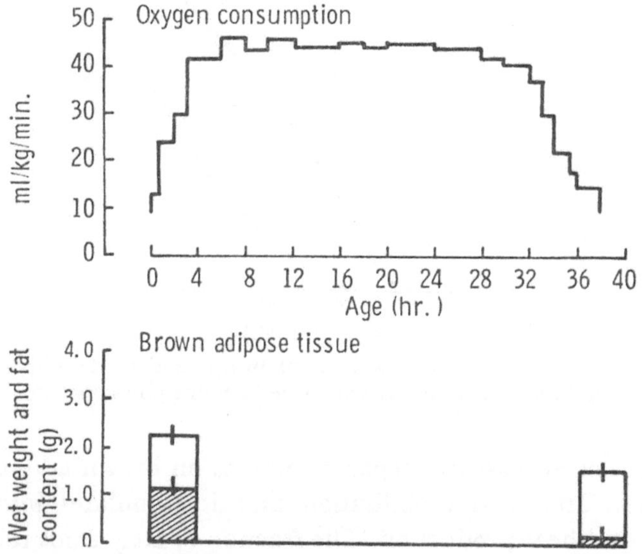

Fig. 2. The upper diagram illustrates the rate of oxygen consumption of a rabbit kept from birth in an ambient temperature (25°C) which stimulates maximal thermogenesis. The lower diagram shows the mean wet weight and fat content (shaded area) of rabbits at birth (n = 12) and aged 32–40 hrs (n = 12) when thermogenesis had fallen due to cold exposure from birth. The vertical line gives the standard error of the mean.

increase in respiratory-cardiac capacity, for during maximum heat production brown adipose tissue's oxygen requirements are such that it takes over a quarter of the cardiac output. In the rabbit immediately after birth thermogenesis is maintained in brown adipose tissue until

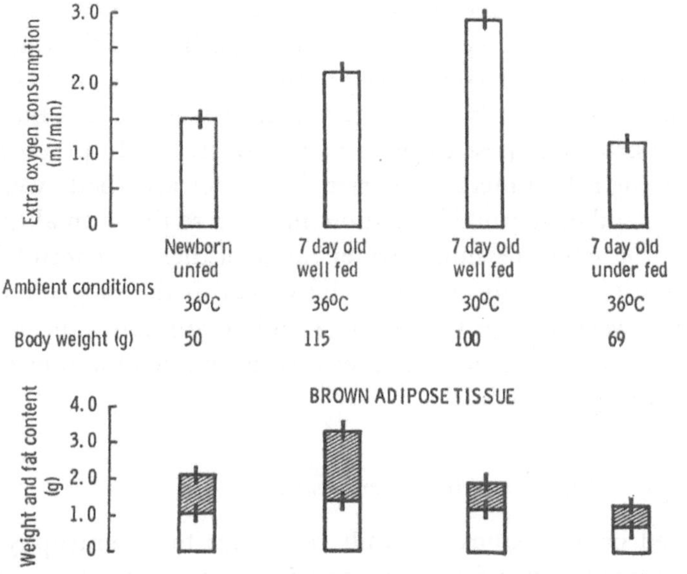

Fig. 3. The maximal increase in oxygen consumption during cold exposure of rabbits on the day of birth is contrasted with the values obtained for rabbits reared to one week of age under differing conditions of nutrition and environmental temperature. The mean wet weight and fat content (shaded area) of the cervical lobes of brown adipose tissue of the four groups of rabbits is also shown. The vertical line gives the standard error of the mean.

the tissue store of fat is exhausted and then thermogenesis falls abruptly. The animal will continue to survive for some time. At this time, glucose feeds are readily absorbed, there is a rise in blood sugar but no return of thermogenesis. On the other hand, after a milk feed, heat production in brown adipose tissue quickly recommences although the tissues fat content does not measurably increase (4). Presumably fatty acids provided by the milk are necessary for thermogenesis.

ADAPTION TO AMBIENT TEMPERATURES AFTER BIRTH

a. *Well fed rabbits reared in a warm environment*

Rabbits reared from birth in a thermoneutral environment grow rapidly and more than double their body weight within the first week of life (5). In contrast, their brown adipose tissue only increases in weight by 50% and this is largely due to the deposition of fat (fig. 3). The maximal response to cold exposure of these animals at 7 days of age was less, expressed per kg./body weight, than it was at birth but the rate per gram brown adipose tissue remained the same. In practical terms, as the young rabbit increases in size, its surface area/body weight ratio improves, and its thermal insulation increases so that a smaller increase in heat production permits a wider range of thermal control (6). This more than compensates for the relative fall in thermogenic capacity, so at one week of age the young rabbit maintains a near constant internal thermal environment over a wider range of ambient temperatures than it did at birth.

b. *Well fed rabbits reared in cold environment*

Prolonged cold exposure of adult rats leads to hypertrophy of their brown adipose tissue with an increase in the capacity of non-shivering thermogenesis (7). In contrast the weight of brown adipose tissue of rabbits reared from birth in cold conditions was less than that of rabbits reared in warm conditions. However, this difference was due largely to its smaller fat content (6) (fig. 3). The thermogenic response to cold exposure of these rabbits at the end of one week was greater than that of rabbits reared in a warm environment, and there are several pieces of evidence to suggest that this was due to increased rates of heat production in their brown adipose tissue. For example, noradrenaline causes a larger increase in the temperature of the tissue and a greater rise in the blood flow through it.

c. *Under-fed rabbits in a warm environment*

Over a surprisingly wide range the rate that rabbits grow is directly proportional to the amount of milk that they receive (8). In rabbits fed so that their body weights increased very little over the first week of life, the maximal rates of heat production were far less than they were at birth. The thermogenic capacity of their brown adipose tissue had fallen considerably, and its wet weight was less than half that normally found at birth (fig. 3). This fall was not due to a fall in triglyceride content alone, for the tissue still contained 50% fat. As we shall see later, this tissue has a greatly increased capacity to supply fatty acids for use elsewhere.

As the young mammal grows not only does the surface area/body weight ratio become more favourable and thermal insulation improve, but also shivering thermogenesis makes an increasing contribution to the animals response to cold (9, 10, 11). Thermogenesis in brown adipose tissue slowly dwindles away; but the tissue remains, in the rabbit it continues to form about 2% of the body weight. We must now consider its performance with respect to its second activity, namely the storage and supply of fatty acids.

BROWN ADIPOSE TISSUE AS A SOURCE OF FREE FATTY ACIDS

On the basis of studies *in vitro* on brown adipose tissue from newborn rabbits DAWKINS and HULL in 1964 (12) suggested that when lipolysis occurred in white adipose tissue the fatty acids were, in the main, released from the cells for oxidation elsewhere, whereas, when it occurred in brown adipose tissue the fatty acids released were largely oxidized in the cell to produce heat. This has now been confirmed by investigations on brown adipose tissue *in vivo* but it is essential to emphasise that it is true only for tissue from newborn animals (13). Experiments on brown adipose tissue in young rabbits has shown that under certain circumstances the tissue releases fatty acids at a rate far greater than has previously reported for brown or white adipose tissue either *in vitro* or *in vivo* (2). This surprising finding must in part be due to the tissues exceptionally generous blood supply (14, 15).

INITIATION OF FATTY ACID RELEASE – THE SWITCH ON

In the uterus, the developing mammal is not only kept warm but also, under normal conditions, does not experience starvation. The weight of evidence at the present indicates that although fatty acids can cross the placenta they do not do so in significant amounts (16). It is probable that glucose forms the main source of cellular energy and that the fat laid down in adipose tissue stores is formed mainly by lipogenesis from glucose.

Studies on the net exchange of metabolites by brown adipose tissue from new-born rabbits within an hour or so of birth show that, whether at rest or whilst producing heat in response to noradrenaline infusion, the tissue takes up glucose but does not release fatty acids. The tissue behaves as though it were under the influence of insulin and indeed the circulating concentration of insulin is high (17).

For the first 48 hours after birth brown adipose tissue is reluctant to release fatty acids in response to starvation (table 1) (18). Only after 48 hours does its fat content begin to fall and the fatty acids escape from the tissue (19). It is relevant to note at this time also, that the tissue is still taking up glucose despite low circulating levels (13). At this time we found that the circulating concentration of insulin was as high as it was in well-nourished does on free feeding at the time of delivery (20).

Table 1. *The rate of fatty acid release from brown adipose tissue in vivo in rabbits before and during noradrenaline infusion. It can be seen that the rate of fatty acid release varies with the age of the animal, and its previous experience of cold conditions, and state of nutrition.*

	Fatty acid release (m-equiv./g. min)	
	At rest	During noradrenaline infusion
Unfed new-born rabbits aged 1–3 hours kept at 36 °C	0.03	0.05
Unfed new-born rabbits aged 48 hours kept at 36 °C	0.22	0.96
Well-fed week old rabbits reared at 36 °C	0.13	0.72
Well-fed week old rabbits reared at 36 °C — then starved for 48 hours	0.33	1.86
Well-fed week old rabbits reared at 30 °C	0.01	0.05
Under-fed week old rabbits reared at 36 °C	0.48	1.60

ADAPTIONS TO NUTRITIONAL PLANE AFTER BIRTH

This slow response in the newborn contrasts with that in well-nourished week old rabbits who had been reared in a thermoneutral environment. In these animals after 48 hours starvation, the tissue had lost half its stored fat and were releasing fatty acids at a considerable rate. This increased further during stimulation with noradrenaline despite an increase in the tissues own fatty acid consumption (table 1). On the other hand, the brown adipose tissue of week-old rabbits reared in a cold environment, which had a lower fat content, was reluctant to release fatty acids either at rest or during infusion of noradrenaline. In this state the tissue needed all it could get for its own metabolic processes. This response is reminiscient of the state in the hibernating animal, which during the starvation of hibernation, slowly depletes its adipose tissue stores. The white adipose tissue fat content falls gradually to zero whereas the fat content of brown adipose tissue falls along with that of white adipose tissue until it reaches 40% and there it stays until arousal. On the other hand, the relative small mass of brown adipose tissue in underfed rabbits, which had the surprising fat content of 50% released fatty acids at a considerable rate without prolonged starvation.

SUMMARY

It would seem that the tissue can adapt to cold or to starvation. The relative deployment of the fuel stores depends on previous conditions. In the immediate newborn period and after prolonged cold exposure the first priority seems to be thermogenesis, and very little is supplied. In the face of prolonged undernutrition the first priority appears to be supply, and the thermogenic capacity of the tissue falls.

Although nonshivering heat production in the young mammal slowly disappears to negligible proportions, brown adipose tissue remains. If it maintains its exceptional ability to supply fatty acids, and preliminary experiments on older rabbits suggest that it does, then its role in the adult may be significant. It has been suspected for some time that the function of storage and supply of fatty acids is by no means equally deployed in the adipose tissue masses and brown adipose tissue may well be a rapid turnover unit.

COMMENT

These experiments pose a number of interesting questions. For example, what mechanisms tune brown adipose tissue towards the end of gestation so that it efficiently produces heat but does not release fatty acids immediately after birth? Do the mechanisms which operate during prolonged cold exposure to increase brown adipose tissue's thermogenic capacity also stimulate its growth? Why does undernutrition reduce the tissue's thermoregulatory role?

Many hormones have been shown to effect brown adipose tissue; for example, insulin increases glucose uptake and reduces fatty acid release but has no effect on thermogenesis (22, 23); catecholamines, like insulin, increase glucose uptake, but they increase the rate of fatty acid release and stimulate thermogenesis. However, the effects of catecholamines varies considerably with the state of the tissue. Thyroxin is one hormone which is known to modulate the effect of catecholamines on adipose tissue. Many other hormones stimulate fatty acid release from brown adipose tissue including growth hormone, corticotrophin, glucogen and other pituitary peptides (23). Many of these also stimulate thermogenesis in newborn animals (24). However it is difficult, from the evidence at present available, to postulate which agents are operating under the varying environmental conditions and to what effect. Further investigations are needed.

REFERENCES

1. WILLIAMSON, J. R., (1970) *J. Biol. Chem.* 245:2043.
2. HARDMAN, M. J. and D. HULL, (1970) *J. Physiol.* 206:263.
3. HULL, D. and M. M. SEGALL, (1965) *J. Physiol.* 181:449.
4. HARDMAN, M. J., E. N. HEY, and D. HULL, (1969) *J. Physiol.* 205:39.
5. HARDMAN, M. J., D. HULL, and J. OYESIKU, (1970) *Biol. Neonat.* (in press).
6. HARDMAN, M. J. and D. HULL, (1970) *J. Physiol.* 210:41.
7. ROBERTS, J. C. and R. E. SMITH, (1967) *Amer. J. Physiol.* 212:519.
8. HARDMAN, M. J., D. HULL, and J. OYESIKU, (1970) *Biol. Neonat.* (in press).
9. BRÜCK, K. and B. WÜNNENBERG, (1967) *Fed. Proc.* 25:1332.
10. ALEXANDER, G., A. W. BELL, and D. WILLIAMS, (1970) *Biol. Neonat.* 15:198.
11. HARDMAN, M. J. and D. HULL, (1970) In: *Brown Adipose Tissue*, Lindeberg, O. ed., Elsevier Publishing Co., New York.
12. DAWKINS, M. J. R. and D. HULL, (1964) *J. Physiol.* 172:216.
13. HARDMAN, M. J. and D. HULL, (1970) *J. Physiol.* (In press).
14. HAUSBERGER, F. X. and M. M. WIDELITZ, (1963) *Amer. J. Physiol.* 204:649.

15. Heim, T. and D. Hull, (1966) *J. Physiol.* 186:42.
16. Myant, N. B. (1970) In: *Scientific Foundations of Obstetrics and Gynaecology.* Philipp, E. E., J. Barnes and M. Newton, eds. Heinemann, London. p. 354.
17. Milner, R. D. G. (1969) *J. Endocr.* 43:119.
18. Hull, D. and M. M. Segall, (1966) *Nature,* 212:469.
19. Heim, T. and M. Kellermayer, (1966) *Excerpta Medica Monograph* p. 249.
20. Hardman, M. J., D. Hull, and A. D. Milner, (Unpublished data).
21. Dole, V. P. (1965) In: *Handbook of Physiology.* Renold, A. E. and G. F. Cahill, eds. American Physiological Society, Washington. p. 13.
22. Hardman, M. J. and D. Hull, (Unpublished data).
23. Joel, C. D. (1965) In: *Handbook of Physiology.* Renold, A. E. and G. F. Cahill, eds. American Physiological Society, Washington. p. 59.
24. Cockburn, F., D. Hull, I. Walton, (1967) *Brit. J. Pharm. & Chem.* 31:568.

DISCUSSION

Prof. Visser: Is there a relation between cold exposure and thyroxin. Would you speculate on the composition of nutritional fats and the building up of brown adipose tissue in the human infant.

Dr. Hull: It was thought that thyroxin was one of the main hormones responsible for the cold-adapting process. However some of the people involved in the work have said that the results were largely due to a higher content of thyroxin in the diet given to the rats.

There is no doubt that thyroxin and noradrenalin activity are closely related. With an increase in thyroxin there is an increased response to noradrenaline. It is attractive to think that in a hyperthyroid state an animal will have a larger thermogenic response to cold exposure.

The fats in brown adipose tissue of newborn mammals are formed larger by lipogenesis from glucose, which determines their fatty acid composition. Afterwards I think brown adipose tissue does not differ from white, other than it more closely reflects what has been eaten recently.

Prof. de Bruyne: Is there much variation within the species in the amount of brown adipose tissue?

Dr. Hull: As far as babies are concerned this is very difficult question. It is not easy to dissect brown adipose tissue out cleanly in lobes, as it is in rabbits. It is intermingled in places with white adipose tissue. Nor can it be distinguished easily either macroscopically or microscopically. When brown adipose tissue is overfilled with fat it is unilocular, just like white adipose tissue.

Dr. Schröter: I should like to come back to the question of small for date babies. Do you think that it is the same whether you have starvation postnatally or in utero?

Dr. Hull: My explanation for the rapid rise in free fatty acids would be that in the animals experienced starvation before birth this would tend to increase the rate with which brown adipose tissue might mobilise fat.

Whether starvation in utero has the same biological effect as starvation afterwards I don't know. I have doubts especially about the effect of insulin. Growth hormone is higher in small for date babies and it is one of the factors which effect lipolysis.

Prof. de Meyer: Do you have any information about the time before birth at which thermogenesis starts? When these animals are delivered one or two days earlier, do you observe the same phenomena? We have been able to show that adipose tissue of rat embryos becomes sensitive to exogenous insulin at the 18th day. Is there any relation between onset of sensivity to insulin and onset of thermogenesis?

Dr. Hull: We have delivered animals more than two days earlier. In sofar as they have the respiratory capacity they respond by heat production. I don't think that particular experiments will answer your question.

As far as insulin in thermogenesis I'm not sure there is any link at all. Insulin is not thermogenetic in itself. In rabbit insulin levels are very high towards the end of term. We wondered whether the explanation for the slow response of brown adipose tissue to the first experience of starvation was a consequence of the high insulin levels. We measured insulin levels after 48 hours of starvation in rabbits. The insulin were still fairly high.

I'm very hesitant to say that is the reason why it is slow to switch on. But it is interesting that there is still insulin around when the rabbit is hypoglycaemic.

THE DEVELOPMENT OF CARBOHYDRATE TOLERANCE

G. W. MEEUWISSE*

It is necessary to make a distinction between the *intestinal* tolerance and the *metabolic* tolerance to carbohydrates. Before I start to describe the development of some important processes I want to give a brief outline of the physiology of the digestion and absorption of carbohydrates.

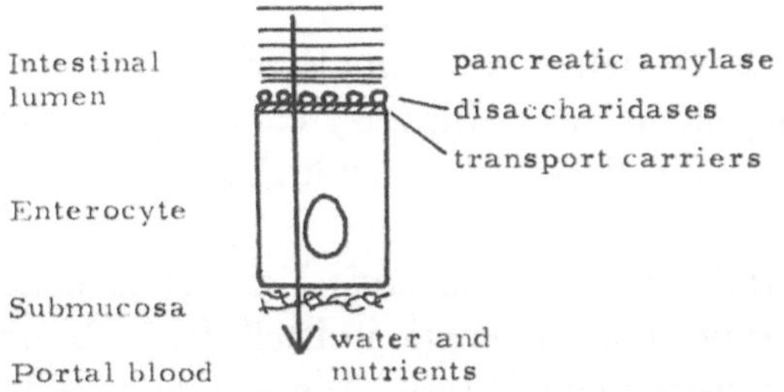

Fig. 1. Topographic relation between enzymes and transport carriers involved in the absorption of carbohydrates.

At the interface between the intestinal fluid and the tissue of the intestinal wall we can distinguish three main steps in the process of digestion and absorption of carbohydrates. As indicated in fig. 1 during absorption there is a stream of water and nutrients from the lumen to the portal blood. Slowly absorbed solutes and unabsorbable material are concentrated in and on a layer of mucopolysaccharides (glycocalix) covering the surface of the enterocytes. Starch is hydrolysed to oligosaccharides by amylase and then further broken down to glucose by disaccharidases. The disaccharidases are firmly attached on or constitute part of the cell membrane. Finally a transport mechanism transfers glucose to the interior of the enterocytes. Although not present in

* Department of Pediatrics, University of Lund, Sweden.

the diet as monosaccharides, glucose and galactose are the physiological fuel for carbohydrate metabolism. The main absorption pathway of the small intestine is identical for these sugars, and it is an active transport mechanism, implying that absorption can occur against a concentration gradient (uphill transport). Fructose, another dietary hexose, liberated by hydrolysis of sucrose, has been considered to be absorbed by a passive process, but according to recent experiments with human (1) and rat (2) tissue, some accumulation of fructose in the intestinal epithelium does take place.

DEVELOPMENT OF GLUCOSE ABSORPTION

To my knowledge measurements of the transport of glucose through the intestinal wall of human foetuses have only been carried out in Koldovský's laboratory in Prague (3). He and his co-workers were able to study foetuses aged between 10 and 20 weeks after conception. At 10 weeks some active transport of glucose and galactose by the jejunum was already demonstrable, and with increasing age there was a steady rise of the transport capacity. Furthermore it was found that active transport, although diminished, was still present after removal of oxygen from the assay system. In adult tissue active transport is not possible in the absence of oxygen. The further development of the intestinal transport mechanism for glucose can only be guessed. Probably there is some further increase in the transport capacity until birth or maybe even thereafter. Experiments by Borgström et al. (4) indicate that glucose disappearance from the gut is slower in premature babies than in full-term newborns. Nevertheless, glucose is often the first nutrient administered to prematures and sick term newborns and it is apparently well absorbed. Studies in rats have shown a postnatal increase in the rate of glucose absorption until the age of about 30 days (3). At least part of this development is a consequence of increasing amounts of dietary carbohydrates. Whether similar changes occur in human babies has not been studied by reliable techniques.

DEVELOPMENT OF DISACCHARIDASES

The important disaccharidases are lactase (a β-galactosidase) and the α-glucosidases sucrase and isomaltase, which together with 2 other

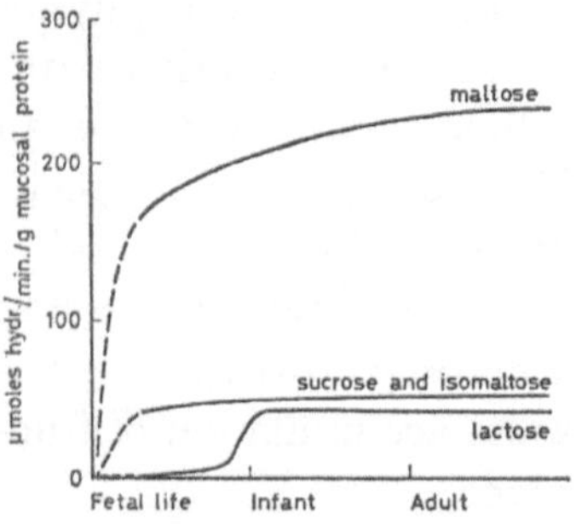

Fig. 2. Development of disaccharidases in the piglet. Data from Bailey et al. (5).

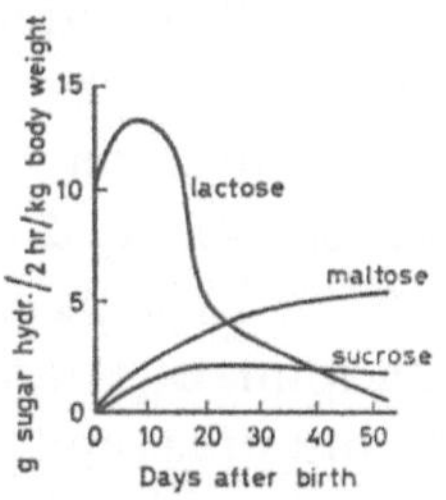

Fig. 3. Development of disaccharidases in the white man. Data from several sources (3, 6, 7).

enzymes hydrolyse maltose. Sucrose is only split by sucrase, and isomaltose only by isomaltase.

Many infant mammals have at birth very low activities of the α-glucosidases. This is exemplified by fig. 2, which shows the development of disaccharidase activities in the pig (5). On the other hand the activity of lactase is high and it remains so during the suckling period. Then, even if lactose feeding is continued, the production of lactase falls and lactose intolerance develops. In guinea pigs, which are rather mature at birth and able to eat adult food, a low activity of intestinal lactase is found and there is little alteration during the weeks following birth. The development of disaccharidases in man has been studied by three groups of investigators (3, 6, 7). The results have been presented schematically in fig. 3. In the foetus of 10 weeks of gestational age, there is already a considerable activity of the α-glucosidases isomaltase and sucrase. If the *whole* small bowel is analysed, there seems to be little increase in these disaccharidase activities, but there is probably an increase in the *jejunal* mucosa (3). A further increase may take place during the last few months of foetal life. The information here upon is still somewhat scarce and, unfortunately, some of the studies have not been done with the best assay techniques.

Lactase activity develops later than that of sucrase and isomaltase. Until 5 months of gestational age only low activities of lactase have been measured. The development of this enzyme occurs mainly during the last 3 or 4 months of foetal life. In one study (6) a further increase of lactase activity during the first 24 hours of life was found. This seemed to be related to the ingestion of food. The question of a postnatal improvement of lactase activity has not been settled definitely. Disappearance of lactosuria, which is often present in newborns (8), is not necessarily due to improved hydrolysis of lactose. The lactosuria of newborns seems rather to reflect an incomplete barrier function of the mucosal epithelium of the upper gastrointestinal tract. There is, however, some evidence that the lactase function is not fully developed at birth and that feeding may have an influence. Studies in premature babies (9) showed increasing rises in blood sugar after oral lactose loads during the first two weeks of life. This could not be attributed to improved absorption of monosaccharides, nor to an altered removal of sugar from the blood stream. In fact, the changing metabolic carbohydrate tolerance ought to result in lower increments of blood sugar concentration with increasing age of the baby. Furthermore, in term infants as well as in premature babies of less than 3 days of age it was possible to obtain significantly larger increments of blood sugar if lactase was administered prior to lactose loading. These studies have shown greater postnatal changes in lactose absorption than one would expect from the measurements of lactase activity in mucosal preparations from foetuses and newborns.

The further fate of lactase of the human intestine is not a subject for this symposium, but I want to make one further remark on fig. 3. In the graph lactase activity is indicated as persisting through childhood and adult life. This is true for this part of the world. In the majority of the world population, however, lactase activity falls to very low levels after the age of 3 or 4 years (10).

The possible influence of dietary changes on the developmental changes of disaccharidase activities has been studied rather extensively in recent years. The current view is that the presence or absence of dietary lactose has no influence on lactase production (11). This contrasts with the stimulation of sucrase and maltase activity by glucose, sucrose and fructose ocurring 2–5 days after the start of carbohydrate feeding.

There are some reports claiming increase in lactase activity after feeding lactose to adult rats (12, 13). The difference, however, seems to be limited to the ileum, and furthermore, it seems likely that the β-galactosidase activity measured was not due to brush border lactase but rather represented the activity of lysosomal β-galactosidase, which is not a functional lactase.

DEVELOPMENT OF α-AMYLASE

Amylase activity of intestinal contents is low in the neonatal period (4). Even at 4 months of age it is still rather low and after a starch meal the degree of carbohydrate polymerisation is correspondingly high (14). A gradual increase in amylase output is seen until about 2 years of age.

DEVELOPMENT OF CARBOHYDRATE TOLERANCE

As this subject has already been dealth with in the first papers of this symposium, I may be allowed to be rather brief on this aspect of carbohydrate tolerance. Fig. 4 represents the alterations in the dis-

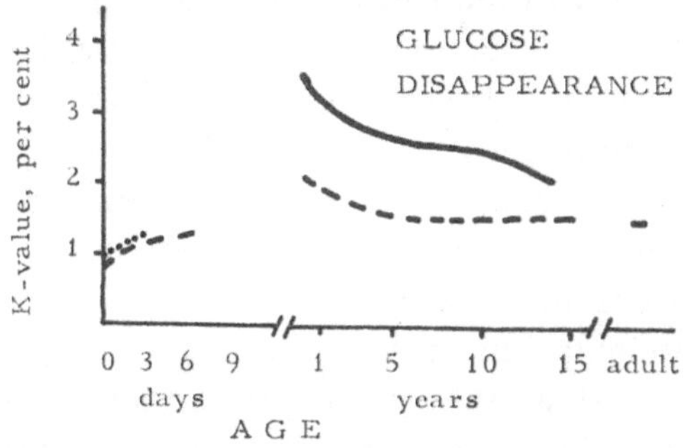

Fig. 4. Disappearance rate of intravenously injected glucose expressed as per cent disappearing per minute (k-value) in relation to age. Data from several sources (15, 16, 17).

appearance rate of intravenously injected glucose during growth (15, 16, 17). The postnatal increase of the glucose removal rate suggests a dietary influence. Starvation and a diet with a low content of carbohydrates is known to reduce the glucose removal rate (18). Galactose is removed from the circulation at a higher rate than glucose (fig. 5). The influence of age has been studied by several authors (19, 20, 21) and the changes resemble those obtained in studies on glucose metabolism. The relatively slow disappearance of galactose during the first days of life is certainly responsible for the frequently observed galactosuria in newborns (22). Acceleration of galactose metabolism during the first weeks of life could of course be due to enzyme induction by

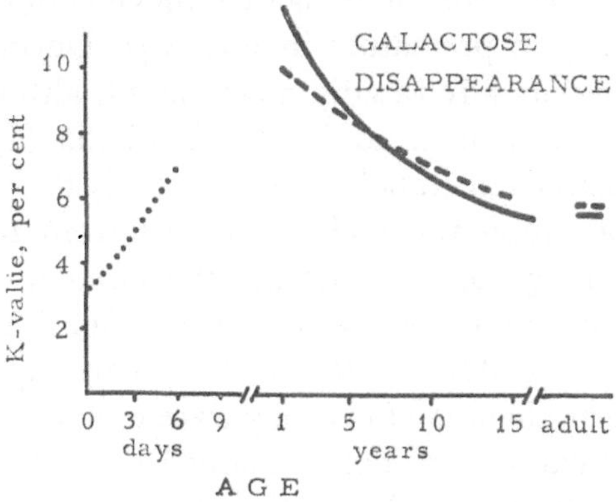

Fig. 5. Disappearance of intravenously injected galactose expressed as per cent disappearing per minute (k-value) in relation to age. Data from several sources (19, 20, 21).

galactose derived from dietary lactose. However, findings in patients with glucose-galactose malabsorption, children who never have absorbed significant amounts of galactose, do not support this assumption. In these patients the removal of injected galactose was as rapid as in normal children (23). Therefore, it seems more likely that the improving galactose metabolism during the newborn period is a consequence of the enlarging total turnover of carbohydrates including, eventually, endocrinologic influences as well.

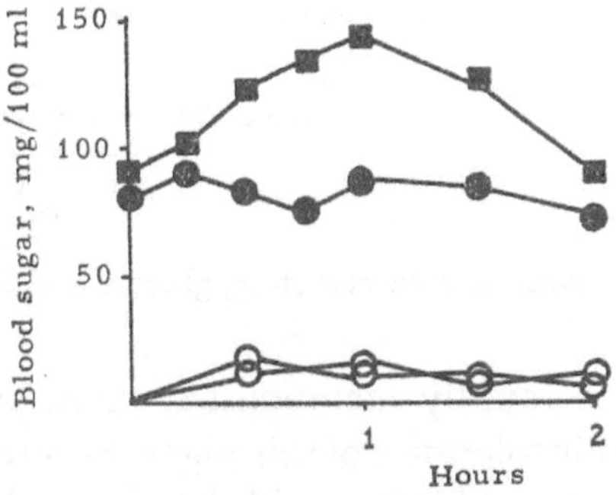

Fig. 6. Influence of nutrition on the fructose tolerance test. Patient with cystic fibrosis. Open symbols, blood fructose. Solid symbols, blood glucose: ●, age 4 months, low-caloric diet and no substitution of amylase; ■, age 5 months, sufficient caloric intake and substitution of pancreatic enzymes (23).

CORNBLATH and collaegues investigated the metabolism of fructose given intravenously to premature infants (24). During the first days of life fructose was already rapidly metabolised, although the process went slightly slower than in adults. In childhood (25) as well as in adult life (26) fructose is metabolised more rapidly than glucose. During carbohydrate starvation removal of fructose from the blood is not affected, but more glucose is entering the circulation than in well nourished individuals (18). As exemplified by fig. 6, the same feature can be observed in children suffering from carbohydrate starvation (23). The observed changes of carbohydrate tolerance after reduction of dietary carbohydrates are best explained by a reduced activity of glucokinase, the enzyme catalysing the phosphorylation of glucose to glucose-1-phosphate (fig. 7).

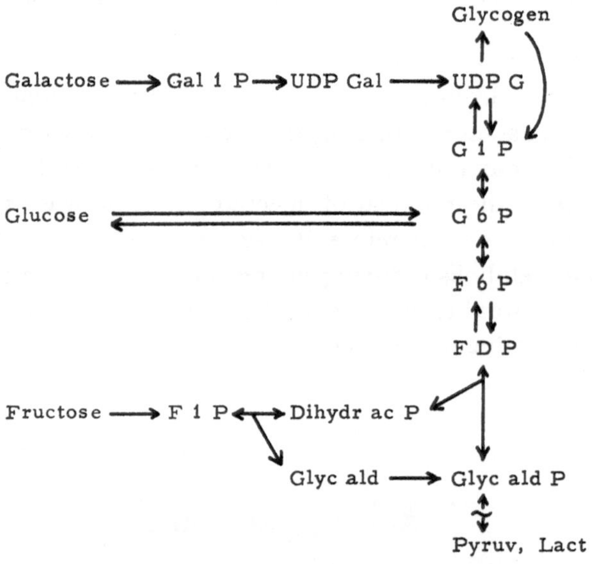

Fig. 7. Main metabolic pathways for galactose, glucose and fructose.

Although fructose is rapidly metabolised, there are certainly limitations in the metabolic tolerance of this sugar. Severe acidosis, probably due to the accumulation of lactic acid, has been observed in children receiving large parenteral infusions of fructose (27). It seems also possible to induce a chronic fructose intoxication. I have seen an infant receiving a therapeutic diet formula containing as much as 10 per cent of fructose, who developed a severe hepatic damage (28), which was similar to the hepato-tubular syndrome observed in some infants suffering from hereditary fructose intolerance (29, 30, 31).

REFERENCES

1. Elsas, L. J., R. E. Hillman, J. H. Patterson and L. E. Rosenberg, (1970) *J. Clin. Invest.* 49:576.
2. Gracey, M., V. Burke and A. Oshin, (1970) Annual Meeting *Europ. Soc. Pediat. Gastroent.* August 22–24, Lund, Sweden.
3. Koldovský, O., (1969) *Development of the functions of the small intestine in mammals and man.* Karger, Basel (Switzerland), New York, p. 168.
4. Borgström, B., B. Lindquist and G. Lundh, (1960) *Am. J. Dis. Child.* 99:338.
5. Bailey, C. B., W. D. Kitts and A. J. Wood, (1956) *Canad. J. Agric. Sci.* 36:51.
6. Auricchio, S., A. Rubino and G. Mürset, (1965) *Pediatrics* 35:944.
7. Dahlqvist, A. and T. Lindberg, (1966) *Clin. Sci.* 30:517.
8. Bickel, H. (1961) *J. Pediat.* 59:641.
9. Boellner, S. W., A. G. Beard and T. C. Panos, (1965) *Pediatrics* 36:542.
10. Bayless, T. M. and N. L. Christopher, (1969) *Amer. J. Clin. Nutr.* 22:281.
11. Rosensweig, N. S. and R. H. Herman, (1969) *Amer. J. Clin. Nutr.* 22:99.
12. Girardet, P., R. Richterich and I. Antener, (1964) *Helv. Physiol. Acta* 22:7.
13. Koldovský, O. and F. Chytil, (1965) *Biochem. J.* 94:266.
14. Auricchio, S., D. D. Pietra and A. Vegnente, (1967) *Pediatrics* 39:853.
15. Bowie, M. D., P. B. Mulligan and R. Schwartz, (1963) *Pediatrics* 31:590.
16. Euler, U. von, Y. Larsson and B. Persson, (1964) *Arch. Dis. Childh.* 39:393.
17. Loeb, H., (1966) *J. Pediat.* 68:237.
18. Craig, J. W., M. Miller, M. S. Mackenzie and H. Woodward Jr., (1958) *J. Clin. Invest.* 37:118.
19. Hjelm, M. and S. Sjölin, (1966) *Scand. J. Clin. Lab. Invest., Suppl.* 92:126.
20. Vink, C. L. J., (1959) *Clin. Chim. Acta* 4:674.
21. Relander, A., (1968) *Scand. J. Clin. Lab. Invest.* 22:196.
22. Dahlqvist, A. and N. W. Svenningsen, (1969) *J. Pediat.* 75:454.
23. Meeuwisse, G. W. and B. Lindquist, (1970) *Acta Paediat. Scand.* 59:74.
24. Cornblath, M., S. H. Wybregt and G. S. Baens. (1963) *Pediatrics* 32:1007.
25. Orsini, M. and T. Stoja, (1951) *Arch. Ital. Pediat.* 15:122.
26. Heinz, F., W. Lamprecht and J. Kirsch, (1968) *J. Clin. Invest.* 47:1826.
27. Andersson, G., J. Brohult and G. Sterner, (1969) *Acta Paediat. Scand.* 58:301.
28. Meeuwisse, G. W. and G. Rohmée (in preparation).
29. Levin, B., G. J. A. I. Snodgrass, V. G. Oberholzer, E. A. Burgess and R. H. Dobbs, (1968) *Amer. J. Med.* 45:826.
30. Lindemann, R., L. R. Gjessing, B. Merton, A. C. Löken and S. Halvorsen, (1970) *Acta Paediat. Scand.* 59:141.
31. Grant, D. B., F. W. Alexander and J. W. T. Seakins, (1970) *Acta Paediat. Scand.* 59:432.

DISCUSSION

Dr. Eggermont: Do you observe satisfactory digestion of starch in the newborn?

Dr. Meeuwisse: Such studies have not been done in children before four months of age. At that age there is still a low digestion of starch I cannot tell you about the development from birth till four months of age.

Dr. Eggermont: We have only data on the amylase content of the pancreas during the first days of life. We do not find any amylase activity in the pancreas at that time of life.

Prof. Fomon: My colleague, Dr. Thomas ANDERSON, has studied carbohydrate tolerance of the newborn. Administration of starch is followed by little change in glucose concentration of the blood. Preliminary studies suggest that if starch is digested by four-month-old infants, the rate of digestion is probably much less than is true of the adult.

EFFECT OF UNDERNUTRITION ON INTESTINAL ACTIVE TRANSPORT OF SUGARS AND AMINO ACIDS

G. WISEMAN*

This series of experiments** (1–6) was begun in 1958, at which time very little critical work had been published on the effect of undernutrition on intestinal active transport, despite its basic interest and the possible value of the results in applied physiology.

Among the early work was that of CORI & CORI (7), who thought that the rate of disappearance of fructose from the gastrointestinal tract of rats was reduced when the pre-experimental period of fasting was increased from 24 to 48 hours. The method employed, introduced by CORI in 1925 (8), required the feeding of strong solutions by stomach tube, washing out the whole of the gastrointestinal tract at the end of the experimental period, and analysing these collected luminal contents for unabsorbed material. By comparison with rats given blank solutions, the amount of the test substance absorbed per 100 g body weight per hour was calculated, and referred to as the 'absorption coefficient'. The use of 'absorption coefficients' derived in this way has been criticized by BURGET, MOORE & LLOYD (9), FEYDER & PIERCE (10), TRIMBLE, CAREY & MADDOCK (11) and FENTON (12) on the grounds that they could find no consistent relationship between body weight and absorption. Nevertheless, FENTON (12) agreed that starvation seemed to reduce sugar absorption, and this was also the opinion of HORNE, MCDOUGALL & MAGEE (13), ALTHAUSEN & STOCKHOLM (14), MARRAZZI (15), MAGEE (16) and LARRALDE (17). On the other hand, FEYDER & PIERCE (10), who used CORI's technique, claimed that a 48-hour fast gave inconsistent results for glucose absorption, and HELLER (18) noted that the decreased absorption produced by fasting rats for 48 hours was not seen in rats fasted for 96

* Department of Physiology, University of Sheffield, England.

** These results were obtained in collaboration with Drs GHADIALLY, HINDMARSH, KERSHAW, KILBY, NEALE, NEAME and ROSS.

hours. HALMI & SPIRTOS (19) reported that the amount and percentage of glucose absorbed by rats was unaffected when the animals were fed only 10 g food per day for 4–6 weeks. Adult rats fed *ad libitum* consume 20–25 g food per day.

In addition to the above observations in under-fed normal animals, work by BLOOR & HAVEN (20) with rats bearing a large Walker Carcinoma 256 (about 50% of the animal's total weight) led to the suggestion that at least some of the loss of weight of the normal tissues was brought about by inadequate digestion and absorption as a result of the intestinal wasting that occurred in such carcinomatous rats. BLOOR & HAVEN (20) did not, however, attempt to measure absorption and they provided no direct evidence about the functional capacity of the intestine in their rats. Theoretical support for BLOOR & HAVEN's speculation came from WISEMAN & GHADIALLY (21) in their account of the probable nutritional events taking place in a tumour-bearing animal. That absorptive function of the rat small intestine might suffer severely during undernutrition was expected because the epithelium is normally replaced every 1½–2 days (22), and according to THAYSEN & THAYSEN (23) starvation in rats caused the intestinal epithelium to become flattened and atrophic. HOOPER & BLAIR (24) stated that during starvation the rat crypt cell mitotic activity was about 80% of normal and was associated with a reduction in the total number of epithelial cells.

It was with this background that we started our investigation into the ability of under-fed small intestine to actively transport sugar and amino acid, chiefly by use of the sac of everted intestine technique of WILSON & WISEMAN (25, 26), but also by some *in vivo* studies.

METHODS

Animals and diets

All the animals were young adult males and were kept in individual cages throughout the experimental period; all (controls and those on a restricted diet) were allowed free access to water. The food was diet 86 for rats and hamsters and diet S.G.I. for guinea-pigs, purchased from Oxoid Ltd., Southwark Bridge Road, London, S.E.I., England.

Control animals were fed *ad libitum* and at the time of experimentation the rats weighed 200–250 g, the hamsters about 100 g, and the guinea-pigs about 320 g.

Rats on a restricted diet were fed 4–10 g food per day for up to 9 days, which caused their body weights fo tall by up to about 30% of their weights at the start of the dietary restriction (initial weight 200–300 g). Some rats were deprived of all food (but allowed water freely) for 4–5 days, resulting in their body weights falling from about 240 g to about 180 g.

Hamsters on a restricted diet were fed 1 g food per day for 7 days, which caused their body weights to fall by about 27% of their weights at the start of the dietary restriction (initial weight about 110 g).

Guinea-pigs on a restricted diet were fed 6 g food per day for 9 days, which caused their body weights to fall by about 18% of their weights at the start of the dietary restriction (initial weight about 300 g).

Chemical estimations

When sugars were used separately they were estimated by the colorimetric method of Nelson (27). When D-glucose plus another sugar were employed, the total reducing sugar content was measured by the Nelson (27) technique and the D-glucose itself assayed by the specific D-glucose oxidase colorimetric method of Huggett & Nixon (28), enabling the amount of the second sugar to be obtained by difference. Sugars do not all reduce the Nelson (27) reagent to the same extent and appropriate allowance for such variation must be made.

Methionine was estimated by the colorimetric method of McCarthy & Sullivan (29) and histidine by the colorimetric method of Macpherson (30).

The amounts of endogenous histidine-reacting and methionine-reacting material released from the intestinal wall during incubation in solutions initially free of these amino acids were measured. No histidine-reacting material was found in the final mucosal fluid; in the final serosal fluid, fully-fed sacs released histidine-reacting material which amounted to 8%, and under-fed sacs 6%, of the total colour producing substance present in experiments in which 2 mM D-histidine had been added initially. In the case of methionine, no significant amount of endogenous methionine-reacting material was released from the intestinal wall during incubation.

The L-glucose was free of D-glucose and L-arabinose.

Estimation of endogenous D-*glucose in rat intestinal wall*

The endogenous D-glucose in the intestinal wall of the rat was measured using the middle two-fifths of the washed out (not everted) unincubated small intestine. The tissue, rinsed free of blood, was dropped into 20 ml boiling water and homogenized using a M.S.E. homogenizer with stainless steel cutting blades operated at 14000 rpm for 3 minutes. The homogenate was deproteinized by the use of $ZnSO_4$ and $Ba(OH)_2$, and 1 ml samples of filtrate from fully-fed rats and 2 ml samples from under-fed rats were analysed by the D-glucose oxidase method (28).

IN VITRO EXPERIMENTS

Preparation of sacs

In some groups of experiments animals were killed by a blow on the head, while in others the animals were anaesthetized with pentobarbitone sodium given intraperitoneally. The abdomen was opened by a mid-line incision and the small intestine washed out with bicarbonate-saline (31) equilibrated with 5% CO_2, 95% O_2 at room temperature. The mesentery was then stripped off the small intestine, the duodenum removed, and the intestine everted with the aid of a glass rod of suitable diameter. In some cases sacs were prepared from only the proximal part of the small intestine, in other experiments sacs were made from equidistant points along the whole small intestine, and in yet other groups of experiments only the mid-small intestine was used. The actual sites from which sacs came for any group of experiments are given in the tables and figures. Sacs from hamsters and guinea-pigs were 4–5 cm long, while rat sacs were 4–5 cm long in some groups of experiments and about 9 cm long in others.

Measurement of initial and final volumes

The initial volume of fluid (serosal) introduced into carefully drained sacs of everted intestine was determined either directly from the 1 ml tuberculin syringe used, or by weighing the sacs before and after filling them. For rats, this initial serosal volume was 0.5–1.0 ml for standard sacs and about 2 ml for extra-distended ones. For hamsters and for guinea-pigs the initial serosal volume was about 0.5 ml. The final volume of the serosal (inner) fluid was estimated by draining the sacs of their contents and weighing the fluid collected. This latter technique enables about 96% of introduced fluid to be recovered from unincubated sacs (32). The volume of outer (mucosal) fluid into which each sac was placed at the beginning of the incubation period was 20 ml.

Almost all standard sacs (initial serosal volume 0.5–1.0 ml) gained serosal fluid, whereas extra-distended sacs usually lost serosal fluid during incubation.

Experimental procedure for transport experiments

A sac, filled with a known volume (initial serosal fluid) of the appropriate solution, was put into a 150 ml Erlenmeyer flask containing 20 ml (initial mucosal fluid) of the same solution as was used for filling it, the air replaced by a gas mixture of 5% CO_2, 95% O_2, and the stoppered flask shaken (80 oscillations per minute for rats and hamsters, 60 oscillations per minute for guinea-pigs; amplitude 5 cm) for 1 hour in a Warburg bath kept at 37 °C. At the end of the hour the sac was removed, its surface drained, and its fluid contents collected. Samples of initial and final mucosal and serosal fluids were analysed for sugar and amino acid concentrations. In some experiments the final solutions needed deproteinization. This was carried out with $ZnSO_4$ and $Ba(OH)_2$ for sugar estimations; for amino acid estimations, samples were deproteinized with equal volumes of 0.6 N perchloric acid, centrifuged at 3000 rpm for 10 minutes, and the supernatants analysed without neutralization for D-methionine but with neutralization with KOH for D-histidine.

The mucosal and serosal fluids were bicarbonate-saline (31) plus the test substrate; the tables and figures indicate the amount and type of substrate studied.

Dry weight

In most experiments sac dry weight was measured directly. After removal of the serosal fluid, the sac was laid on Whatman No. 50 filter paper, and the tissue beyond the ligatures, together with the ligature thread, cut off and discarded. Excess surface fluid was then blotted and the empty sac dried to constant weight at 120 °C.

For some experiments sac dry weight was calculated from the sac's initial wet weight by application of a wet weight/dry weight factor of 19.1 which had been determined experimentally.

Concentration ratios

The *final concentration ratio* was the ratio of the sugar (or amino acid) concentration in the serosal (inner) fluid to that in the mucosal (outer) fluid at the end of the incubation period. The *initial concentration ratio* for all test substances was 1.0.

Rates of transport

The amount of test substance transported into the serosal fluid during an experiment was calculated (the initial and final concentrations and serosal fluid volumes being known) and the transport expressed as μmole entering the serosal fluid per 100 mg dry weight of sac per hour.

The rate of transport of water into the serosal fluid during incubation was calculated in m-mole water per 100 mg dry weight of sac per hour.

L-*glucose recovery experiments*

To test whether L-glucose was lost during incubation, sacs from fully-fed and under-fed rats were made as for standard absorption experiments and filled with 0.8 ml bicarbonate-saline solution with or without 8.33 mM L-glucose and shaken for 1 hour in 10 ml of the same solution as was used for filling them. At the end of the incubation period, each sac was homogenized (as above) and the homogenate added to its pooled final mucosal plus serosal fluids, deproteinized with $ZnSO_4$ and $Ba(OH)_2$, made up to 200 ml, and filtered. One millilitre filtrate was analysed for total reducing sugar by the NELSON (27) method. The amount of reducing sugar found (allowance being made for the initial wet weight of the sac) when no L-glucose had been added ('blank' experiments) was used as a correction factor in determining the amount of L-glucose recovered in experiments in which the sugar had been added. Under these conditions the 'blank' values (no L-glucose added) were about 10% of the recovery values (L-glucose added to the system) with fully-fed rats and about 3% with under-fed rats. For fully-fed rats 96% of added L-glucose (16.2 mg) was recovered at the end of 1 hour incubation, while for under-fed rats the value was 100%.

Analysis of samples with D-glucose oxidase gave no indication of conversion of L-glucose to D-glucose.

IN VIVO EXPERIMENTS

These animals were anaesthetized with intraperitoneal doses of 5 mg pentobarbitone sodium per 100 g body weight and were kept on a warm operating table. The abdomen was opened by a mid-line incision and a transverse cut made in the upper duodenum and at the ileo-caecal junction, so that the whole of the small intestine could be washed out with bicarbonate-saline solution (kept at 37 °C). The duodenum was then ligated about 1 cm distal to the transverse cut and the washing out fluid remaining in the intestine was gently expressed. A ligature was then tightened around the lower ileum and over a blunt needle, attached to a syringe, which had been inserted through the lower transverse cut. Five millilitres of the test solution (containing either D-glucose alone or L-histidine plus D-glucose) was then injected into the intestinal lumen and as the needle was withdrawn the tightened ligature became securely tied. The intestine was then returned to the abdominal cavity for a noted time, at the end of which the animal was killed by opening the chest and incising the heart. The small intestine was then excised, its surface rinsed free of blood, and its contents washed out with bicarbonate-saline solution into a 50 ml volumetric flask, which was then made up to the mark. Samples were analysed for D-glucose or L-histidine in the usual way. The length of the small intestine was measured, care being taken to avoid stretching.

For zero time experiments, the animals were killed as soon as the test solution had been injected into the intestinal lumen, and the latter washed out immediately.

All solutions were gassed with 5% CO_2, 95% O_2 before use.

RESULTS AND DISCUSSION

IN VIVO EXPERIMENTS

The effect of undernutrition (5 g food per day for 9 days; body weight loss 20–25%) on the rates of absorption of D-glucose and L-histidine by anaesthetized rats is shown in figures 1 and 2 respectively. In the case of the sugar, many time intervals from 0–30 minutes were used for measuring absorption rate. For the amino acid, however, it was decided to obtain enough values at zero time and after 10, 20 and 30 minutes to enable a statistical evaluation to be made of the results for each of these experimental periods. The results plotted in figure 2 are the means and 95% confidence intervals for each period of absorption, i.e. it can be said with 95% certainty that the true mean lies within these limits. Testing the significance of the difference of the means of the control and under-fed animals, we found that at zero

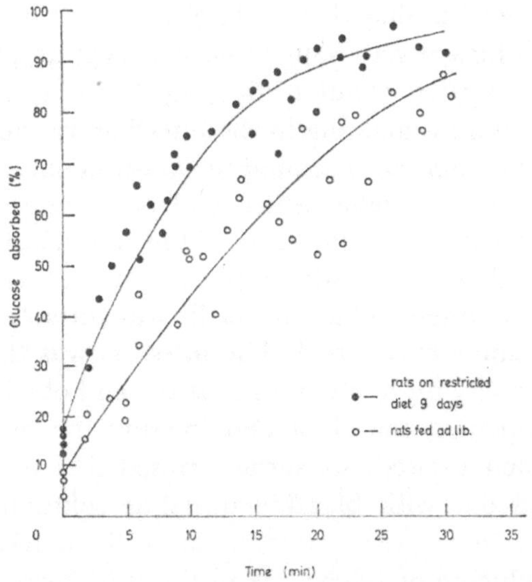

Fig. 1. Effect of undernutrition on the rate of absorption of D-glucose from the whole of the small intestine of rats *in vivo*. Five ml of 22.2 mM D-glucose in bicarbonate-saline solution introduced into each small intestine. O, rats fed *ad libitum*; •, rats restricted to 5 g food per day for 9 days. From KERSHAW *et al.* (3).

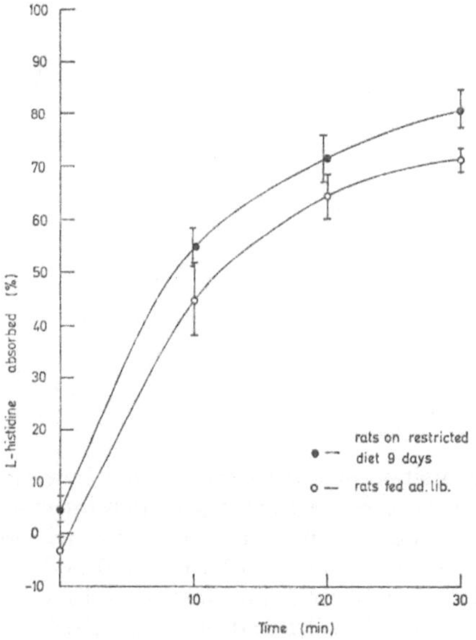

Fig. 2. Effect of undernutrition on the rate of absorption of L-histidine from the whole of the small intestine of rats *in vivo*. Five ml of 1 mM L-histidine with 16.7 mM D-glucose in bicarbonate-saline solution introduced into each small intestine. Ten rats in each group for the estimation of absorption at zero time; eight rats in each group at 10, 20 and 30 minutes. Values are means and 95% confidence intervals. O, rats fed *ad libitum*; ●, rats restricted to 5 g food per day for 9 days. From KERSHAW *et al.* (3).

time $P<0.01$, at 10 minutes $P<0.02$, at 20 minutes $P<0.02$ and at 30 minutes $P<0.01$.

It can be seen that for both D-glucose and L-histidine absorption from the whole of the small intestine was faster in under-fed than in fully-fed rats. Under the conditions employed, the effect was more obvious with the sugar than with the amino acid. After 10 minutes the amount of D-glucose absorbed by the under-fed rats was about 70% of the dose, whereas it was only about 45% for the normal rats; after 20 minutes the values were 90% and 70% for under-fed and normal rats respectively. By about 30 minutes nearly all the D-glucose introduced into the intestinal lumen had been absorbed by both the under-fed and the control animals. For L-histidine, under-fed rats absorbed about 55% of the dose after 10 minutes, in contrast to about 45% for control rats; at 20 minutes the values were about 70% for under-fed

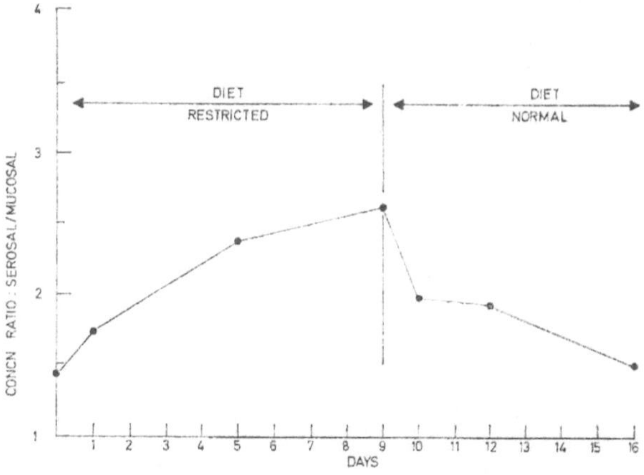

Fig. 3. Effect of undernutrition on the D-glucose final concentration ratio (serosal/mucosal) developed by sacs of everted proximal small intestine of rats restricted to 5 g food per day for up to 9 days. After 9 days on the restricted diet some rats were given food *ad libitum* for up to 7 days. Initial mucosal and serosal fluid contained 16.7 mM D-glucose and 2 mM L-histidine; initial mucosal fluid volume 20 ml; initial serosal fluid volume 0.5–1.0 ml; sac length 3-4 cm; experimental period 1 hour; temperature 37°C. Each point is the mean of 32–36 sacs.

rats and 60% for control ones. For both D-glucose and L-histidine the difference in absorption rates in the two groups of rats was apparent even at zero time.

Although more rapid absorption into the bloodstream is a likely explanation of the enhanced rate of disappearance of substrate from the intestinal lumen of under-fed rats, other possibilities are greater metabolism of the substrate or increased storage in the intestinal wall.

It is interesting to note that the faster uptake of D-glucose and L-histidine in anaesthetized under-fed rats occurred despite the fact that their intestines were somewhat shorter (71 ± 0.7 cm, S.E.M.) than those of fully-fed rats (80 ± 0.8 cm, S.E.M.), had a smaller diameter and hence a decreased surface area, and weighed less.

IN VITRO EXPERIMENTS

a. *Intestinal response to continued under-feeding*

Figures 3 and 4 give the final concentration ratios achieved for D-glucose and L-histidine by sacs made from the upper half of the small intestine of rats restricted to 5 g food per day for up to 9 days (body

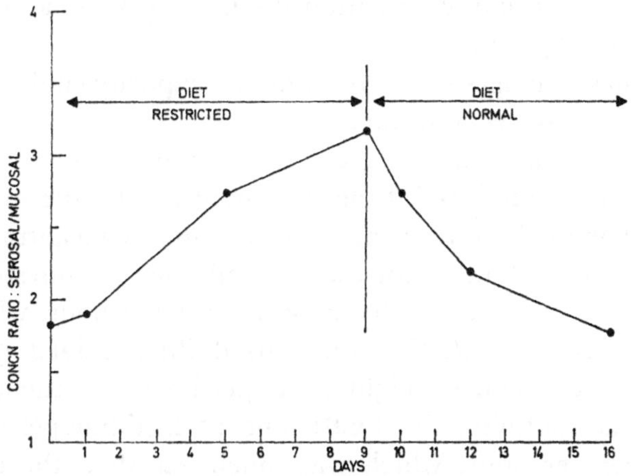

Fig. 4. Effect of undernutrition on the L-histidine final concentration ratio (serosal/mucosal) developed by sacs of everted proximal small intestine of rats restricted to 5 g food per day for up to 9 days. After 9 days on the restricted diet some rats were given food *ad libitum* for up to 7 days. Initial mucosal and serosal fluid contained 16.7 mM D-glucose and 2 mM L-histidine; initial mucosal fluid volume 20 ml; initial serosal fluid volume 0.5–1.0 ml; sac length 3–4 cm; experimental period 1 hour; temperature 37°C. Each point is the mean of 32–36 sacs.

weight loss 20% at 9th day). The final concentration ratio was the ratio of the test substance in the final serosal (inner) fluid to that in the final mucosal (outer) fluid in which the everted intestine had been incubated for 1 hour. The initial concentration ratio for all sacs was 1.0. It was found that whereas normal rat intestine (first point on curve of figure 3) could transfer D-glucose against its concentration gradient to produce a final concentration ratio of 1.44±0.05 (S.E.M.), intestine from rats under-fed for 9 days was able to produce a ratio of as much as 2.63±0.06 (S.E.M.). Similarly, fully-fed intestine (first point on curve of figure 4) gave a final concentration ratio for L-histidine of 1.81±0.05 compared with 3.17±0.13 for intestine from rats under-fed for 9 days. When intestine from rats under-fed for less than 9 days was used, intermediate values were obtained. The final concentration ratios began to rise within the first 24 hours of dietary restriction and from the shape of the curve in figure 3 seemed to be not far from maximum for D-glucose by the 9th day. No attempt was made to under-feed rats beyond 9 days. On re-feeding 9-day under-fed rats with an *ad libitum* diet, the final concentration ratios for both D-glucose and L-histidine fell markedly within the first 24 hours and were back to control levels by 7 days.

None of these changes in active transport capacity could be ascribed to change in net water movement.

Dietary restriction caused greater amounts of D-glucose and L-histidine to be transferred from the mucosal to the serosal fluid concomitant with the improvement in the final concentration ratios. The gain in serosal fluid D-glucose with fully-fed rat intestine was 4.5 μmole D-glucose per 100 mg dry weight of sac per hour, whereas with 9-day under-fed rat intestine the serosal fluid gained 36.6 μmole D-glucose per 100 mg dry weight of sac per hour. For the amino acid, the control serosal fluid gained 2.81 μmole L-histidine per 100 mg dry weight of sac per hour, which was much less than the 8.30 μmole L-histidine per 100 mg dry weight of sac per hour gained by the serosal fluid of 9-day under-fed intestine.

The sudden return to an unrestricted diet had no apparent ill effect on any rat even after 9 days on the reduced diet. This is in agreement with the report of SUN (33), who re-fed starved mice, and in keeping with the observations of LEYTON (34), MOLLISON (35) and MURRAY (36) for semi-starved humans. HEHIR (37) has claimed that in severe starvation there is a point of no return, but his view seems to be incorrect in the absence of disease, gross electrolyte disturbance or avitaminosis, the latter being aggravated or produced especially by large amounts of refined carbohydrate.

b. *Jejunal and ileal response to under-feeding*

Rats: In order to ascertain whether under-feeding affected active transport of one part of the small intestine more than another, the absorption of D-glucose and L-histidine was studied using sacs made from six equidistant points ranging from upper jejunum to lower ileum.

The results for fully-fed rats and those fed 4 g food per day for 7 days (body weight loss 23%), presented in figures 5 and 6, show quite clearly that the final (1 hour) concentration ratios and the total amounts of sugar and amino acid transported to the serosal fluid were much greater for under-fed than for fully-fed intestine, and the phenomenon was evident, for both test substances, throughout the length of

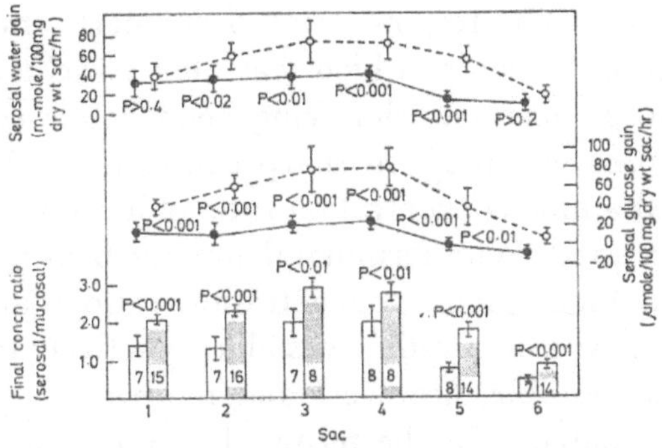

Fig. 5. Effect of undernutrition on the active transport of D-glucose by sacs of everted small intestine of the rat. Rats fed *ad libitum:* open columns and continuous lines. Under-fed rats (4 g food per day for 7 days): stippled columns and interrupted lines. Histogram: ratio of D-glucose concentration in final serosal fluid to that in final mucosal fluid (initial concentration ratio 1.0). Lower two curves: D-glucose entry into serosal fluid. Upper two curves: water entry into serosal fluid. Initial mucosal and serosal fluid contained 16.7 mM D-glucose and 2 mM L-histidine; initial mucosal volume 20 ml; initial serosal volume 0.4–0.5 ml; sac length about 4 cm. Sac 1 = upper jejunum; sac 6 = lower ileum. Experimental period 1 hour. Temperature 37°C. Values are means ± 2 × S.E.M., with number of sacs in each column. From HINDMARSH *et al.* (4).

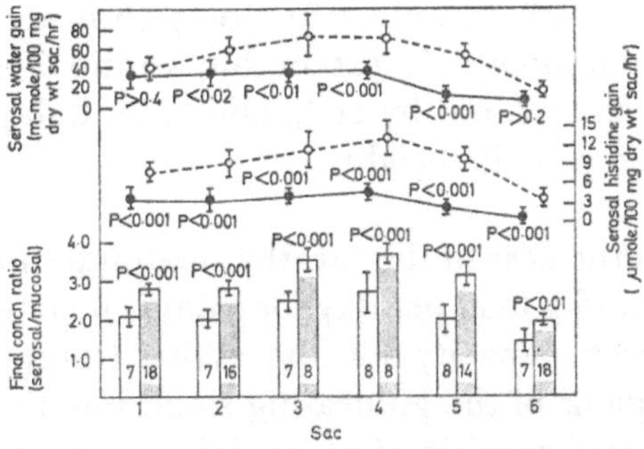

Fig. 6. Effect of undernutrition on the active transport of L-histidine by sacs of everted small intestine of the rat. Rats fed *ad libitum:* open columns and continuous lines. Under-fed rats (4 g food per day for 7 days): stippled columns and interrupted lines. Histogram: ratio of L-histidine concentration in final serosal fluid to that in final mucosal fluid (initial concentration ratio 1.0). Lower two curves: L-histidine entry into serosal fluid. Upper two curves: water entry into serosal fluid. Values are means ± 2 × S.E.M., with number of sacs in each column. Other details as in figure 5. From HINDMARSH *et al.* (4).

the small intestine. The response was particularly impressive for D-glucose absorption by sac 5, which was able to achieve a final concentration ratio of nearly 2, signifying good active transport, when under-fed intestine was used, in sharp contrast to fully-fed intestine which produced a final concentration ratio of less than 1.0, suggesting only passive transport. With terminal ileum, sac 6, although under-fed intestine had a higher final concentration ratio than did fully-fed intestine, neither type of intestine was able to actively transport D-glucose. It remains possible, however, that more prolonged dietary restriction might enable even the terminal ileum to actively transport this sugar. In both groups of rats, active transport of D-glucose was most pronounced with sacs from the middle third of the small intestine. For L-histidine (figure 6), all regions of the rat small intestine transported the amino acid against its gradient, with the middle third once again yielding a peak. Concurrent with the augmented final concentration ratios in the under-fed rats, transport of water into the serosal fluid was enhanced in sacs 2–5 and unchanged in the others. Hence the higher concentration ratios were not a result of decreased net water uptake. The values obtained in these experiments with sacs 1–3 agree well with those reported by KERSHAW *et al.* (3) (figures 3 and 4), who used the proximal half of the small intestine. Also, they are similar to those of SUDA & SHIMOMURA (38), who recorded a L-histidine final concentration ratio of only 1.81 ± 0.17 (S.E.M.) when rats had been fed a diet containing 20% casein, but a ratio of 3.60 ± 0.84 when the casein had been replaced by 20% gluten for 8 days, during which time the rats failed to gain weight.

Guinea-pigs: As in the case of the rat, the small intestine of guinea-pigs on a restricted diet (6 g food per day for 9 days; body weight loss 18%) developed increased capacity for the active transport of D-glucose (figure 7). All regions of the guinea-pig small intestine, including the terminal ileum, were capable of absorbing the sugar against its concentration gradient, and apart from the proximal jejunum (sac 1) all regions had the same final concentration ratio. Net water transport was unaltered by the under-feeding except for sac 1, which gained more water than did normal sacs from this site. Once again, the improved final concentration ratios during under-feeding were not due to a decrease in net water movement.

Hamsters: Unlike the response of rats and guinea-pigs to dietary restriction, golden hamsters fed only 1 g food per day for 7 days (body weight loss 28%) displayed no variation in active transport capacity

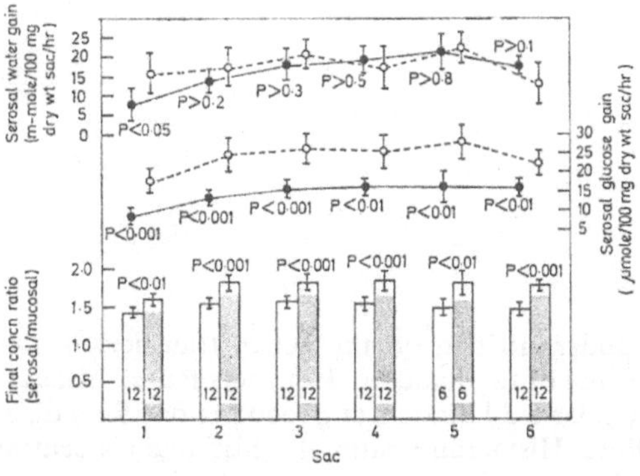

Fig. 7. Effect of undernutrition on the active transport of D-glucose by sacs of everted small intestine of the guinea-pig. Guinea-pigs fed *ad libitum:* open columns and continuous lines. Under-fed guinea-pigs (6 g food per day for 9 days): stippled columns and interrupted lines. Histogram: ratio of D-glucose concentration in final serosal fluid to that in final mucosal fluid (initial concentration ratio 1.0). Lower two curves: D-glucose entry into serosal fluid. Upper two curves: water entry into serosal fluid. The mucosal and serosal fluids had no added amino acid. Values are means ± 2 × S.E.M., with number of sacs in each column. Other details as in figure 5. From HINDMARSH *et al.* (4).

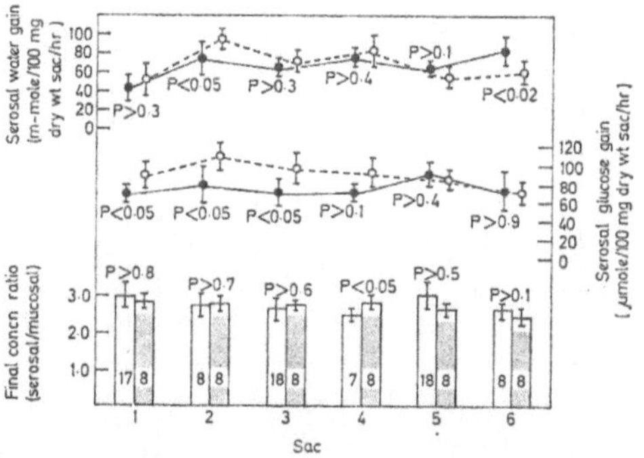

Fig. 8. Effect of undernutrition on the active transport of D-glucose by sacs of everted small intestine of the hamster. Hamsters fed *ad libitum:* open columns and continuous lines. Under-fed hamsters (1 g food per day for 7 days): stippled columns and interrupted lines. Histogram: ratio of D-glucose concentration in final serosal fluid to that in final mucosal fluid (initial concentration ratio 1.0). Lower two curves: D-glucose entry into serosal fluid. Upper two curves: water entry into serosal fluid. Values are means ± 2 × S.E.M., with number of sacs in each column. Other details as in figure 5. From HINDMARSH *et al.* (4).

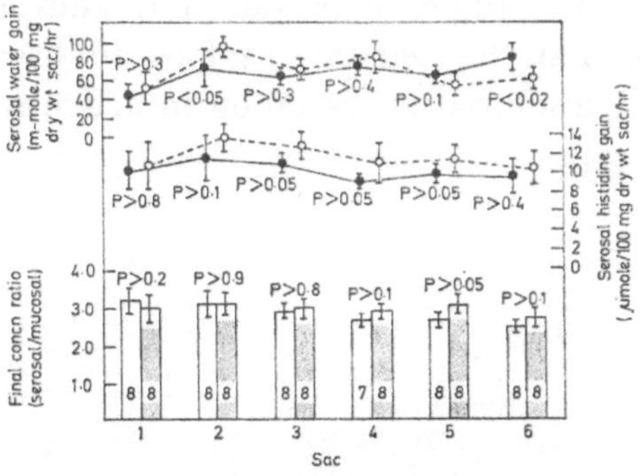

Fig. 9. Effect of undernutrition on the active transport of L-histidine by sacs of everted small intestine of the hamster. Hamsters fed *ad libitum:* open columns and continuous lines. Under-fed hamsters (1 g food per day for 7 days): stippled columns and interrupted lines. Histogram: ratio of L-histidine concentration in final serosal fluid to that in final mucosal fluid (initial concentration ratio 1.0). Lower two curves: L-histidine entry into serosal fluid. Upper two curves: water entry into serosal fluid. Values are means ± 2 × S.E.M., with number of sacs in each column. Other details as in figure 5. From HINDMARSH *et al.* (4).

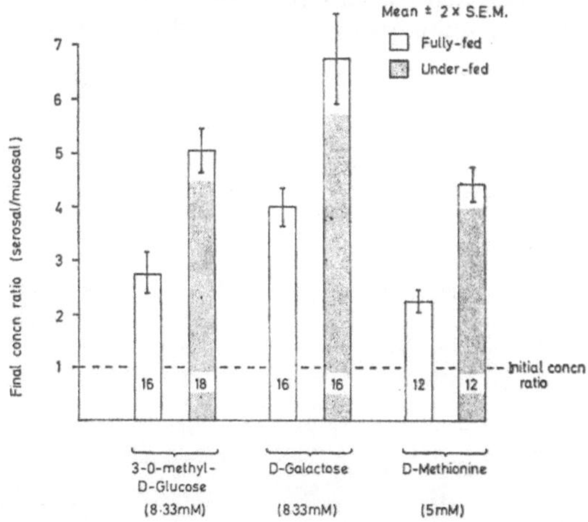

Fig. 10. Effect of undernutrition on the final concentration ratios (serosal/mucosal) of 3-O-methyl-D-glucose, D-galactose and D-methionine developed by sacs of everted mid-small intestine of the rat. The concentration of the substrate in the initial mucosal and serosal fluid is shown in parentheses (each substrate was present alone). Under-fed rats were given 6–10 g food per day for 9 days. Initial mucosal volume 20 ml; initial serosal volume 0.8 ml; sac length about 9 cm; experimental period 1 hour; temperature 37°C. The number of sacs is indicated in each column.

Table 1. *Active transport by standard and extra-distended sacs of everted mid-small intestine of fully-fed and under-fed rats. Underfed rats were given 6–10 g food per day for 9 days. During 1 hour incubation standard sacs gained serosal volume and extra-distended sacs lost serosal volume. Initial mucosal and serosal fluid contained 8.33 mM sugar (initial concentration ratio 1.0); initial mucosal volume 20 ml; sac length about 9 cm; experimental period 1 hour; temperature 37°C. Values are means ± S.E.M., with number of sacs in parentheses.*

	Final substrate concn in serosal fluid (mM)	Final substrate concn in mucosal fluid (mM)	Transport of substrate into serosal fluid (μmole/100 mg dry wt sac/hr)	Gain in serosal fluid water (m-mole/100 mg dry wt sac/hr)	Final concn ratio (serosal/mucosal)
	Fully-fed standard sacs (initial serosal volume 0.8 ml)				
D-galactose	26.6 ± 0.75	6.70 ± 0.11	18.4 ± 1.1	13.3 ± 1.3	4.01 ± 0.17 (16)
3-O-methyl-D-glucose	19.8 ± 0.84	7.25 ± 0.13	14.1 ± 1.5	16.2 ± 2.0	2.78 ± 0.17 (16)
	Fully-fed extra-distended sacs (initial serosal volume 2 ml)				
D-galactose	22.2 ± 0.29	6.45 ± 0.10	29.1 ± 1.3	—3.03 ± 1.08	3.46 ± 0.08 (20)
3-O-methyl-D-glucose	17.6 ± 0.67	6.78 ± 0.11	18.7 ± 1.5	—5.40 ± 1.92	2.61 ± 0.13 (14)
	Under-fed standard sacs (initial serosal volume 0.8 ml)				
D-galactose	39.0 ± 1.80	5.87 ± 0.13	47.4 ± 2.9	20.4 ± 3.4	6.77 ± 0.42 (16)
3-O-methyl-D-glucose	33.3 ± 1.60	6.60 ± 0.14	37.5 ± 2.1	15.5 ± 3.3	5.06 ± 0.21 (18)
	Under-fed extra-distended sacs (initial serosal volume 2 ml)				
D-galactose	34.1 ± 1.80	5.39 ± 0.16	79.4 ± 8.6	—22.4 ± 2.5	6.48 ± 0.49 (14)
3-O-methyl-D-glucose	27.7 ± 0.85	5.80 ± 0.08	50.2 ± 2.2	—16.8 ± 1.4	4.80 ± 0.20 (14)

for either D-glucose or L-histidine (figures 8 and 9). This was despite the fact that the percentage loss of initial body weight (28%) and intestinal dry weight (29%) was as great or greater in the under-fed hamsters as in the under-fed rats and guinea-pigs. Net water movement was also unvaried. As with the guinea-pig, all six sites of small intestine could actively transport D-glucose, and no site was especially endowed for active transport of either the sugar or the amino acid. There is no avaiable explanation for this species difference in intestinal response to under-feeding.

Table 2. *Substrates not actively transported by sacs of everted mid-small intestine of fully-fed and under-fed rats. Under-fed rats were given 6–10 g food per day for 9 days. Initial mucosal and serosal fluid contained 8.33 mM sugar or 2mM D-histidine (initial concentration ratio 1.0); initial mucosal volume 20 ml; initial serosal volume 0.8 ml; sac length about 9 cm; experimental period 1 hour; temperature 37°C.*

Not actively transported by	
Fully-fed intestine	Under-fed intestine
D-arabinose	D-arabinose
D-fructose	D-fructose
D-fucose	D-glucosamine
D-glucosamine	D-mannose
D-mannose	L-arabinose
D-xylose	L-fucose
L-arabinose	L-sorbose
L-fucose	L-xylose
L-glucose	
L-sorbose	
L-xylose	
D-histidine	

C. *Effect of under-feeding on substrates normally actively transported by rat intestine*

In addition to the absorption of D-glucose and L-histidine, already considered in some detail, active transport of 3-O-methyl-D-glucose, D-galactose and D-methionine was studied using sacs of everted mid-small intestine (equivalent to sacs 3 and 4 above) of fully-fed rats and of rats fed 6–10 g food per day for 9 days (body weight loss 32%) (figure 10). All three of these substrates were absorbed against their concentration gradients by normal rats, but the final concentration ratios were very much higher in the under-fed animals. That this phenomenon was independent of net water movement can be seen from the results obtained with standard sacs which gained serosal fluid during incubation and extra-distended sacs which lost serosal fluid during incubation (table 1). Movement of water into or out of a sac made no substantial difference to the final concentration ratio recorded.

d. *Effect of under-feeding on substrates not normally actively transported by rat intestine*

Table 2 gives the substances which were not actively transported by sacs of everted mid-small intestine (equivalent to sacs 3 and 4 above) of fully-fed rats. This was so for standard sacs (initial serosal volume 0.8 ml) which gained serosal volume during incubation and for extra-distended sacs (initial serosal volume 2 ml) which lost serosal volume during incubation. Prevention of water entry into sacs by

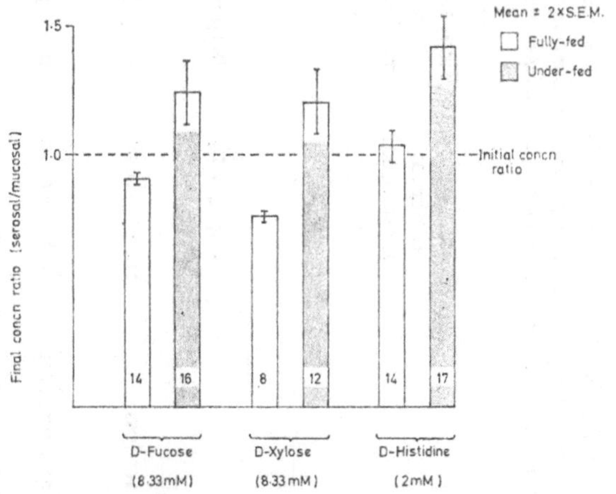

Fig. 11. Effect of undernutrition on the final concentration ratios (serosal/mucosal) of D-fucose, D-xylose and D-histidine developed by sacs of everted mid-small intestine of the rat. The concentration of the substrate in the initial mucosal and serosal fluid is shown in parentheses (each substrate was present alone). Under-fed rats were given 6–10 g food per day for 9 days. Initial mucosal volume 20 ml; initial serosal volume 0.8 ml; sac length about 9 cm; experimental period 1 hour; temperature 37°C. The number of sacs is indicated in each column.

Table 3. *Transport of L-glucose by sacs of everted mid-small intestine of fully-fed, under-fed and completely starved rats. Initial mucosal and serosal fluid contained 8.33 mM L-glucose (initial concentration ratio 1.0); initial mucosal volume 20 ml; initial serosal volume 0.8 ml; sac length about 9 cm; experimental period 1 hour; temperature 37°C. Values are means ± S.E.M., with number of sacs in parentheses.*

	Final L-glucose concn in serosal fluid (mM)	Final L-glucose concn in mucosal fluid (mM)	Transport of L-glucose into serosal fluid (μmole/100 mg dry wt sac/hr)	Gain in serosal fluid water (m-mole/100 mg dry wt sac/hr)	Final concn ratio (serosal/mucosal)
Fully-fed rats (20–25 g food/day)	6.54 ± 0.19	8.19 ± 0.06	0.43 ± 0.20	17.4 ± 1.1	0.80 ± 0.02 (13)
9-day-under-fed rats (6 g food/day: 32% wt loss)	10.53 ± 0.28	8.03 ± 0.06	6.07 ± 0.49	11.7 ± 2.7	1.32 ± 0.04 (15)
5-day-starved rats (given only water: 25% wt loss)	8.85 ± 0.09	8.00 ± 0.03	1.49 ± 0.40	3.74 ± 2.10	1.11 ± 0.01 (12)

extra-distension could not, therefore, convert a non-actively transported substance into an actively transported one.

When sacs from under-fed rats (6–10 g food per day for 9 days; body weight loss 32%) were used, however, active transport did occur for D-fucose, D-xylose, L-glucose and D-histidine (figure 11 and table 3). This first direct demonstration of intestinal active transport of L-glucose and D-histidine (5, 6) substantiated the claim by HINDMARSH, KILBY & WISEMAN (39), who investigated the effect of amino acids on sugar absorption by the fully-fed hamster, that L-glucose and D-histidine movement across the intestine was in some way facilitated. The same authors found that D-fucose was transported against its concentration gradient by fully-fed hamster small intestine. With regard to D-xylose, it has been observed by LARSON, BLATHERWICK, BRADSHAW, EWING & SAWYER (40) that this sugar disappeared from the normal rat intestinal lumen very much more rapidly than did L-xylose, and a special absorption mechanism for it in the fully-fed rat has been suggested by CSÁKY & LASSEN (41) and CSÁKY & HO (42).

The characteristics of D-fucose, D-xylose and L-glucose active transport (need for sodium ions and for oxygen; temperature dependence; inhibition by D-glucose, L-histidine and phlorrhizin) make it most probable that these sugars are transported by the mechanism that actively transports D-glucose.

The sugars which were not actively transported even by under-fed rat intestine are also given in table 2.

e. *Effect of complete starvation*

The ability to actively transport L-glucose after complete deprivation of food (but with freely supplied water) for 5 days was examined in a few rats (table 3). Body weight loss during this period was about 25%, compared with a fall of about 32% for under-fed rats given 6 g food per day for 9 days. Sacs of everted mid-small intestine (equivalent to sacs 3 and 4 above) of these completely starved animals were able to develop a final concentration ratio of 1.11 ± 0.01 (S.E.M.) (indicating active transport), in contrast to a ratio of less than 1.0 (suggesting only passive transport) for fully-fed rats. The rats on the under-feeding programme had a final concentration ratio significantly higher than that of the completely starved rats, possibly because the under-fed rats lost more weight. It may be, though, that enhancement of intestinal active transport is greater with under-feeding than with complete starvation.

f. *Endogenous* D-*glucose in intestinal wall of fully-fed and under-fed rats*

The amount of endogenous D-glucose in the wall of unincubated mid-small intestine of fully-fed and under-fed (6 g food per day for 9 days) rats was measured by means of the specific D-glucose oxidase method (28). Whereas fully-fed intestinal wall had 37.8 mg D-glucose per 100 g wet weight of whole wall, there was only 10.8 mg D-glucose per 100 g wet weight of whole wall for the under-fed rats.

It is possible that the augmented active transport of D-fucose, D-galactose, 3-O-methyl-D-glucose, D-xylose and L-glucose in under-feeding is due, at least in part, to the diminished D-glucose content of under-fed intestine, because D-glucose is a powerful inhibitor of the active transport of these other sugars and its action is greater at higher concentrations. It offers no obvious explanation, however, for the enhanced active transport of D-glucose itself or of the amino acids.

g. *Thinning of the intestinal wall during under-feeding*

Although thinning of the intestinal wall occurs during the under-feeding of rats, guinea-pigs and hamsters, there are a number of reasons for believing that thinning is not the cause of the enhanced active transport:

I. the fall in dry weight, without decrease in length, of the small intestine was as great in under-fed hamsters (29%) as that taking place in under-fed rats (29%) and guinea-pigs (24%), yet hamster intestine showed no change in active transport (4);

II. the distal part of the normal small intestine is thinner than the proximal part (43), yet active transport is no better in the thinner distal part and may be even poorer (4);

III. DOWLING & BOOTH (44) have described enhanced absorption of D-glucose by rat small intestine which had actually hypertrophied as a response to extensive intestinal resection;

IV. stressing the small intestine by feeding a high-bulk low-calorie diet (by adding kaolin) has been reported (45) to cause better absorption of D-glucose and water by the jejunum without change in its thickness;

V. there was faster than normal absorption of both D-glucose and L-histidine from the intestinal lumen of under-fed rats *in vivo* (3). In those experiments the total thickness of the intestinal wall would be irrelevant as the blood vessels carrying away the absorbed substrates lie in close proximity to the epithelial lining.

SUMMARY AND CONCLUSIONS

1. Young adult male rats, guinea-pigs and hamsters were fed a diet deficient only in absolute amount (20–25% of normal intake) but not in its general basic composition. The rats and hamsters lost up to 30% of their body weight at the start of the period of dietary restriction; the guinea-pigs lost about 18%.
2. For rats, under-feeding resulted in faster absorption of D-glucose and L-histidine from the small intestine of anaesthetized animals. It also enhanced the normally occurring active transport, by sacs of everted small intestine, of D-glucose, D-galactose, 3-O-methyl-D-glucose, L-histidine and D-methionine. There was steady improvement in active transport of D-glucose and L-histidine with increasing time of under-feeding over the experimental period of 9 days. In addition, sacs of under-fed small intestine were able to actively transport D-fucose, D-xylose, L-glucose and D-histidine, which sacs of fully-fed rat small intestine could not do. This was the first direct demonstration of intestinal active transport of L-glucose and D-histidine.
3. For guinea-pigs, as for rats, dietary restriction augmented the active transport of D-glucose by sacs of everted small intestine.
4. In contrast to rats and guinea-pigs, under-fed hamsters showed no variation in intestinal active transport capacity for D-glucose or L-histidine. This was despite the fact that the hamsters lost as much as 28% of their initial body weight and 29% of the dry weight of the small intestine. There is no available explanation for this species difference.
5. The final (1 hour) serosal/mucosal concentration ratios produced by sacs for actively transported substrates were independent of net water movement. Causing sacs to lose serosal fluid during incubation

by extra-distending them did not yield a final concentration ratio greater than 1.0 for substrates only passively transported by standard (not extra-distended) sacs.

6. The mid-ileum of the normal rat did not actively transport D-glucose, but it did do so in under-fed rats. The terminal ileum of the rat remained incapable of actively transporting D-glucose even after under-feeding. The whole of the ileum of the guinea-pig and hamster transported D-glucose well.

7. In the rat, D-glucose and L-histidine were transported best by the mid-small intestine. In the guinea-pig, on the other hand, all regions of the small intestine transported D-glucose to the same extent except for the upper jejunum, which was not quite so good as the rest of the small intestine. Similarly in the hamster, no site transported either D-glucose or L-histidine better than any other site.

8. As well as augmenting final concentration ratios, under-feeding caused greater amounts of substrate to enter the serosal fluid.

9. In complete starvation (but with provision of water), as in under-feeding, active transport of L-glucose was stimulated, although it is possible that complete starvation may be less effective than semi-starvation.

10. Neither fully-fed nor under-fed small intestine of rats actively transported D-arabinose, D-fructose, D-glucosamine, D-mannose, L-arabinose, L-fucose, L-sorbose or L-xylose.

11. Fully-fed mid-small intestine of rats had 37.8 mg endogenous D-glucose per 100 g wet weight of tissue, whereas under-fed intestine had only 10.8 mg D-glucose per 100 g. The enhanced active transport of D-galactose, 3-O-methyl-D-glucose, D-xylose and L-glucose by under-fed intestine may be partly explained by this low D-glucose content, since D-glucose is a powerful inhibitor of the active transport of these other sugars. It would not explain, however, the enhanced active transport of D-glucose itself, or of the amino acids.

12. For several reasons, the thinning of the intestinal wall that occurs during under-feeding does not seem to be the cause of the augmented active transport.

13. No apparent ill effect was produced when rats were allowed free access to food after 9 days on a restricted diet.

14. The results show that the small intestine of the rat and the guinea-pig, but not the hamster, has increased active transport capability after a period of under-feeding with a balanced diet.

REFERENCES

1. Neame, K. D. and G. Wiseman, (1959) *J. Physiol.* 146:10P.
2. Wiseman, G., K. D. Neame and F. N. Ghadially, (1959) *Br. J. Cancer* 13:282.
3. Kershaw, T. G., K. D. Neame and G. Wiseman, (1960) *J. Physiol.* 152:182.
4. Hindmarsh, J. T., D. Kilby, B. Ross and G. Wiseman, (1967) *J. Physiol.* 188:207.
5. Neale, R. J. and G. Wiseman, (1968) *J. Physiol.* 198:601.
6. Neale, R. J. and G. Wiseman, (1969) *J. Physiol.* 205:159.
7. Cori, C. F. and G. T. Cori, (1927) *J. biol. Chem.* 74:473.
8. Cori, C. F., (1925) *J. biol. Chem.* 66:691.
9. Burget, G. E., P. Moore and R. Lloyd, (1932) *Am. J. Physiol.* 101:565.
10. Feyder, S. and H. B. Pierce, (1935) *J. Nutr.* 9:435.
11. Trimble, H. C., B. W. Carey, Jr. and S. J. Maddock, (1933) *J. Biol. Chem.* 100:125.
12. Fenton, P. F., (1945) *Am. J. Physiol.* 144:609.
13. Horne, E. A., E. J. McDougall and H. E. Magee, (1933) *J. Physiol.* 80:48.
14. Althausen, T. L. and M. Stockholm. (1938) *Am. J. Physiol.* 123:577.
15. Marrazzi, R., (1940–41) *Am. J. Physiol.* 131:36.
16. Magee, H. E., (1945) *Proc. R. Soc. Med.* 38:388.
17. Larralde, J., (1947) *Rev. esp. Fisiol.* 3:31.
18. Heller, H., (1954) *Br. J. Nutr.* 8:370.
19. Halmi, N. S. and B. N. Spirtos, (1956) *Am. J. Physiol.* 187:432.
20. Bloor, W. R. and F. L. Haven, (1955) *Cancer Res.* 15:173.
21. Wiseman, G. and F. N. Ghadially, (1958) *Br. med. J.* 2:18.
22. Leblond, C. P. and C. E. Stevens, (1948) *Anat. Rec.* 100:357.
23. Thaysen, E. H. and J. H. Thaysen, (1949) *Acta path. microbiol. Scand.* 26:370.
24. Hooper, C. S. and M. Blair, (1958) *Exp. Cell Res.* 14:175.
25. Wilson, T. H. and G. Wiseman, (1954) *J. Physiol.* 123:116.
26. Wiseman, G., (1961) In: *Methods in Medical Research*, Quastel, J. H. ed., Year Book Medical Publishers, Chicago, Ill., p. 287.
27. Nelson, N., (1944) *J. biol. Chem.* 153:375.
28. Huggett, A. St. G. and D. A. Nixon, (1957) *Lancet* 273:368.
29. McCarthy, T. E. and M. X. Sullivan, (1941) *J. biol. Chem.* 141:871.
30. Macpherson, H. T., (1946) *Biochem. J.* 40:470.
31. Krebs, H. A. and K. Henseleit, (1932) *Hoppe-Seyl. Z.* 210:33.
32. Wiseman, G., (1955) *J. Physiol.* 127:414.
33. Sun, T. P., (1927) *Anat. Rec.* 34:341.
34. Leyton, G. B., (1946) *Lancet* 251:73.
35. Mollison, P. L., (1946) *Br. med. J.* 1:4.
36. Murray, R. O., (1947) *Lancet* 252:507.
37. Hehir, P., (1922) *Br. med. J.* 1:865.
38. Suda, M. and A. Shimomura, (1964) *Osaka Univ. med. J.* 16:11.
39. Hindmarsh, J. T., D. Kilby and G. Wiseman, (1966) *J. Physiol.* 186:166.
40. Larson, H. W., N. R. Blatherwick, P. J. Bradshaw, M. E. Ewing and S. D. Sawyer, (1940) *J. biol. Chem.* 136:1.
41. Csáky, T. Z. and U. V. Lassen, (1964) *Biochim. biophys. Acta* 82:215.
42. Csáky, T. Z. and P. M. Ho, (1965) *Proc. Soc. exp. Biol. Med.* 120:403.
43. Wilson, T. H. and G. Wiseman, (1954) *J. Physiol.* 123:126.
44. Dowling, R. H. and C. C. Booth, (1967) *Clin. Sci.* 32:139.
45. Dowling, R. H., E. O. Riecken, J. W. Laws and C. C. Booth, (1967) *Clin. Sci.* 32:1.

DISCUSSION

Dr. Lindblad: This could be of very great importance to the first rehabilitation measures after undernutrition. Our assumption was that the small-for-dates baby was essentially undernourished. We studied the 1 hour post-alimentary increase of leucine in normal fullterm newborns at 4 hours of age and after 48 hours of starvation. At 4 hours of age there was no significant increase of leucine, after 48 hours of starvation there was a significant increase. If we turn to the praemature babies, we had the same results. In the small for dates babies, however, where the mother had hypertension during pregnancy, there was a significant plasma increase of leucine already after the first meal (5 grams of breast milk) at 4 hours of age. It might be, that in small for dates babies the first milk feed means a leucine load.* The same holds true for the newborn starving piglet (CUPERLOVIC, M., (1967) *Acta Met Scand* 8:217).

Dr. Wiseman: There has been some work done on newborn chicks. The ability to actively transport glucose across the wall in newborn chicks is much greater if the chicks are not fed during the first days of life. We have seen that in the hamster we cannot get the same effect as in the rat and in the guinea pig. We were lucky to start our work with the rat and the guinea pig.

Most of the work in the clinical literature shows absorption to be poor in undernourished individuals. I think that most of those individuals were malnourished, not undernourished, and they had disease.

* LINDBLAD, B. S., (1970) *Acta Paediat Scand* 59:13.

METABOLISM OF CARBOHYDRATES AND FAT COMPONENTS IN PREMATURE AND FULL-TERM NEWBORN INFANTS AFTER INFUSIONS OF TRIGLYCERIDES AND GLYCEROL

H. WOLF*

The requirement of the normal newborn infant for energy is high immediately after birth, especially when the environmental temperature is not in the so-called neutral zone. This is very often the case in emergency situations. In premature infants the amount of substrates which provide energy during the first few hours of life is very limited. The carbohydrate reserves are low and the fat deposits do not exceed 5 percent of body weight in infants under 2000 g. In contrast full term normal newborn infants have 16 percent of their body weight as fat (1, 2).

In the past, feeding of prematures was deliberately delayed for two days or longer to prevent aspiration. At the present time most authorities agree that food should be provided as early as possible, and should be predominately in the form of carbohydrate solutions, given initially in the 6th hour of life. As Schröter et al. (3) showed, carbohydrates in appropriate amounts can prevent the keto-acidosis that usually occurs as the result of the highly active fat utilization during the first few days. The ketoacidosis in the newborn infant reaches its highest level on the 3rd day and does not seem to be very harmful. The fact that the respiratory quotient drops to 0.7 also indicates that fat is oxidized in remarkable amounts. The small-for-date infant with nearly no carbohydrate deposits reaches a lower RQ than the normal one in the 12th hour of life (4).

Our studies of enzymes in the liver and in the brown adipose tissue of newborn rabbits revealed a very high activity of hydroxyacyl-CoA-dehydrogenase, the key enzyme in fatty acid oxidation in the brown adipose tissue (fig. 1), (5), as compared with adult values, but not in the liver.

* Department of Paediatrics, Univ. Göttingen, Germany. Supported by the Deutsche Forschungsgemeinschaft, Grant Wo 69/7. Present address: Department of Paediatrics, Kassel, Stadtkrankenhaus.

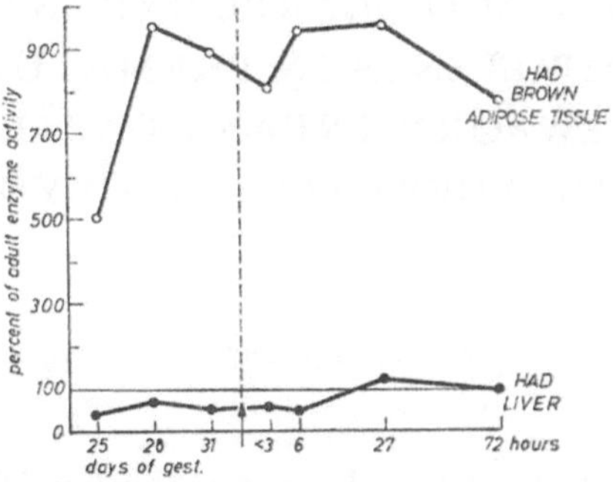

Fig. 1. Activity of hydroxyacyl-CoA-dehydrogenase in the nuchal fat and in the liver of newborn rabbits as percentage of adult values (adult rabbits: activity in nuchal fat or liver = 100%).

Table 1. *Hydroxycyl-CoA-dehydrogenase activity in μ moles of substrate per minute per 100 mg protein in brown adipose tissue of newborn rabbits and white adipose tissue of adult rabbits and newborn infants.*

Brown adipose tissue: (newborn rabbit)	24 to 30 hrs.	57.9
	3 days	46.7
White adipose tissue: (adult rabbit)		6.0
White adipose tissue: (newborn infant)	< 24 hrs.	10.5
	25 to 48 hrs.	14.5
	49 to 66 hrs.	12.1
	4 to 13 days	22.0

We investigated the same enzyme in the white adipose tissue of newborn infants (6), and found that it also had a remarkably high activity, although not nearly as high as in the fat of the newborn rabbit (table 1). Thus we know that fatty acids can be oxidized to a considerable extent in the fat tissue but not to the same extent in other organs (brain, heart, liver).

Although the premature and the small-for-date infant is able to use fatty acids as a source of energy, this ability has not very often been used heretofore in parenteral feeding of such infants. There has been extensive experience with carbohydrate feedings either by the oral or the intravenous route. Only few attempts, however, have been made to provide fat emulsions for parenteral feeding of newborn infants (7, 8). HOLT et al. (9) were the first investigators who showed a decrease in the RQ after fat infusions, indicating that the artifical emulsions had been metabolized. Most of the emulsions produced in the past were not stable enough for use or did not conform to the safety regulations. However, recently fat emulsions from soybean oil (Intralipid®) or cotton seed oil (Lipofundin®) adjusted to isotonicity either with sorbitol or glycerol, have become available.

We investigated a variety of fat emulsions (Infonutrol®, Intralipid®, Lipofundin®) with different admixtures (glucose, glycerol, sorbitol) and different emulsifiers (egg lecithine, soy bean lecithine, soy bean phosphatides).

In short time experiments, we injected 0.5 g of fat emulsion over a 1 to 3 minutes period into premature infants and measured triglycerides, glycerol, free fatty acids, glucose and ketone bodies during the subsequent 4 hours (fig. 2). After a steep rise of triglycerides we observed the slope of the curve very carefully in order to measure the elimination half life time of the triglycerides. The magnitudes of the

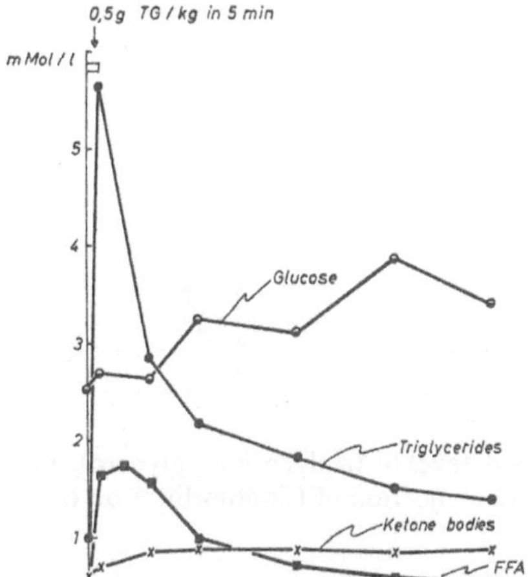

Fig. 2. Blood levels of triglycerides, FFA, glycerol, glucose and ketone bodies (mMol/l) after i.v. injection of 0.5 g triglyceride emulsion per kg into newborn infants.

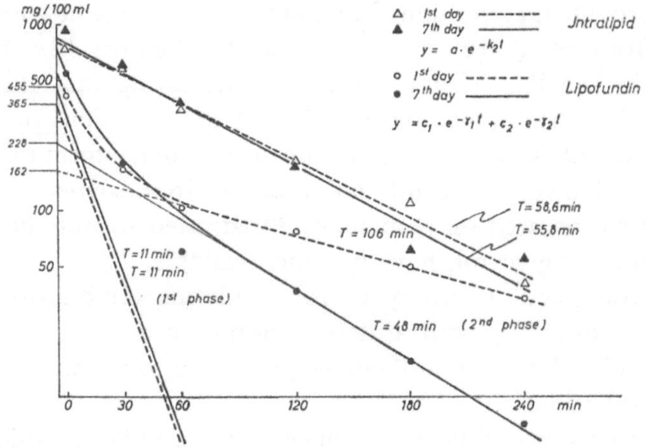

Fig. 3. Elimination of triglycerides in premature infants after injection of Lipofundin ® and Intralipid ® respectively, Y-axis logarithmic scale.

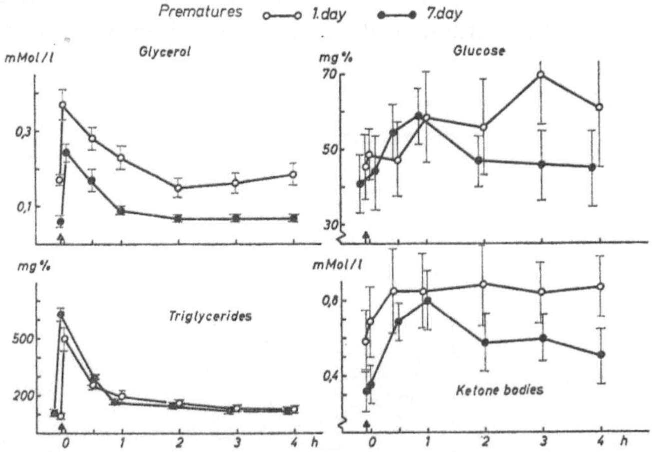

Fig. 4. Changes in blood level of triglycerides, glycerol, glucose and ketone bodies in premature infants after injection of Lipofundin ® on the 1st and 7th day of life.

slope depended on the age of the infant. Only after Intralipid® infusions the slope was identical in the two age groups (1 day and 7 days). With cotton seed oil infusion (Lipofundin®) the older age group (6 to 8 days) was clearly characterised by a shorter elimination time than the younger age group, 1 to 2 days of age. Another difference between these two fat emulsions was the pattern of the elimination curve (fig. 3), Lipofundin® showed an elimination according to a two-compartment-system whereas in Intralipid® this appeared to be a one compartment process and it was slow for both age groups.

The lipolysis was efficient immediately after the injection of the fat emulsion. As shown in fig. 4 glycerol had increased two fold in the one day old infants and 5-fold in the 7 day old ones. In order to calculate the lipolytic rate we used the method of DOST (10). In Intralipid®-infusions we calculated the triglyceride appearance and elimination in the extravascular space (fig. 5 and fig. 6). The rate of lipolysis was 180 mg triglycerides per kg per hour or 4.3 g/kg/day in the one-day-old infants and 296 mg per kg per hour or 7.1 g/kg/day in the 7-days-old ones.

A product of lipolysis and fatty acid oxidation, the ketone bodies, rose soon after the injection of any of the fat emulsions. This increase was much more pronounced in the 7-days-old infants than in the one-day-old ones. The latter maintained a medium ketone level through-

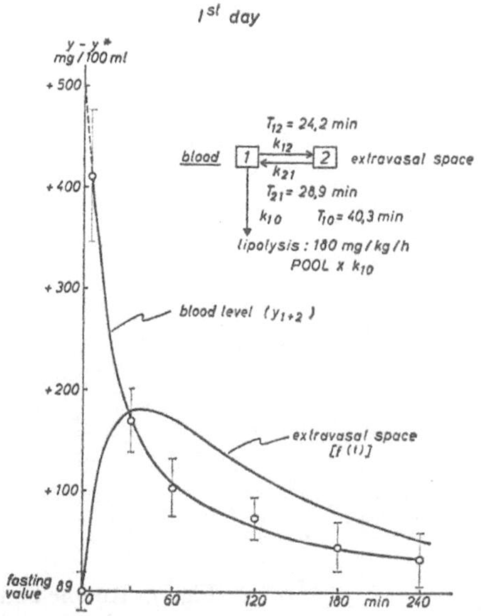

Fig. 5. Elimination of triglycerides from the intravascular and the extravascular space on the first day of life.

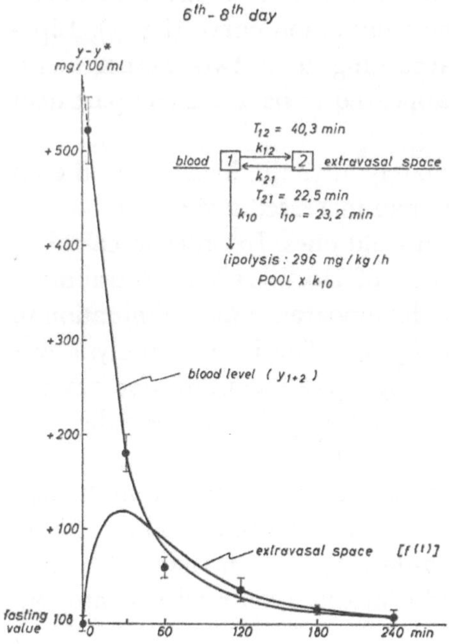

Fig. 6. Elimination of triglycerides from the intravascular and the extravascular space on the seventh day of life.

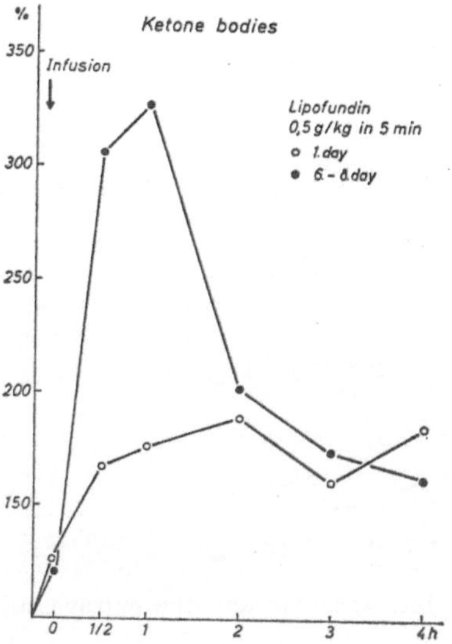

Fig. 7. Ketone bodies in the plasma of 1 day and 7 days old premature infants after injection of 0.5 g triglycerides per kg.

out the experiment (fig. 7). Since the newborn is able to eliminate the ketone bodies in the urine, this behaviour is probably either an expression of the slower oxidation of ketone bodies or failure of extensive ketone bodies production in the very young premature infants, or both.

In order to show to what extent glycerol is metabolized we infused glycerol into newborns of different kinds and ages. Fig. 8 shows that the rate of glycerol elimination is age dependent. We found an elimination of 50% in 40 minutes in one day old infants, 15 minutes in those of 1 week, and 12 minutes in those of 4 weeks of age (11). After infusion of glycerol, the glucose level rose for some time (fig. 9), in all groups. Therefore we have assumed that in infants just as in the animal (12), most of the glycerol is converted to glucose. Taking into account the high needs of small-for-date infants for energy, the rise of blood glucose in this group was very low. It is probable therefore that glycerol is used without conversion to glucose.

We have to be very careful, however, in interpreting those results since in our new studies we saw elevation of glucose after series of heel pricks only without any loading (13).

The elimination of the free fatty acids (FFA) that were produced after the injection of triglycerides was measured in order to calculate

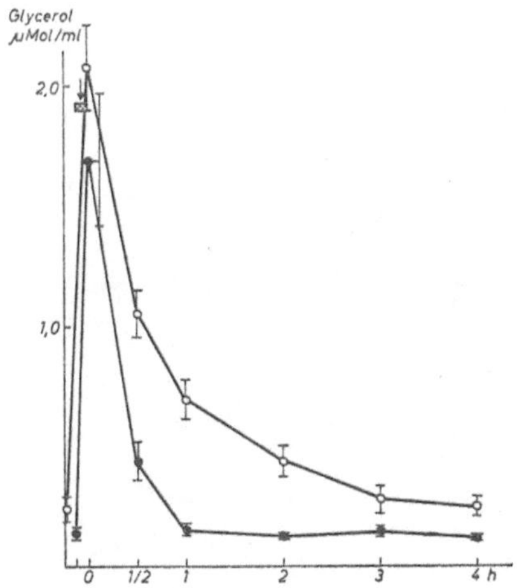

Fig. 8. Elimination of glycerol from the blood stream in full-term infants of 1 day and 4 weeks of age.

the transfer of these metabolites. The formula for the transfer (10) is:

$$T = \frac{D \times k_2 \times y^*}{y1 - y^*},$$

where k_2 is the elimination constant, y^* the fasting level before the infusion and D the dose of FFA given to the infant, calculated from the dose of triglycerides. The turnover or transfer of FFA is highly active in the first few days but it slows down later. The transfer of triglycerides, however, increases. Glycerol shows the same trend as the FFA (fig. 10). The molar ratio between glycerol and FFA is 1.5 on the first, the 7th and 28th day. Thus the infant maintains a constant relationship between recycling and oxidation of FFA in the fat tissue itself, but his rate of production of triglycerides, by digestion of exogenous fat and resynthesis in the intestine increases. The following might be an explanation for the high ketone body production in spite of the lower transfer of FFA: in the first few days FFA–endogenous and exogenous – are used for heat production primarily in the adipose

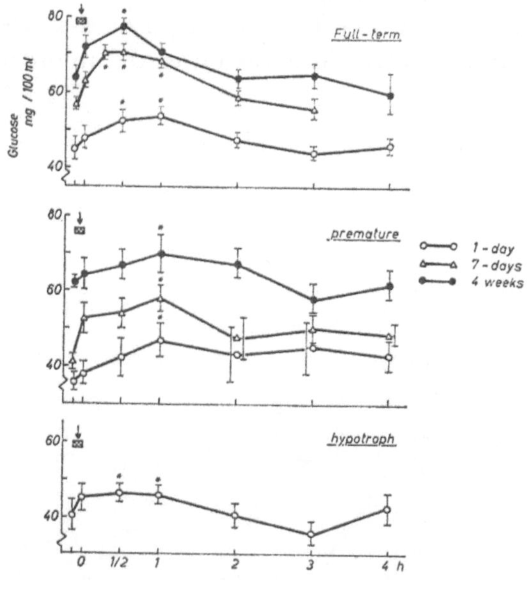

Fig. 9. Changes of blood glucose in newborn infants after infusion of 0.1 g glycerol per kg.

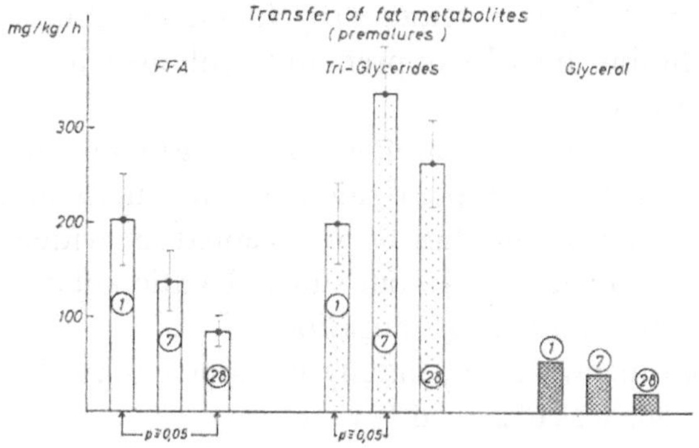

Fig. 10. Transfer of FFA, triglycerides, and glycerol in infants of 1 day, 7 days and 4 weeks of age.

tissue. Transfer of FFA is high without production of ketone bodies since those are produced only in the liver. Older infants with a higher triglyceride turnover because they are fed, produce more ketone bodies since now more FFA enter the liver via portal circulation despite the lower transfer in the body circulation, where we can measure it.

In the light of the new knowledge we tried to adapt the fat emulsions to long term infusion practice. Since the transfer of triglycerides in premature infants is between 180 and 200 mg/kg/hr. on the first day and 300 mg/kg/hr. on the 7th, we administred 2 g/kg during a 6 hour period each day and in older infants a dose of 1.2 to 1.5 g twice a day over a period of 4 hours each time. In some cases with a steady state of glycerol or triglycerides during the infusion we were able to calculate the transfer of the triglyceride glycerol. In one day old prematures and in small-for-date infants the transfer of triglycerides was slightly higher in longterm infusion than with a single dose (265 mg/kg/hour). In infants between ½ and 2½ month the transfer was about 600 mg/kg/hour (14).

The following side effects of triglyceride infusions have been reported:

1. *The overloading syndrome* (13): In certain premature infants smaller than 1000 g at birth who had received infusions we observed by histological examination tiny fat droplets in the cells of the RES in liver and spleen. However, in non-infused small premature infants the fat infiltrations in their tissues were of the same type and even

more frequent (15). AHERNE (16) found fat droplets in several organs including muscles in premature infants who did not receive fat infusions.

2. *Coagulopathy* resulted in animals and occasionally in men after a fat infusion (17). This type of side effect was not seen in our study.
3. *Elevation of transaminases* has been accepted as evidence of cellular damage in the liver (18). In our study elevation of GOT and/or GPT was only slight and of short duration.
4. In some of our own cases, mainly in older infants, brief *elevation of body temperature* was observed (14, 18).

CONCLUSIONS

In premature infants infusions of fat emulsions can be accomplished and are indicated in such conditions as esophagus atresia, atresia of small intestine, malabsorption syndromes, malnutrition, and failure to thrive.

Recommendation: Dose of infusion during the first day of life: 200 mg/kg/hour, not to exceed a total dose of 2 g/kg within a 6 to 10 hour period, and administered only once daily.

Table 2. *Fat infusions to newborn infants.*

Age	Transfer/kg/h	Total dose/kg/day	Time per day
1st day	200 mg	2 g	1×6 hrs
7th day	300 mg	2,5 to 3 g	2×4 hrs
> 2 weeks	500 mg	4–6 g	2–3×4 hrs

Dose on the 7th day: 300 mg/kg/hour, not to exceed 1.5 g/kg over a 4 hour period in 8 hours time intervals given as two infusions a day. Infants older than two weeks: 500 mg/kg/hour; 4–6 g fat per kg/day, 2 to 3 times a day 2 g per infusion period (table 2).

The mixture containing 1 g fat/kg and some carbohydrate provides about 10 calories, and only 5 ml of fluid. This is a great advantage over all other infusion methods for parenteral nutrition.

REFERENCES

1. Shelley, H. J., (1964) *Brit. Med. J.* 1:273.
2. Widdowson, E. M., R. A. McCance and C. M. Spray, (1951) *Clin. Sci.* 10:113.
3. Schröter, W., G. Vogeler and M. Jensen, (1967) *Monatsschr. Kinderhk.* 115:600.
4. Karlberg, P., (1970) *Acta Paediat. Scand*, in press.
5. Stave, U. and H. Wolf, in preparation.
6. Novák, M., E. Monkus, H. Wolf and U. Stave. (1971) xiii. *Int. Congr. Paediatr.* Wien.
7. Fritze, G. and W. Leuterer (1965). *Med. pharm. Mittlg.* 39:19.
8. Schmidt, G. W., (1964) *Fortschr. Med.* 82:87.
9. Holt Jr. L. E., H. C. Tidwell and T. F. M. Scott, (1935) *J. Pediat.* 6:151.
10. Dost, F. H., (1968) *Grundlagen der Pharmakokinetik, 2. Aufl.* G. Thieme Stuttgart.
11. Wolf, H., V. Melichar and R. Michaelis, (1968). *Biol. Neonat.* 12:162.
12. Nikkilä, E. A., and K. Ojala, (1964) *Life Sci.* 3:243.
13. Stubbe, P., and H. Wolf, (1971) *Hormone & Metabolic Res.*, in press.
14. Ley, H. G., (1969). *Fettinfusionen bei Neugeborenen mit niedrigem Geburtsgewicht (Frühgeborene, hypotrophe Neugeborene) und bei jungen Säuglingen.* Thesis, Göttingen.
15. Levenson, S. M., H. L. Upjohn and T. W. Sheehy, (1957) *Metabolism* 6:807.
16. Aherne, W., (1965) *Arch. Dis. Childh.* 40:406.
17. Huth, K., W. Schoenborn and J. Börner, (1967) *Med. u. Ernährg.* 8:146.
18. Otten, A., (1969) *Ketonkörper und Glucose im Blut bei Frühgeborenen und jungen Säuglingen.* Thesis, Göttingen.

In these investigations were involved:

S. Lausmann, Yellow Springs, Ohio, H. G. Ley, München, H. Löhr, Wolfsburg, M. Novák, Miami, Fla., E. Monkus, Miami, Fla., A. Otten, Bremen, U. Stave, Yellow Springs, Ohio, R. Stoltzfus, Yellow Springs, Ohio.

DISCUSSION

Dr. Meeuwisse: At our department we tried to give lipids intravenously to praemature children. Some of the children became acidotic. Do you have any data on acid-base balance during your infusions?

Prof. Wolf: We have measured the ketone-bodies but it does not contribute very much to a change in pH. We measured also the pH, but we found no changes at all.

Dr. Hull: Does the level of circulating free fatty acids influences the rate that the triglyceride is cleared? Do you think there is any point in giving intralipid feeding in the presence of a high level of circulating free fatty acids?

Prof. Wolf: We did not see any difference in the disapperance of triglyceride if we started with high free fatty acids or with low free fatty acids.

CARBOHYDRATE METABOLISM IN THE NEWBORN RAT

R. DE MEYER, P. GERARD AND G. VERELLEN*

The metabolism of newborns is often studied in experimental animals, including the pig, guinea pig, sheep, and cat. Newborn rats, which have the advantage of large litters and can be handled easily, are not suitable for all methods because of their limited size. Nevertheless, it seemed valuable to determine the metabolic parameters of the newborn rat as a basis for research.

Our investigations were limited to carbohydrate metabolism. The animals were obtained by caesarian section on the 21st day of gestation, a few hours before spontaneous delivery would have occurred. For purposes of comparison, we also used 20-day old embryos similarly obtained; these animals survive about 12 to 24 hours if kept under conditions of constant temperature and a high oxygen level of the air, and may be regarded as prematures.

Although there are many data on carbohydrate metabolism in the literature pertaining to experimental neonatology, few concern the newborn rat. The total amount of stored carbohydrates in newborn animals is not known. WIDDOWSON (1), who measured the total amount of glycogen in piglets and newborn infants, obtained values of 9 mg/g and 25 mg/g, respectively, indicating the wide species variation probably related to the degree of differentiation at birth. There are also some data available on the glycogen level in various organs of the newborn rat, as shown in Table I.

The glucose blood levels given in the literature are shown in Fig. 1, from which the increase with increasing gestational age is evident. Lactic acid has been determined by STAFFORD and WEATHERALL (5),

* Laboratory for Teratology and Medical Genetics, Department of Pediatrics, University of Louvain. This study was supported by grants of the 'Fonds de Recherche scientifique médicale' and the 'Fonds médical Reine Elisabeth'.

Table 1. *Glycogen level in four organs of newborn rats (mg/g). Numbers between parentheses indicate references.*

Organs	Alge (days)				
	19	20	21	22	22 1/2
Liver	16 (2) 20 (3)	45 (2) 85 (3)	72 (2) 140 (3)	78 (2) 70 (4) 58 (5)	12 (2) 5 (5)
Heart				26.4 (5)	18 (5)
Lung					6 (2)
Muscle			12 (2)		9 (2)

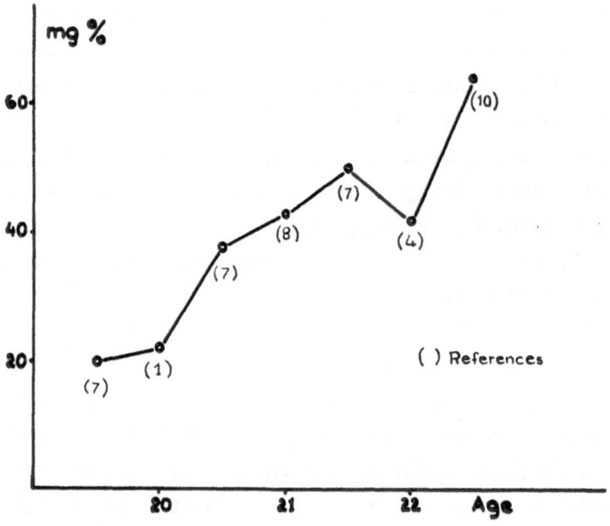

Fig. 1. Glycaemia of rat foetuses.

who found 0.24 mg/g body weight in 22 days old foetuses. Blood values of 73.09 ± 12.07 mg/100 ml have been reported (6).

The changes in these parameters after birth have also been studied. Fig. 2 shows the pattern of glycogen levels in the liver and heart during the first few hours and days after birth.

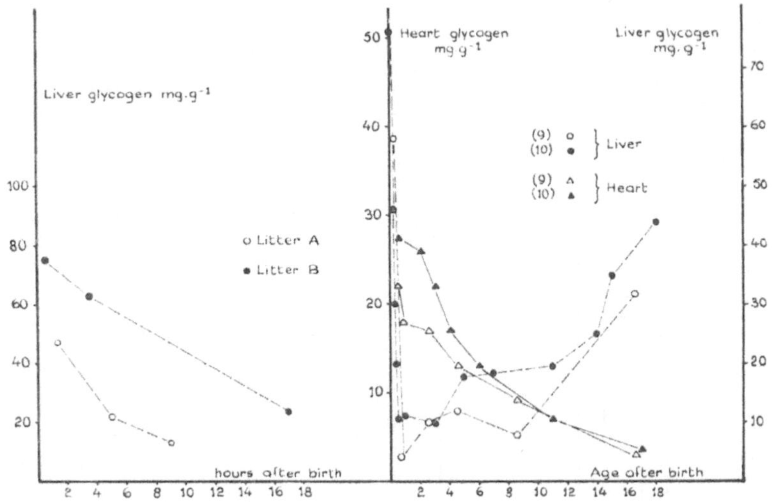

Fig. 2. Glycogen level in newborn rat liver and heart according to STAFFORD and WEATHERALL (1960) and SHELLEY (1961).

Neonatal glucose levels in the blood have been followed by Stafford and WEATHERALL (5); DAWKINS (7); CLARK *et al.* (8); HUNTER (3); and ROUX *et al.* (6). A drop during the first two hours from 40 mg% to 20 mg% is followed by an increase.

The inadequate picture given by the available data led us to perform an extensive investigation of neonatal carbohydrate metabolism. Among the parameters included, some are static, e.g. the body composition at birth, and others dynamic, e.g. the course of the various parameters during the first few hours after birth. Such factors as glycaemia, glycogen and lactic acid contents, oxygen consumption, and carbon dioxide production were considered.

1. CARBOHYDRATE COMPOSITION OF THE RAT EMBRYO

Figure 3 shows the values of glucaemia, lactacidaemia, and total glycogen content. It is clear that as compared with the adult values glycaemia is rather low. No difference is observed between 21 and 22 day old animals.

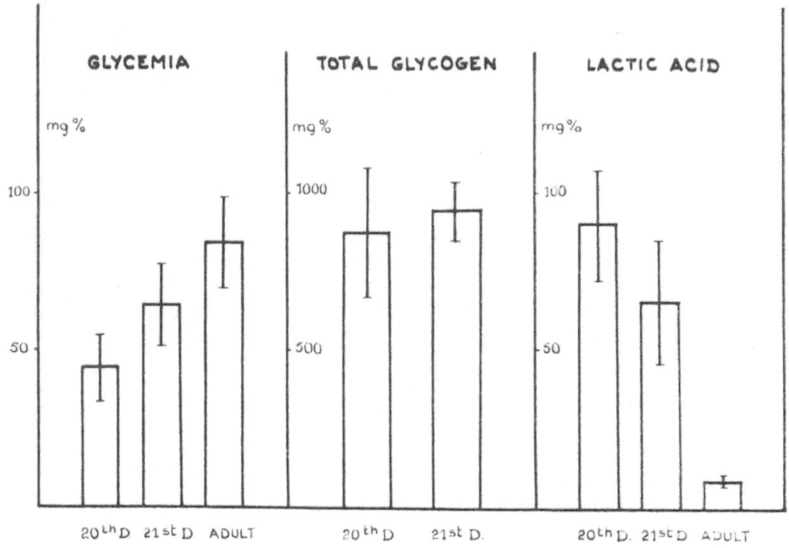

Fig. 3. Carbohydrate metabolism of rat embryo.

On the other hand, lactic acid is rather high on the 20th as well as on the 21st day as compared with the adult level. It is worthwhile to consider the glycogen content of the foetus in more detail, starting with the distribution of glycogen over the different organs as shown in fig. 4.

Although the liver has often been considered the most important source of carbohydrates, it is not the main storage site. Indeed,

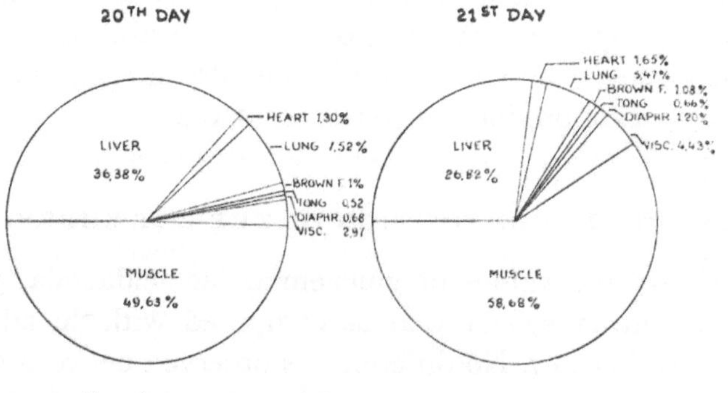

Fig. 4. Glycogen of various organs of the rat embryo.

skeletal glycogen represents a much larger amount, but is nevertheless often neglected in metabolic studies.

From fig. 4, showing the concentration of glycogen in different organs, it is clear that some small organs (heart, lung) have very high concentrations but that, owing to the low weight of these organs, this glycogen represents only a small part of the total stored carbohydrates.

2. CHANGES IN CARBOHYDRATE STORAGE AFTER BIRTH

As can be seen from fig. 5, glycaemia does not decrease during the first hours after birth. In this respect the rat differs completely from human newborns, whose glycaemia tends to decrease progressively.

When very late stages (24 hours after birth) are considered – in animals of the 20th as well as of the 21st day – the glycaemia drops to values far lower than physiological levels. Many animals die at that moment. The glycogen content of certain organs also is lowered, but the decrease is much more marked in the liver than in the other organs. The question will be raised later, whether this glycogen output from the liver is sufficient to prevent hypoglycaemia or whether some other sources of carbohydrates are used to compensate for glucose utilization. Muscle glycogen has to be considered in this connection.

Indeed, CORNBLATH (9) has suggested – at least for human newborns – a mechanism of skeletal glycogen degradation and glucose liberation into the bloodstream from this sketelal source.

Lactic acid, although high at birth in foetuses of the 20th as well as of the 21st day, shows a different pattern in both cases. In the 21 day old foetus, lactic acid decreases very quickly after birth, but, 20 day old animals cannot get rid of their lactic acid.

It is interesting to compare the evolution of these parameters with the survival curves of these animals (fig. 5). Both survival curves show a rapid dip between the 18th and the 24th hour after birth; this phenomenon is probably related in both groups (20th and 21st day) to the exhaustion of carbohydrate stores.

It is not possible to ascertain whether death is related to hypoglycaemia, exhaustion of hepatic glycogen, or exhaustion of cardiac glycogen.

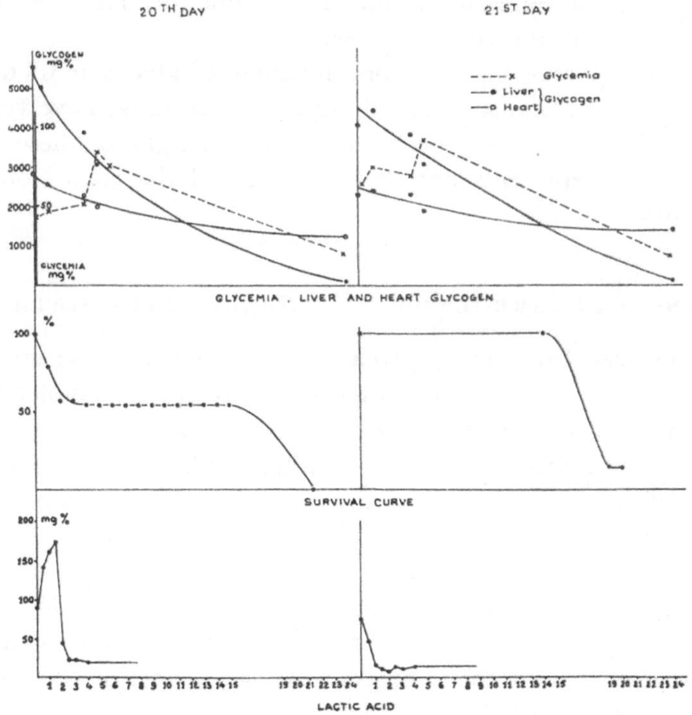

Fig. 5. See text.

Table 2. *Balance of carbohydrate metabolism in rat embryo (20th day).*

Initial glycogen	10.96 mg/g
Residual glycogen (12 hours)	1.35 mg/g
Glycogen disappeared	9.61 mg/g
Initial glycemia	0,45 mg/ml
Residual glycemia (12 hours)	0,56 mg/ml
	Δ —0,10
Glucose space (30% of body weight)	0,80 ml
Glucose gain	0,08
Carbohydrate utilised	9,53 mg/g
Oxygen needed (0,83 ml/mg carbohyd.)	7,91 ml
Oxygen utilisation (observed data)	6,84 ml
Caloric equivalent (4 cal./mg)	37,12 cal/12 h. = 74,24 cal/24 h.
Calculated caloric need	300 cal/24 h.

In the 20 day old foetus another phenomenon – never seen in 21 day old animals – can be observed.

During the first hours after birth, almost 50% of the animals die. This is probably related to an increase of lactic acid concentration, which reflects the incapacity of these foetuses for aerobic catabolism.

Although the next step in our investigation would be to establish a complete metabolic balance, is not possible to elaborate this balance from the data obtained in the above mentioned studies on organs. Therefore, we have also measured the total glycogen content of new-born rats at different times after birth.

Glycogen disappears progressively over a 12-hour period to almost 1/10 of the initial value. On the basis of these data we calculated a metabolic balance, as shown in Table 2. It may be concluded that the caloric expenditure of the new-born rats is low.

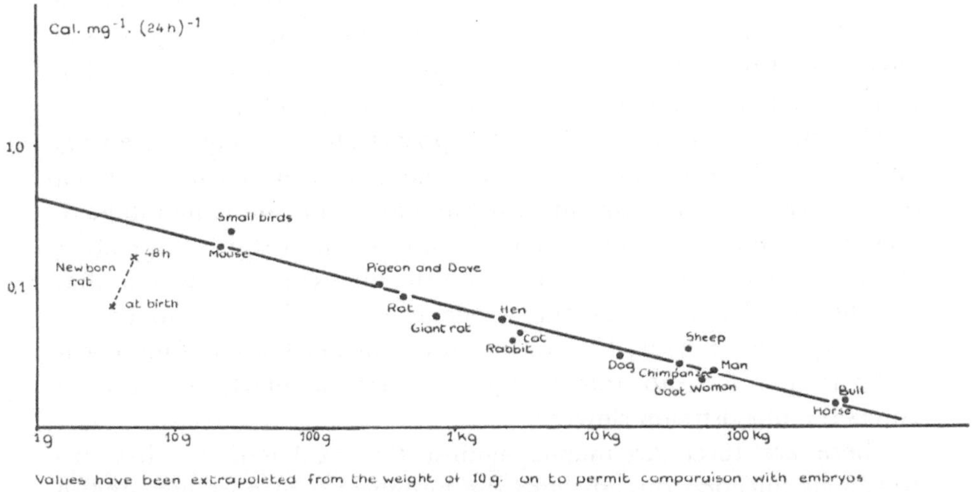

Fig. 6. Average heat production per mg body weight for different species (after Benedict, Carnegie Inst. Wash., Rept. No 503).

Indeed, if we plot this value on a diagram correlating, for different species, caloric expenditure and body weight, we see that the newborn rat lies far below the expected value (fig. 6). A few days after birth, however, a normal value is reached, as was observed in other experiments.

The same changes seem to occur in man, as demonstrated by Cross (10).

3. OXYGEN CONSUMPTION AND CO_2 PRODUCTION

To answer the question of whether any other sources of fuel are used by these newborns, we measured the O_2 consumption and CO_2 production of the newborn rats. The amount of oxygen utilized proved to equal exactly that necessary to oxydize the amount of carbohydrate disappearing from the stores during the same time. On the other hand, the respiratory quotient, calculated from the same data, is almost equal to I, demonstrating that all the energy is derived from carbohydrates.

Production of CO_2 was further investigated by administration of radioactive substrates (glucose-1-^{14}C, glucose-6-^{14}C, or acetate 1-^{14}C) to the newborn, trapping the CO_2 produced, and measuring its radioactivity. We injected these substrates intramuscularly and gave a total dose of about 150,000 cpm. Cumulative values of radioactivity plotted *vs* time gave an –s–shaped curve (fig. 7).

This means that the radioactivity appears progressively in the CO_2 and that the maximum rate of production is achieved only after a dead space. For a certain interval the maximum rate is maintained, giving the middle part of the curve a linear aspect. By extrapolating this linear part, one can determine on the abcissa a certain time that may be considered as a measure of the dead space just mentioned.

The question is now, how to interpret this dead space. One possibility is that the substrate is injected intramuscularly and that it enters the bloodstream slowly.

There are three arguments against this explanation. First, intravenous injection directly into the umbilical vein does not abolish the dead space although it shortens it slightly. Secondly, the radioactivity in the blood after intramuscular injection reaches a maximum after 15 or 20 minutes, demonstrating that there is a good exchange between the intramuscular and the intravascular compartments. The third argument is that the length of the dead space differs with the time of injection (at birth or 90 minutes later) and according to the nature of the substrate injected. Fig. 10 illustrates the length of the dead space under different conditions. For these reasons it may be

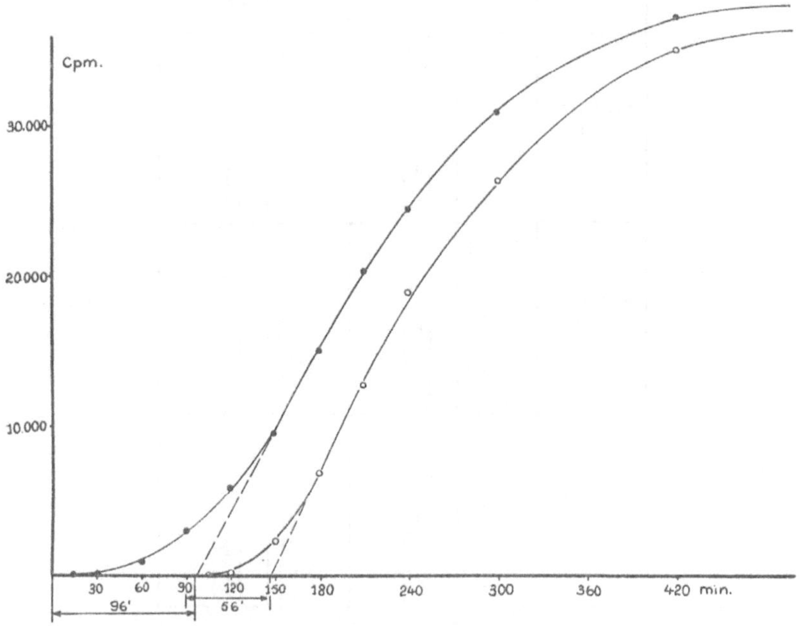

Fig. 7. Radioactive CO_2 produced from glucose-6-^{14}C in the newborn rat.

suggested that this phenomenon is related to special conditions in the metabolic pathways of the newborn rat.

Two points of special interest are to be taken into consideration: 1. for acetate-1-^{14}C, the dead space is long in 20 day old animals injected immediately after birth. Late injection or injection on the 21st day shortens this dead space. This can be explained by supposing that the Krebs' cycle functions slowly in animals born on the 20th day of gestation and that its activity increases rapidly thereafter. This reduced Krebs' cycle activity is not surprising, since it has been found in our laboratory that a similar reduction occurs in younger embryos (11).

2. Radioactivity of glucose-6-^{14}C appeared in CO_2 after a long dead space in all our experiments. This can be explained by the large lactate pool we have observed in newborn animals. Indeed, glucose-6-^{14}C produces radioactive CO_2 when passing through the Krebs' cycle, but before entering this cycle glucose must be transformed into pyruvate,

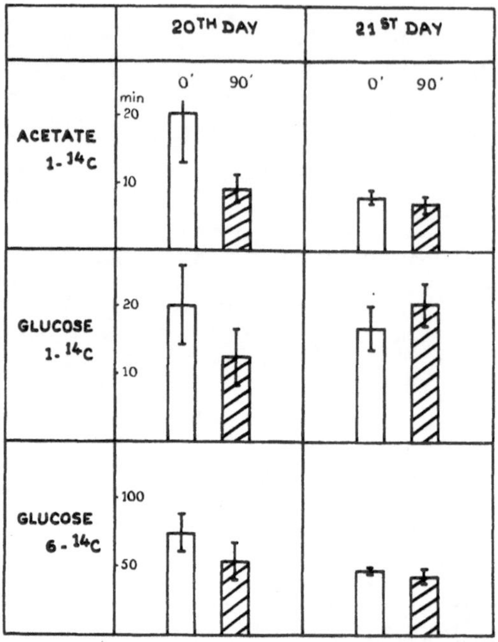

Fig. 8. Dead space between injection of glucose and CO_2 production.

which is linked with the lactate pool. A great deal of the radioactivity is first absorbed in this pool and only when it is saturated does the radioactivity appear in CO_2. The same phenomenon does not occur for glucose-1-^{14}C because part of the CO_2 produced comes from the pentose pathway.

CONCLUSION

1. Metabolism of the newborn rat is characterized by an exclusive utilization of carbohydrates for energy expenditure. This can be concluded from metabolic balance studies, oxygen consumption and RQ determination.
2. Energy requirement is low in the newborn period when compared with that of older animals.
3. Some metabolic pathways (Kreb's cycle) seem to be limited at birth or in prematures.
4. Accumulation of a large pool of lactic acid characterises the metabolism of newborn rats.

REFERENCES

1. Widdowson E. M., (1964) Changes in the composition of the body at birth and their bearing on function and food requirements. In: *The adaptation of the newborn infant to extra-uterine life (Nutricia Symposium)*. Jonxis J. H. P., H. K. A. Visser and J. A. Troelstra (eds.) p. 1–13.
2. Shelley, H. J., (1961) Glycogen reserves and their changes at birth and in anoxia. *Brit. med. bull.*, 17:137–143.
3. Hunter, D. J. S., (1969) Changes in blood glucose and liver carbohydrate after intrauterine injection of glucagon into foetal rats. *J. Endocr.* 45:367–374.
4. Goodner, C. J. and D. J. Thompson, (1967) Glucose metabolism in the fetus in utero: The effect of maternal fasting and glucose loading in the rat. *Pediat. Res. I:* 443:451.
5. Stafford, A. and A. C. Weatherall, (1960) The survival of young rats in nitrogen. *J. Physiol.* 153:457–472.
6. Roux, J. M., C. Tordet-Caridroit and C. Chanez, (1970) Studies on experimental hypotrophy in the rat. I. Chemical composition of the total body and some organs in the rat foetus. *Biol. Neonat.* 15:342–347.
7. Dawkins, M. J. R., (1963) Glycogen synthesis and breakdown in fetal and newborn rat liver. *Ann. N. Y. Acad. Sci.* III:203.
8. Clark, C. M., Jr, G. F. Cahill, Jr, and J. S. Soeldner, (1968) Effects of exogenous insulin on the rate of fatty acid synthesis and glucose C-14 utilization in the twenty-day rat foetus. *Diabetes* 17:362.
9. Cornblath M., E. Y. Levin and H. H. Gordon (1956) Studies of carbohydrate metabolism in the newborn. I. Capillary-venous differences in blood sugar in normal newborn infants. *Pediatrics* 18:167–176.
10. Cross K. W., (1965) Respiration and oxygen supplies in the newborn. In: *Handbook of Physiology*, Respiration. Washington D.C. American Physiological Society, sect. 3, vol 2, 52:1329–1344.
11. De Plaen J. L., (1969) *Aspects dynamiques du métabolisme glucidique chez l'embryon de rat. Action de substances hypoglycémiantes et tératogènes*, pp. 250. Maloine Paris—Arxia Bruxelles.

DISCUSSION

Dr. Sereni: There has been much discussion which factors after birth induce gluconeogenetic enzyme systems. One of the speculations was that the sharp drop of glucose in the blood causes an increased glucagon secretion. You have demonstrated that this theory is probably not correct.

Prof. de Meyer: In our experiment we did not observe a drop of glucose level but we did not see either gluconeogenesis; we just observed a glycolysis.

Dr. Hull: We have kept newborn rabbits in a thermoneutral environment after birth. We found no fall in blood glucose levels. If they are exposed to cold, the glucose goes up for the first few hours and then slowly goes down. I would not be surprised if the same was true in the human baby.

Could I make another comment. We have measured glycogen levels in newborn rabbits in different organs, including the muscle and found that the glycogen in the liver fell according to the ambient temperature. The glycogen in the heart, diaphragm and skeletal muscle, varied with the temperature, presumally because of the amount of work they had to do. The glycogen in the muscle is not available outside the muscle, it has to be used in the muscle itself. Have you found the same in your rats?

Prof. De Meyer: Our experiments have all been performed on the same temperature of 32 °C. What you say about glucose utilization has been confirmed by our experiments. When we calculate the amount of glycogen disappearing from the liver and the amount of glucose leaving the bloodstream, we see that these two values are nearly the same. So we must admit that the glycogen disappearing from the muscle is utilized in loco to keep the blood glucose level constant.

Dr. Hull: I would agree. In the animals we have starved for 48 hours, we found still good glycogen levels in the muscles, but the liver was totally depleted and the blood glucose level was nearly zero.

Dr. Widdowson: At the first Nutricia Symposium, I showed a table giving the total amount of glycogen in the muscle of the newborn pig, and an estimate of the amount in the muscle of the human baby.

Prof. De Meyer: But I am not aware of any experiment giving these data for the rat.

GENERAL DISCUSSION

Prof. Villee: We tend to think of glucose transport as involving some sort of carrier molecules that can cross membranes. I wonder if Dr. Wiseman would think that the increased glucose transport in the underfed individuals results either from an increased number of transport molecules or some sort of increased activity of a constant number of molecules.

Dr. Wiseman: One of the speculations is that the number of sites per cell is increased. No one can say why it does increase. But it is equally possible that more sites become available. It has been suggested that when the metabolic rate in the cell decreases, the use of glucose in the cell goes down, this leaves more glucose over to be transported. That would account for the D-glucose, but it would not account for L-glucose which is not metabolised or converted and also not for the aminoacids.

Prof. McCance: I am going to ask a question. The last paper of Prof. de Meyer about the amount of glycogen in muscle. I know muscle is not supposed to break down its glycogen to glucose, but is it not a fact that muscle glycogen can be broken down to lactic acid, which is transported to the liver and there converted to glucose? I know this can happen in anaerobic conditions, but I am not sure to what extent this can happen in aerobic conditions.

Prof. De Meyer: Indeed muscle glycogen can be broken down to lactic acid and then utilised elsewhere or converted to glucose by the liver. But when we calculate our data we see that this does not happen.

Prof. Bickel: I would like to ask Prof. Wolf to give us his opinion about the clinical application of these fat emulsions. Every paediatrician want to have an infusion which has an high calorie value/100 ml. So far one has had many troubles with those fat emulsions with untowards effects. I would like to know a little more about your indications for using these emulsions and about the side-effects.

Prof. Wolf: We use them where normal feeding is impossible, for instance malabsorption syndrome, surgical cases and so on. We can use these emulsions without any side-effect if we avoid overloading as mentioned in my paper.

Prof. Bickel: It doesn't give you so much calories if one follows your scheme.

Prof. Wolf: To obtain sufficient caloric intake we are giving fat emulsions twice a day. In the older children we could give about 40 calories per kg per day. In the one day old infants we came up to 15 calories per kg per day only as fat.

Dr. Schröter: I have a question to Dr. MEEUWISSE, concerning the limited tolerance for fructose in newborn infants. I think you know that Schwartz prefers fructose in the infants of diabetic mothers. We too infused fructose in those infants and we have found that fructose can be converted very quickly into glucose. I would like to ask Dr. Meeuwisse if he can give us the dose of fructose for a newborn infant. Is there a difference between normal newborns and infants of diabetic mothers?

Dr. Meeuwisse: I don't think I can answer your question. As I said it is known that fructose is more rapidly metabolised at all ages. Fructose has also been recommended in the treatment of diabetics of all ages. This is to my opinion a consequence of a misunderstanding. What has been said is that fructose can be metabolised without the aid of insulin. It is true that you get more glycogen, but to utilize it you must have insulin. I don't think it is of any use to give fructose. The infants of diabetic mothers have an increased disappearance of glucose and an increased release of insulin. I must say I see no the reason to give fructose in such cases.

Dr. Schröter: It has been said that the release of insulin may be smaller after infusion of fructose.

Dr. Eggermont: We could analyse the aldolase activity of the liver of 5 praemature infants. The aldolase activity was more active on fructose-diphosphate than on fructose-1-phosphate and resembles therefore the activity found in children with fructose intolerance. Before fructose infusions can be recommanded in newborn infants, more information on the developmental pattern of liver aldolase should be available.

Prof. Villee: During these two days there has been frequent reference to babies that are small-for-date. It has been suggested that those babies are starving or partially starving in utero. Is there any real evidence that this is the case? Some of my friends in Boston even refer to placental insufficiency and blame the placenta for this, again I think without any real evidence.

Can anyone tell me of real evidence that the small for date baby is nearly starving?

There is general feeling that small is bad and big is better. If a baby is small we should feed him to make him bigger and better? Perhaps we are overfed. At least in experimental animals rats that are slightly underfed live longer, and have less tendency to get arterosclerosis than fully fed animals.

Dr. Hull: When you ask about the small-for-date baby do you ask: is it starved in utero or does it experience more severe starvation afterwards.

Prof. Villee: Yes.

Dr. Hull: That is difficult. There are just babies who definitely show more symptoms of starvation and sooner after birth than others. They show a rapid rise in free fatty acids and a rapid drop in blood sugar. I think that is established. But whether in fact they are suffering from starvation before birth I would leave to others to answer.

Dr. Young: The first question of Dr. VILLEE's might be answered by an experiment, which could you give some idea of the maternal placental blood flow relative to the weight of placenta and the weight of the conceptus throughout gestation.

At the present moment Dr. WIDDOWSON and I are involved in some simple observations, which might help. We are injecting into the maternal circulation alpha-amino-isobutyric acid, and measuring its uptake relative to placental weight and relative to foetal weight. That gives you of course an uptake measurement at that special moment of time. What is really needed is a longitudinal study.

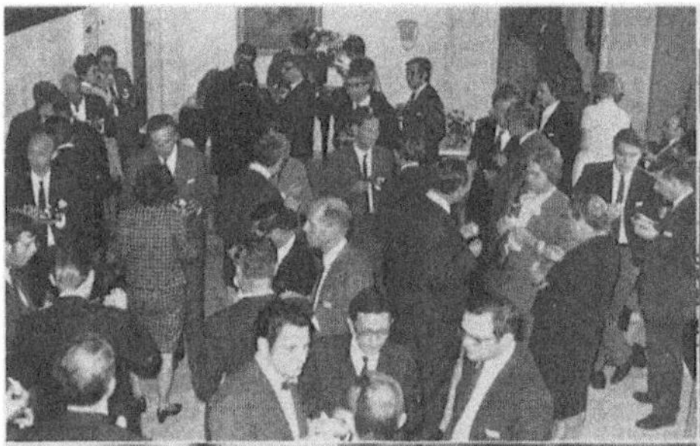
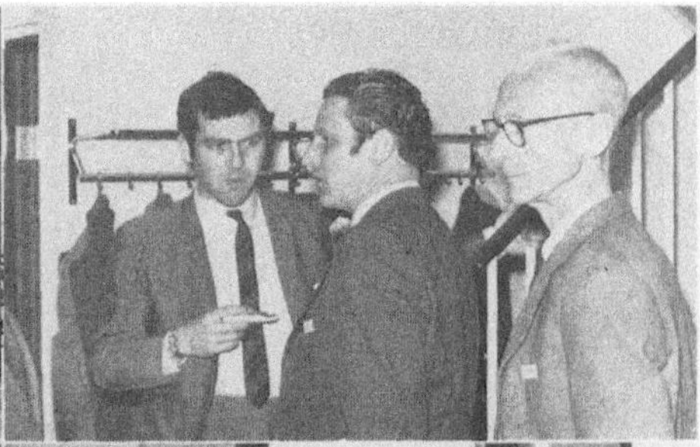
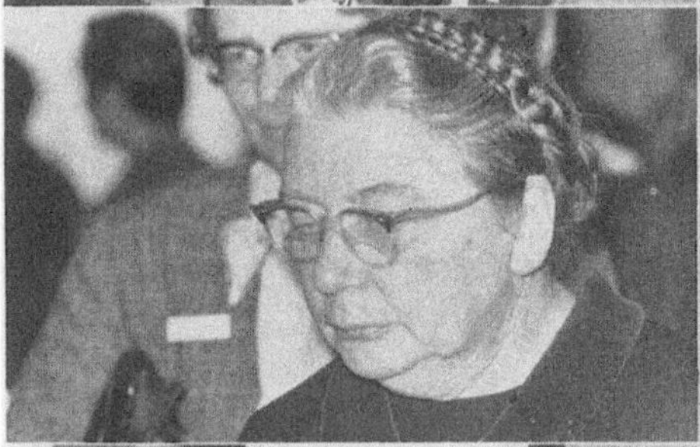
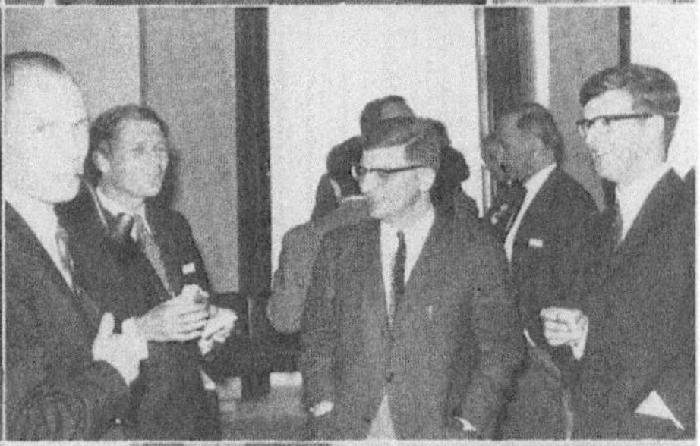
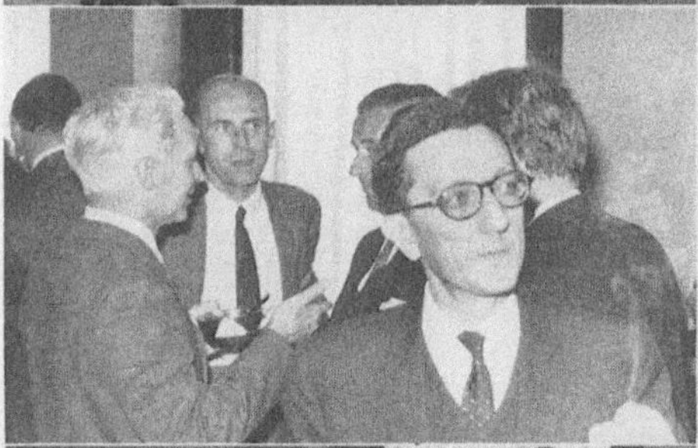
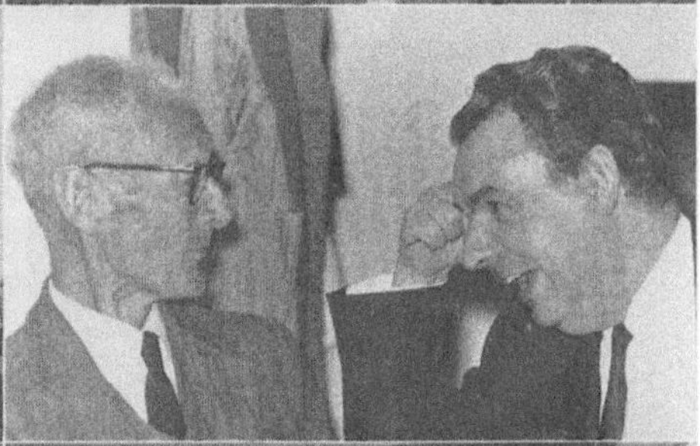
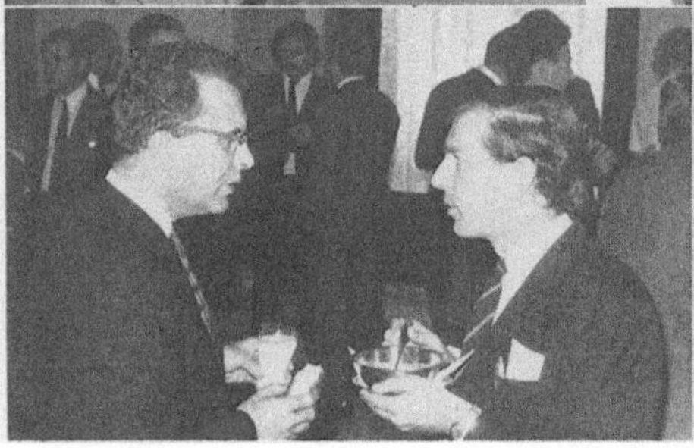
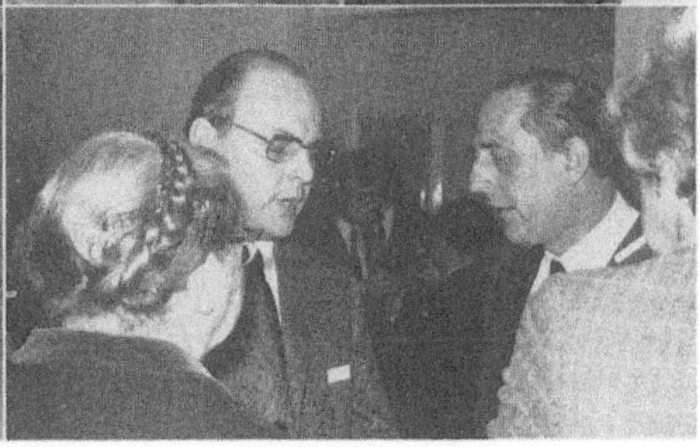

INDEX OF AUTHORS

INDEX OF SUBJECTS